Psoriasis

Psoriasis

Diagnosis and Management

EDITED BY

Wolfram Sterry, MD, PhD

Department of Dermatology and Allergy
University Hospital Charité
Berlin, Germany

Robert Sabat, MD, PhD

Head of Psoriasis Research and Treatment Center
Department of Dermatology and Allergy/Institute of Medical Immunology
University Hospital Charité
Berlin, Germany

Sandra Philipp, MD, PhD

Psoriasis Research and Treatment Center
Department of Dermatology and Allergy/Institute of Medical Immunology
University Hospital Charité
Berlin, Germany

WILEY Blackwell

This edition first published 2015, © 2015 by John Wiley & Sons, Ltd.

Registered Office
John Wiley & Sons, Ltd., The Atrium, Southern Gate, Chichester, West Sussex, PO19 8SQ, UK

Editorial Offices
9600 Garsington Road, Oxford, OX4 2DQ, UK
The Atrium, Southern Gate, Chichester, West Sussex, PO19 8SQ, UK
111 River Street, Hoboken, NJ 07030-5774, USA

For details of our global editorial offices, for customer services and for information about how to apply for permission to reuse the copyright material in this book please see our website at www.wiley.com/wiley-blackwell

Library of Congress Cataloging-in-Publication Data

Psoriasis (Sterry)
Psoriasis : diagnosis and management / [edited by] Wolfram Sterry, Robert Sabat, Sandra Philipp.
p. ; cm.
Includes bibliographical references and index.
ISBN 978-0-470-65736-2 (cloth)
I. Sterry, Wolfram, editor. II. Sabat, Robert, editor. III. Philipp, Sandra, editor. IV. Title.
[DNLM: 1. Psoriasis–diagnosis. 2. Psoriasis–therapy. WR 205]
RL321
616.5′26–dc23

2014029373

A catalogue record for this book is available from the British Library.

Wiley also publishes its books in a variety of electronic formats. Some content that appears in print may not be available in electronic books.

Cover image: Charité
Cover design: meadencreative.com

Set in 9.5/13pt Meridien by SPi Publisher Services, Pondicherry, India
Printed and bound in Malaysia by Vivar Printing Sdn Bhd

1 2015

Contents

List of contributors

Frank Bachmann, MD, PhD
Department of Dermatology and Allergy, University Hospital Charité, Berlin, Germany

Marina Backhaus, MD, PhD
Department of Rheumatology and Clinical Immunology, Charité-Universitätsmedizin Berlin, Berlin, Germany

Simone Cazzaniga, MD, PhD
Bergamo General Hospital, Bergamo, Italy

Kenneth B. Gordon, MD, PhD
Professor of Dermatology, Northwestern University, Feinberg School of Medicine, Chicago, IL, USA

Erhard Hölzle, MD, PhD
Department of Dermatology and Allergology, Klinikum Oldenburg, Oldenburg, Germany

Georgios Kokolakis, MD, PhD
Psoriasis Research and Treatment Center, Department of Dermatology and Allergy/ Institute of Medical Immunology, University Hospital Charité, Berlin, Germany

Knud Kragballe, MD, PhD
Department of Dermatology, Arhus University Hospital, Arhus, Denmark

Peter C.M. van de Kerkhof, MD, PhD
Department of Dermatology, Radboud University Nijmegen Medical Centre, Nijmegen, Netherlands

Alan Menter, MD, PhD
Department of Dermatology, Baylor University Medical Center, Dallas, TX, USA

Luigi Naldi, MD, PhD
Bergamo General Hospital, Bergamo, Italy

Steven M. Nwe, MD, PhD
Department of Dermatology, Northwestern University, Feinberg School of Medicine, Chicago, IL, USA

Sandra Philipp, MD, PhD
Psoriasis Research and Treatment Center, Department of Dermatology and Allergy/Institute of Medical Immunology, University Hospital Charité, Berlin, Germany

Giovanna Rao, MD, PhD
Bergamo General Hospital, Bergamo, Italy

Caitriona Ryan, MD, PhD
Department of Dermatology, Baylor University Medical Center, Dallas, TX, USA

Hans-Joachim Röwert-Huber, MD, PhD
Department of Dermatology and Allergy, University Hospital Charité, Berlin, Germany

Robert Sabat, MD, PhD
Psoriasis Research and Treatment Center, Department of Dermatology and Allergy/Institute of Medical Immunology, University Hospital Charité, Berlin, Germany

Wolfram Sterry, MD, PhD
Professor, Department of Dermatology and Allergy, University Hospital Charité, Berlin, Germany

Ellen Witte, PhD
Psoriasis Research and Treatment Center, Department of Dermatology and Allergy/Institute of Medical Immunology, University Hospital Charité, Berlin, Germany

Kerstin Wolk, PhD
Psoriasis Research and Treatment Center, Department of Dermatology and Allergy/Institute of Medical Immunology, University Hospital Charité, Berlin, Germany

Preface

Research in psoriasis has come to a point where we understand the framework of genetic background, eliciting factors, and molecular pathogenesis, thus allowing for new and very effective treatments. Nevertheless, without knowing the clinical presentations in all their variations and being able to entertain differential diagnostic considerations, optimal care for the patient is not possible. This also includes a detailed understanding of the mode of action of the various treatments currently available, and the optimal use in a particular patient. We are grateful that our friends and colleagues from the international psoriasis field have agreed to share their knowledge and to contribute the many excellent chapters on all relevant aspects of psoriasis. We do hope that this book satisfies your expectations and helps you to provide better care and gain a better understanding of your patients suffering from psoriasis.

PART I

Epidemiology and economic aspects

CHAPTER 1
Epidemiology and economic aspects

Luigi Naldi, Simone Cazzaniga, and Giovanna Rao
Bergamo General Hospital, Bergamo, Italy

Epidemiology

Epidemiologic research should be understood in the light of its main interest, that is, prevention of the disease and its consequences in man.

Descriptive epidemiology

The measures employed are incidence and prevalence. A first step in descriptive epidemiology is to obtain a valid definition of what constitutes a "case." Quite surprisingly, up to now, no widely employed diagnostic criteria have been developed for clinical and population based studies of psoriasis. The first diagnosis made by a physician and the first appearance of skin lesions as reported by the patient have both been taken as markers of "onset" in epidemiologic studies.

Incidence—there are few studies

In a pilot study conducted in Rochester, Minnesota, in the period 1980–1983, incident cases were defined as patients requiring, for the first time in their life, medical care for a condition diagnosed as psoriasis. The age- and sex-adjusted (1980 US white population) annual incidence rate was 60.4 per 100,000 people. The crude rates were 54.4 for men and 60.2 for women. In another study from the United States, a cohort of 1633 adult subjects was followed up from 1970 to 2000. Rates adjusted to the 2000 US population increased significantly over time from 50.8 in the period 1970–1974, to 100.5 per 100,000 in the period 1995–1999. In a third study from the United States, a cohort of people younger than 18 years was followed up between 1970 and 1999. The overall incidence of psoriasis age- and sex-adjusted to the 2000 US population was 40.8 per 100,000. The incidence increased steadily with increasing age. Moreover, incidence increased in most recent years in both boys and girls. In a study based on data from the United Kingdom General Practice Research Database (UKGPRD) where cases were recorded by general practitioners from January 1996 to December 1997, a rate as high as 14 per 10,000 person-years was estimated, much higher than rates in the United States.

Psoriasis: Diagnosis and Management, First Edition. Edited by Wolfram Sterry, Robert Sabat, and Sandra Philipp.

Prevalence

Each new case (incident case) enters the prevalence pool and remains there until either recovery or death. If recovery and death are not frequent, even low incidence rates (such as those calculated for psoriasis) produce a high prevalence. Prevalence measures may be relative to a point in time (point prevalence) or to a longer period (period and lifetime prevalence). Prevalence of psoriasis "ever experienced" in the past at any age (i.e. lifetime prevalence) approximates the cumulative incidence in that age group, that is, the proportion of the birth cohort developing the disease until the time of survey, provided that psoriasis does not affect mortality per se and that the recall of past episodes is complete.

Results of selected studies of the prevalence of psoriasis in defined populations provide estimates ranging from 0.05% in China to 4.8% in Norway (Table 1.1). Besides geographic variations, these estimates are expected to change according to the period considered, that is, point prevalence vs "lifetime prevalence." In addition, variations may be expected to arise from differences in case definition and ascertainment, and from differences in age distribution of dynamic populations.

Ethnic and geographic variations

It appears that Mongoloid races in the Far East of Asia have remarkably low prevalence rates. Lower prevalence rates have also been documented in African Americans compared with Caucasians in United States. Duffy *et al.* analyzed cumulative incidence in 3808 twin pairs and documented significantly higher prevalence rates in southern states of Australia with respect to northern areas. Geographical variations were also described in Norway with the northern regions of Troms and Finmark showing higher rates, and Hedmark and Oppland regions in the south of the country showing lower rates.

Sex and age variations

Most prevalence studies suggest that psoriasis tends to be slightly more prevalent among men than among women. The few studies available providing age-specific incidence rates of psoriasis suggest that incidence increases more or less steadily with age up to the seventh decade of life. If psoriasis appeared throughout life, then both point prevalence and lifetime prevalence would increase with age. However, prevalence estimates in several studies do not increase with age and even decrease, suggesting higher mortality rates in older psoriatics compared with the general population. It has been reported that age at onset in large series of psoriatic patients has a bimodal distribution. This has been taken as evidence for etiologic heterogeneity, and type I and type II psoriasis have been proposed. In fact, variations in numerator data, that is, the number of people experiencing onset at different ages, may simply reflect the age distribution of the population of origin.

Table 1.1 Selected estimates of the prevalence of psoriasis.

Country	Ascertainment method	No. of subjects (age)	Measure[a]	Estimate ×100
Faroe Islands	Clinical examination	10,984	PT	2.8
Norway	Questionnaire	14,667 (20–54 years)	LT	4.8
Norway	Questionnaire	10,576	PT	1.4
Sweden	Monitoring of diagnoses	159,200	PP	2.3
Denmark	Questionnnaire	3892 (16–99 years)	LT	4.2
Croatia	Clinical examination	8416	PT	1.5
USA	Clinical examination	20,749 (1–74 years)	PT	0.8–1.4[b]
China	Monitoring of diagnoses	670,000	PT	0.05–0.84
England	Questionnaire and clinical examination	2180	PT	0.6–1.6[b]
Australia	Questionnaire and clinical examination	1037 (adults)	PT	2.3
Italy	Questionnaire	3660 (>44 years)	LT	3.1
Germany, working adults	Examination	90,880	PP	2.0
USA	Questionnaire	10,122	LT	3.1
Sweden, male conscripts	Examination	1,226,193 (20 years)	LT	0.5
United Kingdom UKGPRD	Examination	7,533,475	PP	1.5
USA (Caucasians vs African Americans)	Questionnaire	21,921 vs 2443	LP	2.5 vs 1.3
Spain	Questionnaire	12,938	LP	1.17–1.43
Portugal	Questionnaire and clinical examination	1000	PP	1.9

[a] LT: lifetime prevalence; PP: period prevalence; PT: point prevalence.

[b] Different estimates are provided according to severity indexes, or age groups.

Familial aggregation

A history of psoriasis in first degree relatives is given by 20–30% of psoriatics. In a study, the prevalence of psoriasis increased with the number of first-degree relatives affected from 3% with no relative affected to about 40% with two relatives affected.

Analytic epidemiology

The causative model of psoriasis involves interaction between genetic predisposition and environmental factors.

Genetic factors

Heritability quantifies the overall role of genetic factors when a multifactorial model of inheritance is postulated. Measures of the heritability of psoriasis have been provided based on population data and the analysis of concordance of twins. The estimates ranged from 0.5 to 0.9.

Personal habits

Smoking has been consistently linked with psoriasis. Studies that examine the exposure before the onset of psoriasis and control for confounding factors offer the more convincing evidence. There are indications that the risk for smoking may vary according to gender, with it being higher in women. Smoking and alcohol may alter the expression of psoriasis (e.g. pattern distribution, clinical varieties) and its clinical course. Smoking has been linked with acral lesions. Alcohol has been associated with severity of psoriasis and treatment failures.

Body weight and diet

It is well established that increased body mass index (BMI) and increased waist circumference are risk factors for developing psoriasis (Table 1.2). The association has been documented also in infantile psoriasis. Scanty data are available concerning diet. In an Italian case-control study, the risk of psoriasis increased with increasing BMI and was inversely related to the consumption of carrots, tomatoes and fresh fruit, and to the index of beta-carotene intake.

Drugs and infections

Several drugs, such as lithium salts, beta-adrenergic blocking agents, and antimalarials, have been reported to be responsible for the onset or exacerbation of psoriasis, but the evidence is inconclusive. An infection with β-haemolytic streptococci often precedes the first manifestation of guttate psoriasis. Furthermore, a cohort study in the United States, involving 265,000 members of the Harvard Community Health Plan, demonstrated that chronic HIV infection is linked to a higher risk of psoriasis (relative risk 3.5). The risk increases with the progression of the disease from the asymptomatic phase to full-blown AIDS.

Psychosocial factors

Psychosomatic factors are deemed to play a role in psoriasis, and stressful life events have been linked with the risk of incident psoriasis. A major problem in this area is that virtually all the research is based on the recall of past events. People have a strong tendency to seek explanations in order to account for what happens to them, and stress is commonly used for this.

Table 1.2 Summary of main recent epidemiologic studies on risk factors for incident psoriasis.

Country (year)	Study design	Study subjects	Factors analyzed	Results
Italy (2005)	Case-control	560 newly diagnosed cases and 690 controls with other skin diseases	Alcohol, smoking, BMI, stressful life events	OR increased in smokers and ex-smokers, 1.7 and 1.9 respectively. Stronger association in women as compared with men and in pustular psoriasis. OR 1.6 and 1.9 for overweighed and obese, respectively. OR increased for increased stressful life-event score.
UK (2007)	Cohort and nested case-control	3994 cases and 10,000 controls	Skin infection, smoking	Infection OR 2.1. Smoking OR 1.4.
UKGPRD				
USA (2007)	Cohort	79,722 nurses	BMI, waist circumference, weight change	RR increases from 1.40 for BMI 21.0–22.9, to 2.69 for BMI >35.0. Weight gain from the age of 18 years, higher waist circumference, hip circumference, and waist–hip ratio were all associated with a higher risk of incident psoriasis.
Nurse Health Study II				
USA (2007)	Cohort	78,532 nurses	Smoking	RR 1.78 for current smokers and 1.37 for past smokers. Increased risk with increased number of cigarettes smoked per day. The risk in former smokers decreases almost to that of never smokers 20 years after cessation.
Nurse Health Study II				
UK (2008)	Case-control	36,702 cases and matched controls	Beta-blockers and other anti-hypertensive drugs	No association.
UKGPRD				
Sweden (2009)	Case-control	373 cases and matched controls	Smoking, BMI, alcohol	Smoking OR 1.7. BMI 9% increased risk per unit increase.
Denmark (2010)	Cohort	309,152 school children	Increase in BMI	Psoriasis in adulthood associated with increased BMI at age 12 and 13 in females only.
Turkey (2011)	Case-control	537 cases and 511 controls younger than 18 years	Passive smoking, BMI, stressful life events	Passive smoking OR 2.9. Life events OR 2.9. BMI (>26) OR 2.5.

Natural history and prognosis

Limited data are available concerning long-term outcome and prognosis. An analysis over a 20-year follow-up period of patients enrolled in the psoralen and ultraviolet-A light (PUVA) cohort study documented that, on average, individuals with moderate to severe disease remained at these same levels for 11 or more years, and that, in spite of looking for a cure, consistent control of their psoriasis often had not been achieved.

Although psoriatic arthritis in clinical series represents up to 25% of all patients, population-based estimates suggest that no more than 5–10% of psoriatic patients present seronegative arthritis as an associated feature. Modifiable risk factors for psoriasis, namely smoking and obesity, may influence clinical severity, comorbidities, or response to treatment, and may even be responsible for an increased mortality among psoriatics as compared with the general population. Established psoriasis has been associated with the many components of the metabolic syndrome, including hypertension, dyslipidemia, obesity, and impaired glucose tolerance. Besides cardiovascular disease, a number of other conditions partly associated with smoking or obesity have been linked with psoriasis, including inflammatory bowel disorders, and tumors of specific sites, such as lung cancer, colonic cancer, and kidney cancer. A rare but well-defined association is with celiac disease.

In spite of the need for their continuous use, limited data are available on the long-term impact of treatment modalities for psoriasis. A model example are cohort studies of PUVA therapy which, among the others, enabled elevated risks for nonmelanoma skin cancer (including male genital tumors) to be estimated in PUVA-treated patients. Similar studies are needed for most new therapies, and registries of systemic treatments for psoriasis have recently been established in several countries. A merging of data from these registries to assess the risk for rare events would be desirable.

Social and economic impact

Negative feelings and moral evaluation are associated with skin manifestations. For centuries in many different cultures, skin diseases have been associated with disgrace and danger. A notable association is the connotation of dirtiness, bound up with fears of infection or contagion. The available surveys document that patients with psoriasis commonly experience social stigmatization and overt public rejection. These rejection experiences may result in greater sensitivity to the attitudes of others and further anticipation of rejection. A 1-year prospective study documented that improvement in skin condition did not correlate with feeling less stigmatized in women over 1 year. Feelings of embarrassment or lack of self-confidence can reduce social and even employment opportunities. One study in the United States, using data from the National

Psoriasis Foundation database, showed that the probability of a low income (<US$30,000) was significantly greater among patients with severe disease than among those with mild psoriasis ($P = 0.0002$). It must also be conceded that low income may lead to behaviors (such as unhealthy alimentary habits and poor compliance) that further exacerbate disease and poor socioeconomic outcomes. The negative impact of psoriasis on relationships is similar to that of other chronic conditions, with relatives of patients reporting social disruption (55%), limitations to holiday plans and leisure activities (44%), and deterioration of close relationships (37%).

Economic cost

A systematic literature search dealing with cost-of-illness analyses in psoriasis, that is, analyses assessing direct, indirect and intangible costs, retrieved a total of seven papers. All studies but one were performed before biologics became available. The total annual costs per patient ranged between €1079 and about €23,000. The studies may have underestimated some psoriasis costs not included in their protocols, such as comorbidities and reduction in productivity by families and caregivers. Data from the studies show that the more severe the plaque psoriasis, the higher the direct and indirect costs for its management. Direct costs were higher than indirect costs, hospitalization representing the most significant item. There were considerable discrepancies between the results obtained in the different studies. Reasons for these discrepancies are manifold including differences in the selection of the sample, as well as in the methods for calculating costs. Only the adoption of a common methodology would help to discern differences attributable to different healthcare systems and to identify areas where intervention to optimize costs should be directed. Interestingly, an analysis of trends in the average wholesale price of brand-name psoriasis therapies from 2000 to 2008 demonstrated an average increase of 66%; thus, costs of several brand-name psoriasis drugs greatly outpaced the rates of inflation for all items and all prescription drugs.

Further reading

Jobling, R. and Naldi, L. (2006) Assessing the impact of psoriasis and the relevance of qualitative research. *Journal of Investigative Dermatology*, **126**, 1438–1440.

Naldi, L. (2004) Epidemiology of psoriasis. *Current Drug Targets—Inflammation & Allergy*, **3**, 121–128.

Naldi, L., Conti, A., Cazzaniga, S., *et al.* (2014) Diet and physical exercise in psoriasis. A randomized trial. *British Journal of Dermatology*, **170**, 634–642.

Naldi, L. and Mercuri, S.R. (2010) Epidemiology of comorbidities in psoriasis. *Dermatologic Therapy*, **23**, 114–118.

Parisi, R., Symmons, D.P., Griffiths, C.E., Ashcroft, D.M. and Identification and Management of Psoriasis and Associated ComorbidiTy (IMPACT) Project Team (2013) Global epidemiology of psoriasis: a systematic review of incidence and prevalence. *Journal of Investigative Dermatology*, **133**, 377–385.

Pouplard, C., Brenaut, E., Horreau, C., *et al.* (2013) Risk of cancer in psoriasis: a systematic review and meta-analysis of epidemiological studies. *Journal of the European Academy of Dermatology and Venereology*, **27**(Supplement 3), 36–46.

Raho, G., Koleva, D.M., Garattini, L. and Naldi, L. (2012) The burden of moderate to severe psoriasis: an overview. *Pharmacoeconomics*, **30**, 1005–1013.

Samarasekera, E.J., Neilson, J.M., Warren, R.B., Parnham, J. and Smith, C.H. (2013) Incidence of cardiovascular disease in individuals with psoriasis: a systematic review and meta-analysis. *Journal of Investigative Dermatology*, **133**, 2340–2346.

Setty, A.R., Curhan, G. and Choi, H.K. (2007a) Obesity, waist circumference, weight change, and the risk of psoriasis in women. Nurses' Health Study II. *Archives of Internal Medicine*, **167**, 1670–1675.

Setty, A.R., Curhan, G. and Choi, H.K. (2007b) Smoking and the risk of psoriasis in women—Nurses' Health Study II. *American Journal of Medicine*, **120**, 953–959.

CHAPTER 2

Cost-effective psoriasis management

Luigi Naldi, Simone Cazzaniga, and Giovanna Rao
Bergamo General Hospital, Bergamo, Italy

There has been mounting pressure on the medical profession in recent years to stem the rise in national health-care expenditures. One result of that pressure has been the popularization of the term "cost-effective." Different meanings are attached to such a term. Some use the term as a synonym for "effective," while others translate it as "cost saving." In pharmacoeconomic analyses, the term is used to describe a management strategy that, when compared with another, is (1) less costly and at least as effective; (2) more costly and more effective, but the added efficacy is worth paying for at the price offered; (3) less effective and less costly, but the additional cost of the alternative is too high for the added benefits provided. Cost-effectiveness studies may help make the best use of limited resources. They put the highly individualized physician–patient relationship in a wider social context and impose new responsibilities on physicians for their decisions. Clinicians should be aware of health-economics issues and should balance them with effectiveness data and patient instances. Before discussing cost-effectiveness analyses in psoriasis, a brief overview of methods in health economics is provided.

Health economics in a nutshell

The aim of health economics is to identify the interventions that produce the best health output with the available resources. An economic evaluation analysis compares at least two alternative interventions or activities with regard to costs and consequences. There are five commonly used forms of economic evaluation of medical procedures (Table 2.1):

- cost–benefit analysis;
- cost-effectiveness analysis;
- cost–utility analysis;
- cost-minimization analysis;
- decision analysis.

Psoriasis: Diagnosis and Management, First Edition. Edited by Wolfram Sterry, Robert Sabat, and Sandra Philipp.

Table 2.1 Main methods of analysis in health economics.

Type of analysis	Costs	Benefits	Applications
Cost-benefit	All relevant costs associated with the intervention	Benefits valued in monetary terms (e.g. willingness to pay)	To compare alternatives that produce quite different benefits
Cost-effectiveness	All relevant costs associated with the intervention	Benefits expressed by some common measure of effect (e.g. saved life years)	To compare alternatives where the outcome can be expressed in a common natural unit
Cost-utility	All relevant costs associated with the intervention	Benefits expressed by changes in patient utility, usually a composite of the extension of life weighted by an index of quality (QALY)	To compare alternatives where the outcome can be expressed in the same measurement of QALY
Cost-minimization	All relevant costs associated with the intervention	Benefits assumed to be identical	When two alternatives have the same outcome
Decision analysis	No measure	Benefits measured in units comparing different types of medical interventions	When only the results of the intervention are important

A *cost–benefit analysis* evaluates benefits of healthcare, comparing competing alternatives of medical procedures in monetary terms. It is most commonly applied when the benefits of competing investments are quite different, for example, preventing melanoma vs treating psoriasis. Expressing benefits such as saving life or of pain relief in monetary terms in this mode of analysis is a very complicated problem. One way of addressing it is by using willingness-to-pay analyses, expressing how much the individual is able to pay for an improvement in their state of health. Medical applications of cost–benefit analysis are rather in the experimental stages in comparison with other modes of economic analysis.

A *cost-effectiveness analysis* contrasts the relative costs and outcomes (effects) of two or more courses of action for the same health problem. Typically the analysis is expressed in terms of a ratio where the denominator is a gain in health from a measure (years of life, premature births averted, months on PASI 75), and the numerator is the cost associated with the health gain. The incremental cost-effectiveness ratio is one of the most general ways to compare a newly emerging strategy with an existing one. This ratio compares the difference in costs between the two strategies, divided by the difference in their effectiveness.

A *cost–utility analysis* is similar to a cost-effectiveness analysis but incorporates "utilities," that is, strength of preference values for patients' own health, into outcome measure. The measure employed is called quality-adjusted life years, that is, a combination of the duration of life and the health-related quality of life (HRQoL). HRQoL is measured on a preference scale anchored at 1 (perfect or best imaginable health) and 0 (a quality of life as bad as being dead). It is not easy to measure the value of a healthy state, and there are different methods used for this purpose, such as asking individuals to trade off improvements in their health status against either life expectancy (time trade-off) or risk of death (standard gamble). The results of these exercises are called "utilities."

A *cost-minimization analysis* is used when the health effects of two alternative interventions are known to be equal, and only the costs need to be analyzed. For example, comparing phototherapy at home with phototherapy in a hospital setting.

A *decision analysis* is applied when only the health effects of medical interventions are important, the alternative intervention has the same cost, or costs are not important in a particular decision situation.

To conduct an economic analysis, data from randomized controlled trials or observational studies are used. Unfortunately, clinical studies do not always follow up patients for long enough after intervention, and modeling is needed. Modeling techniques enable the clinical outcomes (such as survival) to be extrapolated beyond a point observed in a trial. However, they may pose artificial conditions to the analyses. It is very important to state the *perspective* from which the study will be valued, since costs may vary greatly if one considers the patient or the hospital, or the societal perspectives. Studies based on different perspectives are not comparable. The societal perspective is the most pragmatic choice because it represents the public interests rather than those of any particular group. Costs are generally divided into three categories: *direct, indirect,* and *intangible costs*. Direct costs include all resources associated with the provision of an intervention. Indirect costs refer to productivity loss incurred by an illness. Costs-of-illness studies have shown that indirect costs may be many times higher than direct costs. Most recently published studies use a human capital approach, which broadly encompasses both paid and unpaid work (e.g. parenting or housekeeping) to estimate indirect costs. Intangible costs are defined as pain and sufferings of patients because of a disease, and are usually measured by using the reduction in quality of life.

In many medical interventions, benefits and costs may occur in the future. For example, melanoma surgery may provide benefits for patients in the future, but also may create additional future costs, such as consultations of specialists and sequelae. Costs and benefits that occur in the future should be reduced (*discounted*) to their present value because of "time preference," that is, we would rather have something now than in the future, because the present time has more value for us.

Cost-effectiveness and cost–utility analyses in psoriasis

There is no definitive cure for psoriasis. All the available therapies are able to suppress disease activity temporarily, but once they are stopped, the disease usually relapses. As a consequence, both effectiveness data and economic analyses should focus on a relevant time frame that is not days or weeks but rather months and years. Psoriasis affects a significant proportion of the general population. If all patients were to be treated, the costs would likely involve a substantial use of resources. A number of issues make a cost-effectiveness evaluation of psoriasis treatment difficult. Among the others, are the possibility of combining and personalizing treatment, poor adherence to therapy (especially topical), and the need to consider social and psychological issues. The long-term nature of psoriasis and potential for prolonged use of systemic treatment bring about associated related costs concerning adverse reactions and their monitoring. Finally, interpreting costs in the context of different healthcare systems may represent an enormous challenge. Direct costs may vary according to country. In the USA, for example, there are direct financial costs to the patient, which are not appreciated by patients treated under the National Health Systems of most European countries.

A selection of cost-effectiveness analyses conducted on psoriasis in recent years is summarized in Table 2.2. Treatment for psoriasis includes topical, ultraviolet light-based, and systemic therapies. Costs may vary greatly according to disease severity and previous response to treatment. A step-by-step hierarchical strategy based on levels of disease severity, which starts with topical agents in mild psoriasis and moves to phototherapy and systemic agents in moderate to severe psoriasis, appears to make the best use of resources, and it is expected to be the most cost-effective. Unfortunately, no systematic evaluation of the advantages and drawbacks of this kind of strategy in a real-life situation is available. There are common limitations in the current cost-effectiveness studies of psoriasis. Since evidence from trials comparing treatments head to head is generally lacking, one should rely on indirect comparisons based on estimates from studies that may be heterogeneous and poorly comparable. Due to limited data on long-term outcome, modeling is usually performed which may be prone to uncertainties and arbitrary assumptions. Observational studies with large sample sizes of patients (through, for example, initiatives such as the Psonet collaboration) are required to demonstrate that beneficial effects are maintained over time and to monitor safety profiles. Much debate concerns new biological agents. The cost-effectiveness profile of biologics changes according to the population studied and the amount of money the society is willing to pay for unit of incremental effectiveness. Biologics have been documented to be most cost-effective in people with severe plaque psoriasis when conventional therapies have failed. With an improved knowledge of long-term effectiveness and safety, cost-effective profiles may change significantly in the near future.

Table 2.2 Summary aspects of recent studies on cost-effectiveness in psoriasis.

Country, year	Comparators	Outcome	Cost per outcome unit
The Netherlands, 2002	Inpatient treatment vs short contact dithranol vs UVB phototherapy	Clearance-days	ICER between inpatient and short contact was €6065 to increase response rate by 28%. The response rate for short contact was comparable with UVB, but the latter was less expensive (mean costs €1776 vs €1273)
UK, 2008	Infliximab vs etanercept continuous use or efalizumab or supportive care	QALYs (mapping changes in DLQI score, conditional on PASI response, to changes in EQ-5D)	ICER for infliximab against etanercept varied from £44,000 to £49,000 per QALY gained and from £42,000 to £47,000 against efalizumab (ERG estimates)
UK, 2008	Adalimumab vs etanercept, or efalizumab or infliximab or supportive care	QALYs (mapping changes in DLQI score, conditional on PASI response, to changes in EQ-5D)	ICER for adalimumab vs intermittent etanercept was £36,700 per QALY gained (ERG estimates)
UK, 2009	Ustekinumab vs etanercept, or efalizumab or infliximab or supportive care	QALYs (mapping changes in DLQI score, conditional on PASI response, to changes in EQ-5D)	ICER for ustekinumab vs supportive care and vs etanercept (25 mg intermittently), £27,105 and £29,587, respectively, per QALY gained. Adalimumab and etanercept given continuously were dominated by ustekinumab (manufacturer's estimates).
The Netherlands, 2010	Home vs outpatient phototherapy	Number of days with a relevant treatment effect (≥50% improvement of the baseline SAPASI). QALYs	ICER of €20 per additional day with a relevant treatment effect on home vs outpatient phototherapy. Incremental costs per QALY gained €4646 by one year
Germany, 2010	Biologicals to obtain clearance after 12 weeks of treatment vs placebo	Cost per patient achieving PASI-75 relative to placebo	Infliximab 3 mg/kg was the most cost-effective agent, followed by adalimumab, infliximab 5 mg/kg, and ustekinumab. The least cost-effective agent was etanercept 50 mg/week. Sensitivity analysis showed considerable overlap of the cost-effectiveness ratios

(Continued)

Table 2.2 (*Continued*)

Country, year	Comparators	Outcome	Cost per outcome unit
UK, 2011	Etanercept vs infliximab vs adalimumab for psoriatic arthritis not responding to DMARD treatment	QALYs taking into account Psoriatic Arthritis Response Criteria (PsARC), ACR 20, PASI and functional status	In psoriatic arthritis with mild-to-moderate skin disease, the ICER of etanercept vs palliative care was £18,000 per QALY, and the ICER of infliximab vs etanercept was £44,000 per QALY. Adalimumab was extensively dominated. In psoriatic arthritis with moderate to severe skin disease, the ICER of adalimumab vs palliative care was £16,000 per QALY, the ICER of etanercept vs adalimumab was £21,000 per QALY, and the ICER for infliximab vs etanercept was £26,000 per QALY
USA, 2011	Phototherapy and systemic therapies	Cost per patient achieving DLQI minimally important difference and PASI 75	Lowest cost for phototherapy and methotrexate highest cost for alefacept
USA, 2013	Ustekinumab 45 and 90 mg vs etanercept 50 mg	Costs and QALYs, estimated from the US societal perspective. All costs were adjusted to 2011 US dollars.	The ICER for ustekinumab 90 mg vs etanercept 50 mg was US$384,401 per QALY gained. Ustekinumab 45 mg dominated etanercept 50 mg for the same time horizon
UK, 2013	Topical therapies for localized plaque psoriasis	Costs and QALYs	The use of twice-daily potent corticosteroids was the most cost-effective first-line strategy for both trunk/limbs and scalp psoriasis

ERG: evidence review group; ICER: incremental cost-effectiveness ratio, comparing the difference in costs between the two strategies, divided by the difference in their effectiveness; QALY: combination of the duration of life and the health-related quality of life.

Further reading

Hartman, M., Prins, M., Swinkels, O.Q. *et al.* (2002) Cost-effectiveness analysis of a psoriasis care instruction programme with dithranol compared with UVB phototherapy and inpatient dithranol treatment. *British Journal of Dermatology*, **147**, 538–544.

Koek, M.B.G., Sigurdsson, V., van Weelden, H. *et al.* (2010) Cost effectiveness of home ultraviolet B phototherapy for psoriasis: economic evaluation of a randomised controlled trial (PLUTO study). *BMJ*, **340**, c1490.

NICE (2008a) Adalimumab for the treatment of adults with psoriasis [WWW document]. NICE Technology Assessment Guidance 146. URL www.nice.org.uk/TA146 [accessed on June 15, 2014].

NICE (2008b) Infliximab for the treatment of adults with psoriasis [WWW document]. NICE Technology Assessment Guidance 134. URL www.nice.org.uk/TA134 [accessed on June 15, 2014].

NICE (2008c) Ustekinumab for the treatment of adults with moderate to severe psoriasis [WWW document]. NICE Technology Assessment Guidance 180. URL www.nice.org.uk/TA180 [accessed on June 15, 2014].

Rodgers, M, Epstein, D., Bojke, L. *et al.* (2011) Etanercept, infliximab and adalimumab for the treatment of psoriatic arthritis: a systematic review and economic evaluation. *Health Technology Assessment*, **15**, i–xxi, 1–329.

Sawyer, L., Samarasekera, E.J., Wonderling, D. and Smith, C.H. (2013) Topical therapies for the treatment of localized plaque psoriasis in primary care: a cost-effectiveness analysis. *British Journal of Dermatology*, **168**, 1095–1105.

Schmitt-Rau, K., Rosenbach, T., Radtke, M.A. and Augustin, M. (2010) Cost-effectiveness of biological therapy in remission induction of moderate to severe plaque psoriasis. *Dermatology*, **221**, 236–242.

Staidle, J.P., Dabade, T.S. and Feldman, S.R. (2011) A pharmacoeconomic analysis of severe psoriasis therapy: a review of treatment choices and cost-efficiency. *Expert Opinion on Pharmacotherapy*, **12**, 2041–2054.

Villacorta, R., Hay, J.W. and Messali, A. (2013) Cost effectiveness of moderate to severe psoriasis therapy with etanercept and ustekinumab in the United States. *Pharmacoeconomics*, **31**, 823–839.

PART II
Etiology and pathogenesis

Robert Sabat
Psoriasis Research and Treatment Center, Department of Dermatology and Allergy/Institute of Medical Immunology, University Hospital Charité, Berlin, Germany

Owing to the efforts of innumerable scientists and physicians who, since the early 1950s, have been performing numerous experiments, investigations, and studies, as reflected by about 36,000 psoriasis-related scientific publications, we have been obtaining an increasingly complete picture of the etiology and, especially, the pathogenesis of psoriasis. This gain in knowledge has also benefited enormously from the great advances in immunology, particularly with respect to our understanding of the course of immune reactions, novel cytokines, and newly discovered immune cell populations and their functions. Naturally, the psoriasis research has also contributed continuously to the progress in immunology.

Currently, we think that the etiology of psoriasis involves genetic and environmental factors. At the beginning of psoriasis pathogenesis, exogenous triggers initiate an immune reaction that leads to the development of a small number of certain immune cells (specific T-cell populations) able to migrate to and act in the skin. Upon later local skin damage or other kinds of disturbance, resident immune cells are stimulated and produce small proteins called cytokines that attract blood immune cells into the skin. Infiltrating immune cells are activated and produce other cytokines that stimulate tissue cells. The activated tissue cells support the inflammation so that the evolving vicious circle normally does not stop without therapeutic intervention. A specific cytokine cocktail finally changes the functions of keratinocytes, endothelial cells, and fibroblasts, so that the characteristic skin alterations, including the thickening of the epidermis and the elongation and contortion of the dermal capillaries, become obvious. The development and maintenance of this pathogenetic cascade are favored by genetic, lifestyle-related, and environmental factors, too.

Psoriasis: Diagnosis and Management, First Edition. Edited by Wolfram Sterry, Robert Sabat, and Sandra Philipp.

CHAPTER 3

Microscopic skin alterations

Kerstin Wolk[1], Hans-Joachim Röwert-Huber[2], and Robert Sabat[1]

[1] *Psoriasis Research and Treatment Center, Department of Dermatology and Allergy/Institute of Medical Immunology, University Hospital Charité, Berlin, Germany*

[2] *Department of Dermatology and Allergy, University Hospital Charité, Berlin, Germany*

The microscopic alterations of the lesional psoriatic skin reveal very impressive features that mainly concern the epidermis and the papillary dermis. In many aspects they are characteristic for psoriasis and, in connection with specific staining methods, allow a differential diagnosis regarding other cutaneous diseases such as *Tinea corporis*, subacute and chronic eczemas, and *Pityriasis rubra pilaris*, although the distinction from psoriasiform drug reactions may remain challenging.

To understand the histological changes that manifest in the psoriatic lesions, it is necessary to understand the structure and dynamics of healthy skin. This chapter will provide details regarding normal skin before focussing on the manifold histological alterations observed with psoriatic skin. Since there are slight variations concerning the macroscopic and microscopic pictures of different psoriasis forms, we will focus on the most common form: psoriasis vulgaris.

The human skin: a multilayered, dynamic barrier to the environment

The skin is composed of three main layers: the epidermis representing a cornifying epithelium that forms a direct barrier to the environment; the dermis, which ensures the nutrition of the epidermis and harbors the appendages of the skin; and the subcutaneous adipose layer called the subcutis (Figure 3.1). The epidermis is mostly composed of keratinocytes. It is attached to the underlying basement membrane and builds projections into the dermis called rete ridges, a property that causes a tight toothing of the epidermis and the dermis. The keratinocytes are not uniform but form different epidermal strata: the outermost *stratum corneum*, the *stratum lucidum* (only in the palms of the hands and soles of the feet), the *stratum granulosum*, the *stratum spinosum*, and the basement membrane-associated *stratum basale*. Apart from the keratinocytes, melanocytes, Merkel cells, and immune cells

Psoriasis: Diagnosis and Management, First Edition. Edited by Wolfram Sterry, Robert Sabat, and Sandra Philipp.

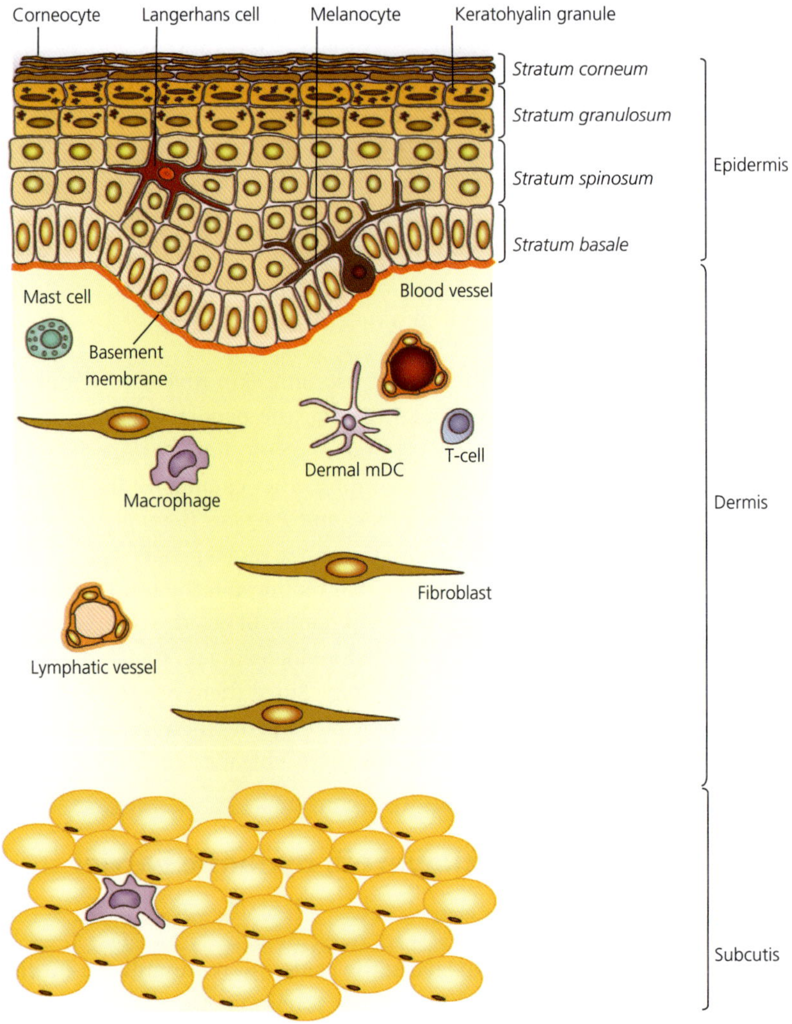

Figure 3.1 Schematic depiction of normal skin structure.

including Langerhans cells (CD1a+CD207+), and very few T-cells (CD3+) are also present in the epidermis. The epidermis is not vascularized but is nourished by diffusion from dermal blood capillaries. The dermis comprises the upper papillary region between the epidermal rete ridges and the lower reticular region. It mainly consists of connective tissue composed of collagenous and elastic fibers as well as fibroblasts. Apart from the blood vessels, the dermis contains many nerve fibers and mechanoreceptors, hair follicles, perspiratory, sebaceous, and apocrine glands, as well as lymphatic vessels. It also harbors immune cells such as immature myeloid dendritic cells (mDCs; CD11c+CD1c+), plasmacytoid dendritic cells (pDCs; CD11c–CD123+CD303+), mast cells (CD117+, tryptase+), macrophages (CD11c+CD68+), and some T-cells. Most of the T-cells have a memory phenotype (CD45RA–CD45RO+) and are distributed perivascularly. The subcutis attaches the skin to underlying bone and muscle, and supplies it with blood vessels and nerves. It consists of clusters of adipocytes lying between connective tissue strands. Fibroblasts and macrophages are also present.

Throughout our whole life, the epidermis is a highly regenerative tissue, even without notable damage. Under normal conditions, it is in an equilibrium state created by the coordination of three processes: the generation of new cells in the *stratum basale*, their upward movement and differentiation, and their final apoptosis and exfoliation.

The *stratum basale* contains proliferating (interfollicular epidermal stem cells) along with differentiating cells. The level of β-1 integrin expression determines their strength of adherence to extracellular components of the basement membrane. The mitosis of a stem cell produces proliferating as well as differentiating daughter cells.

When the newly produced cells lose their ability to adhere to the basement membrane, they move up the strata, thereby changing composition and shape. In the overlaying *stratum spinosum*, the expression of basal cell keratins (K5, K14, K15) is replaced by suprabasal keratins (K1, K10). Formed K1/K10 filaments favor the mechanical strength of the layer. Moreover, these filaments are essential for a process called terminal differentiation, which finally leads to the cornification of the keratinocytes and the production of the *stratum corneum*. During this process, cells start to synthesize numerous proteins that are encoded by the epidermal differentiation complex on chromosome 1 (1q21). Their intracellular acquisition of keratohyalin granules containing profilaggrin means that they have a granular appearance (*stratum granulosum*). Profilaggrin encodes a protein precursor molecule that is proteolytically processed providing the N-terminal peptide and several copies of filaggrin. Filaggrin bundles K1/K10 filaments into macrofibrils, a process that promotes a flattened cell shape. Underneath the plasma membrane, further newly synthesized proteins (such as involucrin, loricrin, and small proline-rich proteins) covalently and irreversibly associate with the keratin–filaggrin aggregations and finally form the so-called cornified envelope that replaces the cytoplasmic membrane. The enzymes catalyzing these covalent associations include transglutaminases such as TG3. Lipids including ceramides, cholesterol and free fatty acids are synthesized as precursers, stored within the cells in the form of laminar bodies, extruded into the extracellular space, and processed. While some of these lipids become covalently attached to the cornified envelope, most of them form intercellular lamellae. After the dissolution of the cell nuclei, a process that is supported by the profilaggrin-derived N-terminal peptide, the final corneocytes lie in a lipid matrix and are tightly attached to each other by corneodesmosoms. However, in the uppermost *stratum corneum*, the corneodesmosomal proteins are cleaved by proteases of the kallikrein and the cathepsin families to allow physiological desquamation. The number of corneocytes that are (almost unnoticeably) desquamated by the healthy individual has been estimated to be around 50,000 million daily. All these processes are strongly impaired in the diseased skin of patients suffering from psoriasis.

The psoriatic skin: inflammation with epidermal and vascular remodeling

The microscopically visible skin alterations in psoriasis concern the interfollicular areas. Already at the onset of a psoriatic plaque, changes are visible, although they are first very subtle and nonspecific, and predominantly restricted to the upper dermis. They include dermal edema, the dilatation of blood vessels of the papillae, and perivascular cell infiltrations composed of lymphocytes (mostly T-cells) and monocytes/macrophages. The detailed analysis of experimentally induced lesions in psoriasis patients revealed that the first cells reaching the skin are CD4+ T-cells, followed by CD8+ T-cells and macrophages a few days later.

As the disease progresses, the density of the immune infiltrates increases, and besides mononuclear cells, neutrophilic granulocytes can be found, first in the dermis and then in the epidermis. Initial alterations of the skin architecture include a slight thickening of the living epidermis, whereas the *stratum corneum* appears normally.

In the fully developed lesion, the living epidermis is strongly thickened, a feature that is called acanthosis and causes the visible elevation of the skin surface (Figure 3.2). While the suprapapillar epidermis thickness is, if at all, only slightly increased, this thickening is mainly due to the enlargement and elongation of the epidermal rete ridges. The rete ridges form long downward projections into

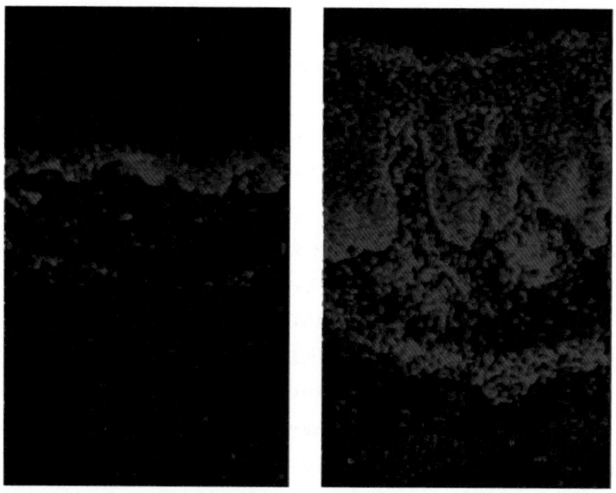

(a) (b)

Figure 3.2 Histological pictures with nuclear staining (fluorescent dye DAPI) of (left) non-lesional and (right) lesional skin of a psoriasis patient.

the dermis, thereby also expanding the papillary portion of dermis (papillosis). At least in evolving lesions, the *stratum granulosum*, representing the ongoing terminal keratinocyte differentiation, is lost. In addition to the changes in the living epidermis, the appearance of the *stratum corneum* is altered. This layer is massively thickened (called hyperkeratosis) and rather loosened, resulting in the generation of large, visible scales. Moreover, remaining cell nuclei are highly prominent within the corneocytes, a condition called parakeratosis.

These epidermal alterations have two causes: the massively increased proliferation of basal keratinocytes, which can be confirmed by staining of Ki-67, and the inhibited and in some way also abnormal terminal differentiation of keratinocytes of the upper layers, which is indicated among others by decreased staining for K1 and K10 (early terminal differentiation markers) and increased staining of K16 (marker of a regenerative state). Both increased proliferation and inhibited terminal differentiation are reminiscent of a regenerative state, as they are transiently observed also during wound repair but appear to be uncontrolled in psoriasis.

The proliferation rate of basal keratinocytes is strongly raised in psoriatic lesions compared with that in the normal epidermis. In fact, most cells of the *stratum basale* are proliferative, and the cell cycle time is shortened in that situation. The aberrant proliferation is thought to increase the two-dimensional extension of the *stratum basale* and, therewith, to elongate the rete ridges. The increased generation of epidermal cells in turn induces a general growth of the suprabasal, differentiating cell layers. It has been proposed that the two-dimensional increase in the size of the proliferative layer (*stratum basale*) is proportional to the three-dimensional increase in the size of the differentiating compartment (mainly *stratum spinosum* in psoriasis).

Although one could suggest that in the psoriatic lesion, the massive production and decreased turnover time of keratinocytes in the epidermis are the reasons for the reduced terminal differentiation of these cells, we will show in the next chapter that the terminal differentiation is regulated at least partially independently of the hyperproliferation. As a consequence of the inhibited terminal differentiation, which normally starts in the *stratum spinosum*, the generation of the cytoplasmic keratohyalin granules, the flattening of the cell shape, and the dissolution of the cell nuclei do not take place properly. This in turn is responsible for the loss of the *stratum granulosum*, the thickening of the *stratum spinosum* (acanthosis), and the parakeratosis, respectively. Moreover, the inhibited terminal differentiation does not allow the accurate production of the intercorneocyte lipid layers, impairing the normal intercorneocyte lipid structure and water-permeability barrier of the *stratum corneum*. In addition, the hyperkeratosis is generated as a result of the excessive generation of keratinocytes, which, although not properly following the terminal differentiation program, finally die in a premature state in the uppermost layers. As the degradation of corneodesmosomal proteins such as corneodesmosin and desmoglein in the upper *stratum corneum*, which is necessary for normal desquamation, is impaired in psoriatic lesions, the hyperkeratosis is further strengthened, and large, lamellar scaling occurs. It is, however, interesting to note that despite the highly increased proliferation and the incomplete terminal differentiation of generated cells, the epidermis of established psoriatic lesions seems to have reached a new equilibrium state between cell generation and cell loss, keeping the special thickened form.

The psoriatic alterations further include changes in the architecture of the blood vessels in the papillary dermis. These vessels are contorted and elongated, spreading along the extended papillary dermal region between the outstretched epidermal rete ridges. Their increased Ki67 staining indicates an increased angiogenesis. Moreover, the dermal vessels are dilated. These changes explain the visible redness of the psoriatic lesions. Regarding the molecular level, the endothelial cells are activated, as demonstrated by their increased staining for molecules such as CD54, CD106, and P-selectin, which facilitates the continuous immigration of immune cells into the skin tissue.

Massive immune infiltrations are indeed present in the psoriatic lesions (Figure 3.3). Most striking are accumulations of mixed mononuclear cells in the epidermis and, even more prominently, in the dermis. They are mostly composed of mDCs, macrophages, T-cells, innate lymphoid cells, neutrophile granulocytes, and some mast cells. Interestingly, the numbers of T-cells, macrophages, and dendritic cells are similar. Whereas CD4+ T-cells are present in both the epidermis and dermis, CD8+ T-cells are more preferentially found in the dermis. A large subset of the T-cells expresses the so-called cutaneous lymphocyte-associated antigen (CLA), known to guide leukocytes to inflamed skin. Furthermore,

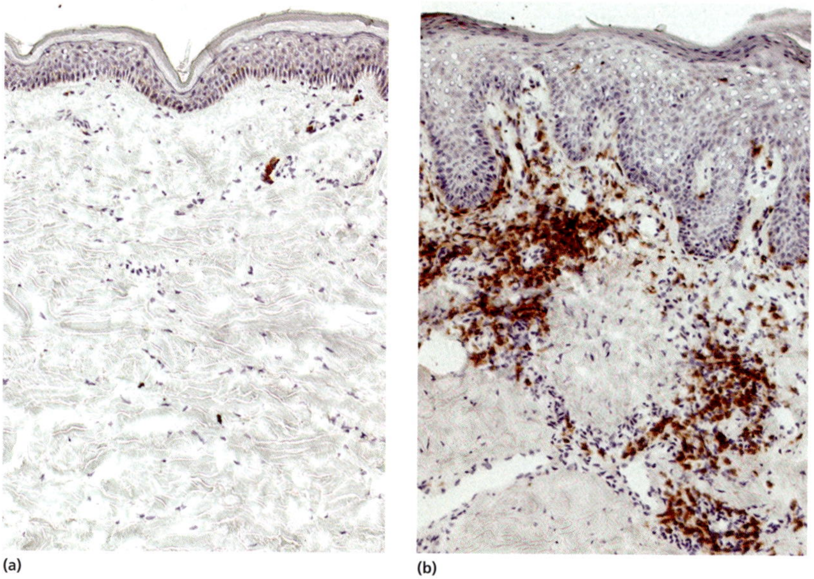

(a) (b)

Figure 3.3 Immunohistochemical CD3+ T-cell staining of (left) non-lesional and (right) lesional skin of a psoriasis patient.

they have memory (CD45RA–CD45RO+) and activation (HLA-DR+, CD69+) phenotypes. Corresponding to their successful entry in the skin tissue, T-cells also show positive staining for integrins. In fact, it has been shown that most intraepidermal T-cells in psoriatic skin lesions expressed CD11a/CD18, and 58% of CD4+ and 85% of CD8+ T-cells expressed VLA-4. Functional polarization of the present T-cells is evidenced by their effector cytokine expression, pointing to the dominance of Th17-, T22-, and T1-cells (see Chapter 4). The close neighborhood between antigen-presenting cells and T-cells in the aggregates suggests functional interaction as a prerequisite of the local reactivation of the infiltrated T-cells. The population of dendritic cells, present in high numbers in the lesional skin, mostly comprises myeloid subsets including those that are known from normal skin (see above) as well as inflammatory cells. The latter include the epidermal inflammatory mDCs (CD1a+CD207–) and the dermal inflammatory mDCs (CD1c–CD11c+). The number of pDCs does not seem to be different from that in healthy skin. Apart from the mononuclear cells, neutrophilic granulocytes are present in the inflamed skin of the psoriasis lesion. In the fully evolved lesions in patients with psoriasis vulgaris, they form small foci of the epidermis underneath and within the *stratum corneum*, known as Munro's microabscesses.

Further reading

Candi, E., Schmidt, R. and Melino, G. (2005) The cornified envelope: a model of cell death in the skin. *Nature Reviews Molecular Cell Biology*, **6**, 328–340.

Clark, R.A. (2010) Skin-resident T cells: the ups and downs of on site immunity. *Journal of Investigative Dermatology*, **130**(2), 362–370.

Creamer, D., Sullivan, D., Bicknell, R. and Barker, J. (2002) Angiogenesis in psoriasis. *Angiogenesis*, **5**(4), 231–236.

Iizuka, H., Takahashi, H. and Ishida-Yamamoto, A. (2004) Psoriatic architecture constructed by epidermal remodeling. *Journal of Dermatological Science*, **35**(2), 93–99.

Ragaz, A. and Ackerman, A.B. (1979) Evolution, maturation, and regression of lesions of psoriasis. New observations and correlation of clinical and histologic findings. *American Journal of Dermatopathology*, **1**(3), 199–214.

Zaba, L.C., Krueger, J.G. and Lowes, M.A. (2009) Resident and "inflammatory" dendritic cells in human skin. *Journal of Investigative Dermatology*, **129**(2), 302–308.

CHAPTER 4
Pathogenesis of psoriasis

Robert Sabat and Kerstin Wolk
Psoriasis Research and Treatment Center, Department of Dermatology and Allergy, and Institute of Medical Immunology, University Hospital Charité, Berlin, Germany

The pathogenesis of psoriasis resembles in many aspects an adaptive immune reaction that leads to an overshot regeneration-like response of the skin tissue cells. Adaptive immune reactions proceed in two main phases: the sensitization phase and the effector phase (Figure 4.1). During the sensitization phase, professional antigen-presenting cells (APCs) like myeloid dendritic cells (mDCs) and macrophages capture locally present antigens (Ags) and are activated. Subsequently, they degrade these Ags intracellularly and present fragments of them on special proteins at their surface. These matured and activated APCs then induce the development of Ag-specific, skin-directed effector and memory Th17-, T22-, and T1-cells. It is important to note, that this part of psoriasis pathogenesis is normally not accompanied by any skin alterations. The sensitization phase can be followed by a silent phase of variable length. The subsequent effector phase is provoked by exogenous triggers that activate skin-resident immune cells, such as macrophages or mast cells. As a result of this activation, these cells secrete small proteins like chemokines and other inflammatory cytokines that lead to the infiltration of various immune cells [neutrophilic granulocytes, various subpopulations of T-cells, monocytes/macrophages, and various subpopulations of dendritic cells (DCs)] into the skin. The infiltrated immune cells are enabled to produce further cytokines that activate local cells to further secrete chemokines and other inflammatory mediators, and together support the immune-cell infiltration process. Over time, the cocktail of cytokines that are secreted by activated immune and tissue cells is altering the biology of keratinocytes and endothelial cells, resulting in a reaction that is reminiscent of an overshot regeneration process (like wound healing). Finally, the simultaneously occurring effector phase processes including immune-cell infiltration, immune-cell activation, tissue-cell activation, and alteration of tissue cell biology amplify each other, making the effector phase becoming self-reliant. It is important to note that only the last part of effector phase creates the visible psoriasis-typical skin alterations. After a successful treatment, the effector phase largely stops. However, a weak exogenous trigger can again initiate the effector phase.

Psoriasis: Diagnosis and Management, First Edition. Edited by Wolfram Sterry, Robert Sabat, and Sandra Philipp.

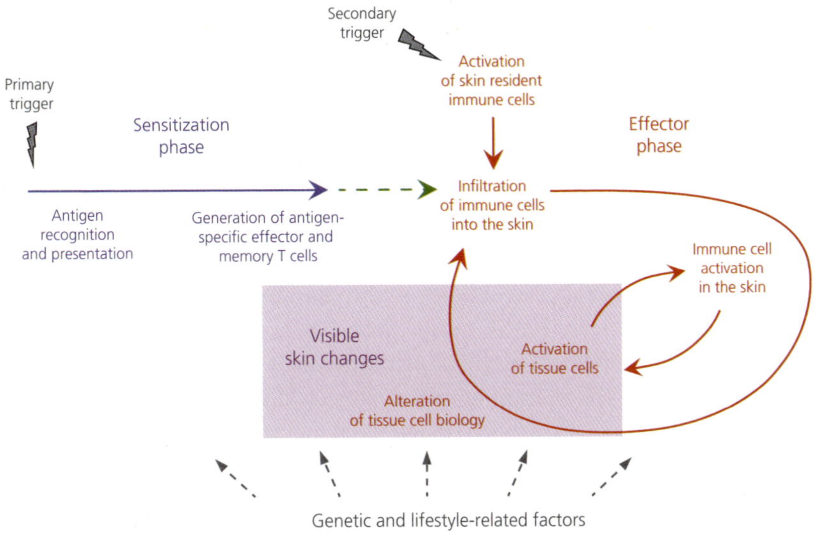

Figure 4.1 Phases of the psoriasis pathogenesis. The pathogenesis of psoriasis proceeds in the context of the underlying genetic predisposition and life-style-related factors. Resembling an adaptive immune reaction, the pathogenesis can be subdivided into the sensitization and the effector phase. During the sensitization phase that is triggered by primary exogenous factors, antigen-presenting cells guide the generation of specific effector and memory Th17-, Th22-, and Th1-cells in secondary lymphatic organs. The effector phase is triggered by secondary exogenous triggers, which activate skin-resident immune cells. Their release of inflammatory proteins leads to the infiltration of generated T- and other immune cells into the skin where they activate each other and tissue cells. The continuous presence of inflammatory mediators induces a regeneration-like state of the tissue cells and, eventually, the skin structure alteration characteristic for the psoriatic lesion.

Sensitization phase: antigen processing and presentation

The initial steps of every adaptive immune reaction are performed by professional APCs and include: (i) the recognition and uptake of an (exogenous) Ag by immature mDCs, (ii) the migration of these cells to the T-cell areas of secondary lymphoid organs, (iii) the intracellular degradation of the incorporated Ag into peptide fragments, and (iv) the presentation of selected Ag fragments on the major histocompatibility complex class II (MHC) molecules on the DC cell surfaces.

Immature mDCs are located within and beneath epithelia as well as in most organs, where they monitor the tissue for incoming Ags. Dermal immature mDCs preferentially settle along the blood vessels. In this state, they are not able to form stable complexes of MHC II molecules and antigenic fragments because of the absence of incorporated Ag and minimal cellular lysosomal activity. Instead, the MHC II molecules in immature mDCs preferentially reside intracellularly in specialized endo-/lysosomal compartments where they are associated with the chaperonic invariant chain. In addition, these compartments contain protease inhibitors and inactive proteases. The invariant chain stabilizes the conformation of MHC II molecules, protects them from premature peptide loading, and retains them in the endosomal compartments. An additional mechanism accounting for the low MHC II expression and antigen presentation in immature mDCs is the increased endocytosis of these molecules, which leads to their very short half-life on the cell surface.

After the uptake of Ag, mDCs undergo a maturation process if they receive a stimulus through cytokines like TNF-α or through Toll-like receptor-stimulating microbial products. As an initial result, they begin to express the chemokine receptor CCR7 on their surface, and follow the gradient of CCR7-activating chemokines (CCL19, CCL21) to afferent lymphatic vessels. In fact, depositions of CCL21 complexed with collagen are located on the basal membrane on afferent lymphatic vessels, and activated mDCs recognize these complexes and migrate through membrane gaps into the lymphatic vessel lumen. Here, they crawl along endothelial cells and later switch to passive drifting into the T-cell area of the regional lymph nodes. At the same time, they are carrying the previously uptaken Ag insight them and drastically reduce their capacity to incorporate further Ags. Furthermore, several changes happen in the MHC II pathway. The maturation of mDCs is accompanied by a decreased production of protease inhibitors and by activation of the vacuolar ATPase that reduces the pH value in the endosomal/lysosomal compartments towards the optimum for proteases. The resulting increased protease activity leads to splitting of both the invariant chain and incorporated Ags. The degradation of the invariant chain takes place in a defined sequence of steps. In the final step, its endosomal retention signal sequence is split off, and only the invariant chain fragment (named CLIP) that blocks the peptide-binding cleft of the MHC II molecule remains intact. Interestingly, this limiting step is operating in mDCs by a unique cysteine endopeptidase named cathepsin S. The degradation of incorporated Ags is a process in which numerous proteases, including cathepsins and legumain, are involved, and which produces peptides of approximately 12–25 amino acids in length. If these peptides have a high affinity for the peptide-binding cleft of a special MHC II molecule, they are substituted for CLIP. This substitution is facilitated by means of the nonclassical MHC II molecule HLA-DM. The peptide-loaded MHC II complex is then transported to the surface of the mDC.

After a transient upregulation during the beginning maturation, the further synthesis of MHC II molecules is inhibited in mature mDCs. This is caused by the reduced expression of the transcriptional regulator class II transactivator due to the epigenetic modulation of the promoter of the encoding gene. Both the extenuated Ag uptake and the reduced MHC II molecule synthesis prevent the presentation of further Ags that the DC could meet, for example, in lymph nodes. This prevention in connection with the increased half-life of the MHC II molecule–Ag peptide complexes on the cell surface of mature mDCs guarantees that these cells present (for a very long time) the same fragments of previously uptaken Ag. The presented MHC II molecule–Ag peptide complex is recognized by CD4+ T-cells via the T-cell receptor (TCR) given that this TCR is specific for that respective MHC II molecule–Ag peptide complex. This recognition in combination with further events that are described below leads to the generation of specific effector and memory CD4+ T-cells. Importantly, the compositions of the Ag-processing proteases in DCs as well as the DC's MHC types determine the nature of the presented peptides and thereby, in the end, the specificity of the effector and memory T-cells that are generated in the sensitization phase.

In addition to the activation of CD4+ T-cells via MHC II molecule–Ag peptide complexes, mDCs also present Ag fragments on MHC I molecules to stimulate CD8+ T-cells. Most Ags whose fragments appear on MHC I molecules were primarily intracellular Ag; however, some DCs (e.g. CD1c+mDCs from skin) have the ability to cross-present extracellular Ags on MHC I molecules (e.g. parts of microbes).

At this point, a question arises that is crucial for understanding the pathogenesis of psoriasis, namely which Ag is responsible for initial T-cell priming. Unfortunately, we cannot currently answer this question for the majority of patients. The identity of the psoriatic Ag(s) should be revealed when the reactivity of T-cells in psoriatic lesions is identified. Interestingly, some reports have described how T-cell lines established from psoriatic lesions, in particular from patients suffering from psoriasis guttate, proliferate and produce IFN-γ in the presence of APCs and isolates from streptococci. A streptococcal origin of the primary Ag(s) would be in line with the fact that first manifestation and relapses and aggravations of psoriasis guttate are often linked to infections with streptococci, especially β-hemolytic *Streptococcus pyogenes*. However, it seems that only a very small proportion of epidermal CD8+ T-cells (approximately 2–3%) recognize streptococcal Ags (probably the M protein, an element of streptococcal cell membrane) and in only two-thirds of patients with chronic plaque psoriasis. In addition, some of the dermal CD4+ T-cells might react against peptidoglycans from the streptococcal cell wall. However, neither the proportion of such CD4+ T-cells within the whole CD4+ T-cell infiltrate nor the proportion of psoriasis patients with dermis infiltrated T-cells against streptococcal Ags is currently known. Furthermore, T-cells reacting against streptococcal Ags are often also present in the blood of control patients, thus prompting the question of which Ag is responsible for initial T-cell priming in the majority of psoriasis patients remains unanswered.

Sensitization phase: generation of effector and memory T-cells

In secondary lymphoid organs, mature, Ag fragment-presenting mDCs induce and govern the development of effector and long-living memory T-cells from naïve T-cells. This evolution is necessary for the T-cells to gain substantial functions and for the ability to migrate into tissues, and comprises the following steps: recognition of the MHC moelcule–Ag peptide complexes, initial activation, proliferation, and differentiation.

The naïve, L-selectin- (CD62L) and CCR7-expressing T-cells circulate continuously between blood and secondary lymphoid organs, such as lymph nodes, spleen, and tonsils. In T-cell areas of these organs, they foregather with mature mDCs. If the TCR of a naïve CD4+ T-cell has an adequately high affinity for binding a MHC II molecule–Ag peptide complex, this T-cell will stick to the respective mDC. Importantly, this interaction ensures the specificity of the developing effector T-cells because (1) the structure of the portion of the MHC II–Ag peptide complex that is recognized by the TCR is unique, (2) a naïve T-cell expresses only one type of TCR, and (3) this TCR type is transmitted to its offspring.

The interaction between TCR and the MHC II–Ag peptide complex is stabilized by a T-cell transmembrane molecule named CD4 that binds to a nonpolymorphic region of the MHC II molecule. In so doing, a tyrosine kinase (Lck), which is intracellularly attached to the CD4, is moved towards the TCR and the TCR-associated proteins: CD3 and ζ-chain. Lck phosphorylates special tyrosines of the intracellular parts of the CD3 and the ζ-chain, and initiates the activation cascade as follows: The phosphorylated ζ-chain acts as a docking site for the ZAP-70 molecule, which, after phosphorylation, acquires its own tyrosine kinase activity and enables large cytoplasmatic signaling molecules and transcription factors. These translocate to the nucleus where they bind to the promoters of numerous genes and induce their transcription.

Interestingly, the stimulation of around 100 TCRs is already sufficient to start the T-cell activation. However, in order to be completely activated, the T-cell needs two additional signals: the signal given by adhesion molecules and, in particular, costimulatory molecules and the signal delivered by soluble mediators from the DC (Figure 4.2).

The specific contact area between a T-cell and mDC is named immunological synapsis and represents a unique arrangement of molecules within it. The initial interaction between the T-cell and the mDC is stabilized by nonspecific binding through adhesion molecules that actively form a ring around the clustered MHC II molecule–Ag peptide–TCR complexes. Simultaneously, the large CD45 molecules are moved to an outer ring. The most important adhesion molecules are: the intercellular adhesion molecule 1 (ICAM-1; CD54) on the DC that interacts with lymphocyte function-associated antigen-1 (LFA-1; CD11a/CD18; αL:β2) on the T-cell and the lymphocyte function-associated antigen 3 (LFA-3; CD58) on the DC that binds CD2 on the T-cell. Interestingly, the signal received via the TCR induces a conformation change of LFA-1 that results in a tighter binding to CD54.

Further important components of immunological synapsis include the costimulatory molecules. In fact, the activation of T-cells in the absence of

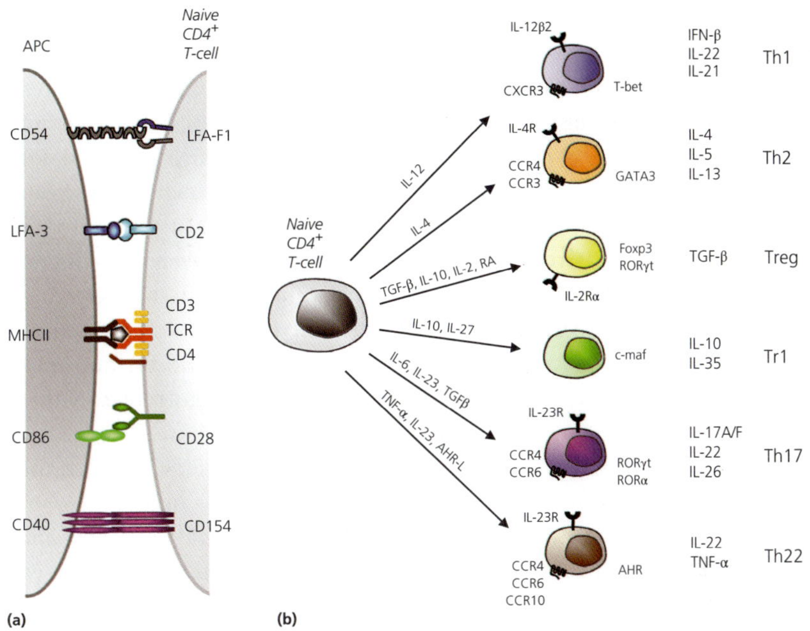

Figure 4.2 Requirements for effector and memory T-cell generation. For the development of effector and memory Th-cell subsets from naïve CD4+ cell precursors, different levels of interaction with the antigen-presenting cells are necessary. Facilitated by nonspecific stabilizing interactions with the APC through adhesion molecules (e.g. ICAM1–LFA-1, LFA-3–CD2), the naïve T-cell needs three APC signals: The specificity of interaction is based on the recognition of the APC's MHC II–Ag peptide by the TCR complex. Costimulatory signals (e.g. from the DC's CD86, CD80, and CD40) ensure full activation and prevent anergy of the T-cell. Specific polarizing cytokines secreted by the APC are essential for the proliferating T-cell to obtain its effector function, that is, to become polarized into a Th1-cell, Th2-cell, Th17-cell, Th22-cell, inducible regulatory T-cell (iTreg), or type 1 regulatory T-cell (Tr1).

costimulatory signals leads to the development of unresponsive T-cells. The most potent costimulatory molecules expressed by DCs are those of the B7 family: CD86 (B7–2), CD80 (B7–1), B7h, PD-L1, and PD-L2 as well as CD40. CD86 and CD80 interact with the T-cell molecules CD28 and CD152 (cytotoxic T-lymphocyte-associated protein 4, CTLA-4). The T-cell counterpart for B7h is a molecule named ICOS, the counterpart for PD-L1 and PD-L2 is PD-1, and that for CD40 is CD154. CD28 shows a large constitutive expression in T-cells, particularly in naïve T-cells. Engagement of CD28 reduces the number of triggered TCRs required for T-cell activation and allows activation of T-cells by low-affinity ligands. Additionally, it is important for stable IL-2 production and the expression of the IL-2 receptor α-chain component (IL-2Rα; CD25). Furthermore, engagement of CD28 prevents induction of anergy and apoptosis of T-cells after TCR stimulation. Hence, CD86 in DCs functions as a major costimulatory molecule and is critical for full activation, particularly of naïve T-cells. CD152 is not expressed on resting T-cells, but is transported from intracellular clatherin vesicles to the cell surface following TCR stimulation. Engagement of CD152 inhibits TCR- and CD28-mediated signal transduction, increases the threshold for activation of these cells, represses the cell cycle, and blocks IL-2 production. Therefore, it counteracts acute T-cell responses but is also essential for the formation of memory T-cells (otherwise all cells would differentiate into effector cells with short lifetimes). The biological significances of CD28 and CD152 might be time-dependent: On naïve T-cells constitutively expressed CD28 initially interacts with CD86/CD80 and potentiates activation. Later, stimulated T-cells express CD152, which, based on its higher affinity to CD86/CD80, terminates the T-cell proliferation and supports the development of effector and memory T-cells. Interestingly, the interactions of costimulatory molecules with their ligands not only induce T-cell activation but also stimulate the mDCs. For example, the binding between CD40 and CD154 enhances the Ag presentation by mDCs.

As a result of the stimulation from the MHC II–Ag peptide complex and the costimulatory molecules, T-cells secrete large amounts of IL-2 for 1–2 days and express the CD25 on their surface. On resting T-cells, only the low-affinity IL-2R composed of β- (IL-2 binding chain) and γ-chain (signaling unit) is present. The occurrence of CD25 during activation leads to formation of the high-affinity IL-2R (affinity about 10^{-11} M). The interaction of IL-2 with this receptor complex results in activation of receptor-associated kinases and, finally, in cell division and clonal expansion of the T-cell. Furthermore, other mDC cytokines contribute to the T-cell proliferation. For example, IL-1β enhances the expression of CD25 and thereby assists T-cell proliferation. Over time, some of the progeny of the proliferating T-cells differentiate into effector cells.

The third signal mentioned above is essential for the proliferating T-cells to obtain their effector function (polarization). According to current knowledge, naïve CD4+ T-cells can be polarized into six different directions: Th1-, Th2-, Th17-, Th22-, inducible regulatory T-cells (iTreg), and type 1 regulatory T-cells (Tr1; Figure 4.2).

If IL-12 (p35/p40 heterodimer) is present, the T-cells are polarized into Th1-cells through activation of the transcription factors: signal transducer and activator of transcription (Stat)4 and T-bet. The generation of Th1-cells is further supported by interferon (IFN)-γ, which increases the expression of the specific receptor chain for IL-12 (IL-12Rβ2). During repeated activation, Th1-cells primarily secrete IFN-γ, IL-22, and TNF-α.

If IL-4 is present, naïve T-cells are polarized into Th2-cells through activation of the transcription factors Stat6 and GATA-3. These T-cells secrete IL-4, IL-5, and IL-13 during repeated activation.

The activation of naïve T-cells in the presence of transforming growth factor (TGF)-β, IL-6, and IL-1β induces Th17-cell development and upregulates the receptor for IL-23 (IL-23R). Importantly, IL-23 (p19/p40 heterodimer) plays an essential role in the maintenance and survival of these cells. Th17-cell development is dependent on retinoic acid-related orphan receptor (ROR)γt, RORα, and IRF4. Th17-cells primarily produce IL-17, IL-26, and GM-CSF.

Interestingly, the Th1-cell inducing cytokines IL-12 and IFN-γ actively suppress the development of Th2- and Th17-cells. Conversely, the Th2-cell inducing cytokine IL-4 inhibits the development of Th1- and Th17-cells. Furthermore, strong Th17-cell development in experimental animals prevents the appearance of Th1- and Th2-cells.

In the presence of TNF-α, IL-6, and activators of the hydrocarbon receptor (AHR), naïve T-cells are polarized towards Th22-cells. These cells primarily secrete IL-22 during repeated activation.

The development of iTreg cells that constitutively carry high levels of CD25 is dependent on IL-2 and TGF-β. As mentioned above, TGF-β is simultaneously essential for the generation of Th17-cells because it induces RORγt in T-cells. Retinoic acid, the ligand of RORγt, acts as a cofactor and enhances the TGF-β-mediated induction of Foxp3 expression. Foxp3 prevents the RORγt functions in the Th17-cell generation and is essential for the suppressive features of iTreg. However, when IL-6 is present, it overcomes the effect of Foxp3 and, together with IL-1β, creates the programming of Th17-cells that is RORγt-dependent. Thus, inflammatory conditions tilt the balance between iTreg and Th17 towards Th17 direction. Tr1-cells develop from naïve T-cells under the influence of IL-27 through activation of the transcription factor c-maf. These cells primarily secrete IL-10 and IL-35 during repeated activation. Tr1- and iTreg-cells are jointly responsible for limiting T-cell immune responses, partly by production of immunosuppressive cytokines such as TGF-β, IL-10, and IL-35 and by cell surface molecules such as CD152 and CD25.

Interestingly, the different Th-cell subsets display distinct patterns of chemokine receptors on their surface. CXCR3 and CCR5 expression characterizes Th1-cells, and CCR3 and CCR4 are present on Th2-cells. Th17-cells express CCR4 and CCR6 but not CXCR3, and Th22-cells bear CCR4, CCR6, and CCR10.

The polarization into Th1-, Th2-, Th17-, or Th22-cells is accompanied by the differentiation of naïve T-cells into effector T-cells (TE), effector memory T-cells (TEM) or central memory T-cells (TCM). TE-cells immediately home into the inflamed tissue to which they are directed, display their effector functions, and die. The memory populations are generally responsible for the secondary, accelerated immune response to the same (or very similar) Ag during the subsequent contact. TEM-cells recirculate between blood and peripheral tissues and can demonstrate immediate effector functions such as (for CD4+ T-cells) the production of effector cytokines, but they have a limited proliferative capacity. Probably, epigenetic modifications, such as cytosine methylation at cytosine/guanine-rich DNA regions (CpG) by DNA cytosine-5-methyltransferase 1, and the presence of pivotal transcriptions factors, such as T-bet and GATA3, are the major determinants of the cytokine memory of these cells. In contrast to TE- and TEM-cells,

TCM-cells mainly recirculate between blood and lymph nodes. Normally, they do not produce any of the prototypic cytokines of the effector cell lineage immediately after stimulation through the TCR, although they secrete IL-2. Instead, they proliferate extensively and produce their primed effector cytokines only later. However, TCM-cells show moderate flexibility regarding the cytokine profile that they secrete. The differentiation of naïve T-cells into effector TE-cells is also accompanied by changes in their adhesion molecule equipment. Indeed, the levels of CD62L strongly decrease, and the expression of CD44, integrins, and ligands for E- and P-selectins increases, and this strongly favors their infiltration in inflamed tissue. Accordingly, the expression of the lymph-node homing receptors CCR7 and CD62L in combination with CD45 expression allows the phenotypical distinction between peripheral blood CD4+ T-cells: CD45RA+/CCR7+/CD62L+ cells represent the naïve compartment, CD45RA–/CCR7–/CD62L– cells represent the TEM compartment, and CD45RA–/CCR7+/CD62L+ cells represent the TCM compartment. Among CD8+ T-cells, TE-cells seem to add to the CD45RA+/CCR7–/CD62L– fraction.

A subset of successfully activated T-cells expresses the so-called cutaneous lymphocyte-associated antigen (CLA). CLA, a defined carbohydrate epitope [so-called sialyl-Lewis(x)], guides leukocytes to the inflamed skin. In line with that, the majority of CLA + T-cells are located in the skin, and only a small fraction of these cells circulate in the blood. With the help of fucosyltransferase VII, CLA can be placed on top of P-selectin glycoprotein ligand-1 (PSGL-1). PSGL-1 is a cell-surface molecule expressed constitutively on all peripheral T-cells. Moreover, CD43, a sialomucin that is also constitutively expressed on T-cells, can coat the CLA epitope. Interestingly, CLA-modified PSGL-1 binds both E- and P-selectin, whereas CLA-modified CD43 only binds E-selectin. However, the mechanisms by which DCs induce the expression of CLA on a defined subset of activated T-cells are still widely unknown. DCs and stromal lymph node cells may induce the expression of tissue-specific homing receptors on T-cells in dependence on the organ from which the DC comes and the respective local lymph node the DC monitors. An exception may be made for tonsillar DCs that present streptococcal Ags corresponding to the localization of streptococcal infection in the upper respiratory tract and the tonsils. These DCs seem to generate some skin-addressed T-cells as well. In fact, approximately 5–10% of tonsillar T-cells express CLA, and some of them might migrate into psoriatic lesions.

Effector phase: infiltration of immune cells into the skin

The detailed analysis of experimentally induced lesions (Koebner's response) in psoriasis patients revealed that the first cells reaching the skin are CD4+ T-cells, followed by CD8+ T-cells and macrophages a few days later. In line with this, the superficial perivascular infiltrates of lymphocytes and monocytic cells, and the dilation of the blood vessels in the dermal papillae are the first microscopically visible events during the developing of psoriatic plaques. These alterations occur before epidermal changes become visible. The processes occurring after mechanical influence might be as follows. Minimal injuries that lead to the entry of small numbers of microbes colonizing the body surface into the skin and the destruction of single keratinocytes are probably the triggers that initiate the extravasation of immune cells into the dermis and, thereby, the effector phase of psoriasis pathogenesis. The entered microbes might stimulate tissue-resident Langerhans cells, macrophages, and mast cells via Toll-like receptors to secrete inflammatory cytokines such as TNF-α and IL-1β. The damaged keratinocytes release self-RNA, which forms complexes with the antibacterial peptide cathelicidin (LL37). These complexes are able to activate mDCs via Toll-like receptor 8 and stimulate them to secrete TNF-α and IL-6. Importantly, owing to their expression of P- and E-selectin, the nonlesional skin of psoriasis patients is already predisposed to guide immune cells into the skin tissue. However, secreted TNF-α might first launch and then amplify this process by several mechanisms described below. Over time, the infiltrating neutrophils and later T-cells and monocytes strengthen the original minimal inflammation and enhance further immune-cell infiltration.

The passage of leukocytes from the blood vessels into the tissue occurs in five steps: rolling, triggering, adhesion, diapedesis, and migration (Figure 4.3). In the first step, leukocytes roll along the blood-vessel wall. Rolling reduces the flow velocity of the leukocytes and is mediated by the interaction between P- and E-selectin expressed by endothelial cells and selectin ligands expressed by leukocytes (PSGL-1, CLA-modified PSGL-1, and CLA-modified CD43). In healthy skin, endothelial cells of cutaneous postcapillary venules express low amounts of P-selectin molecules. In the uninvolved skin of patients with psoriasis, endothelial cells express both P- and E-selectin, and its expression is much more enhanced in psoriatic skin. One of the actions of TNF-α is the early release of so-called Weibel–Palade bodies containing P-selectin. Additionally, TNF-α induces the synthesis and surface expression of E-selectin molecules and the production of vasodilator substances (e.g. prostaglandins).

Very important for the tissue homing is the presence of chemokines that are produced by activated endothelial cells, macrophages, and keratinocytes. Most chemokines possess two binding sites, for their specific transmembrane receptor and for carbohydrate groups on proteoglycans, and exist as soluble mediators but also bound to glycosaminoglycans on endothelial cells at the site of inflammation. In the second step of skin infiltration, the immune cells rolling along the blood vessel wall recognize chemokines presented by endothelial cells and are activated. It seems that the interaction between CCL17 and CCR4 expressed by T-cells is highly relevant for their migration into the psoriatic skin. In line with this assumption, in psoriasis lesions, the majority of CD4+ T-cells and

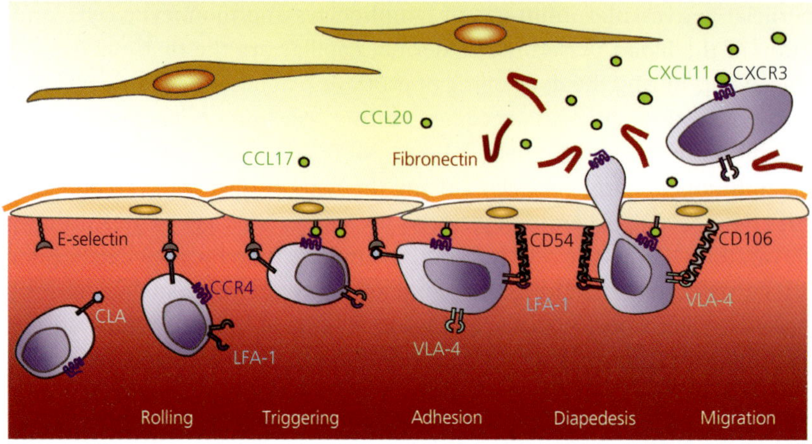

Figure 4.3 Leukocyte skin infiltration. The passage of leukocytes from the blood vessels into the tissue occurs in five steps: rolling, triggering, adhesion, diapedesis, and migration. Leukocyte rolling along the blood-vessel wall reduces the flow velocity of the leukocytes and is mediated by the interaction between P- and E-selectin expressed by endothelial cells and selectin ligands such as CLA expressed by leukocytes. Chemokines produced by activated endothelial cells, macrophages, and keratinocytes, and bound to glycosaminoglycans on endothelial cells, activate the immune cells via their specific chemokine receptors and induce an increased affinity of their integrins to the endothelial integrin ligands (triggering). The integrin-dependent interaction with the endothelial cells (e.g. LFA-1–ICAM-1, ICAM-2) causes the tight adhesion to the blood vessel and the rapid arrest of the immune cells in the blood flow. The passage of immune cells through the endothelial wall, called diapedesis, is also dependent on integrins such as VLA-4 and LFA-1.

about half of the CD8+ T-cells express CCR4. Interestingly, CCL17 is produced by TNF-α or IFN-γ stimulated dermal endothelial cells but not by activated keratinocytes. CXCR3 and its ligands (CXCL9, CXCL10, CXCL11) represent the second chemokine/chemokine receptor pair with great significance for T-cell migration into the skin. CXCR3 may be particularly important for the migration of Th1- and CD8+ T-cells into the epidermis, since its ligands CXCL9 and CXCL10 are expressed by TNF-α or IFN-γ stimulated keratinocytes. The third pair is composed of CCR6 and CCL20, and is particularly responsible for the skin infiltration of Th17-cells, Th22-cells, and mDCs. Keratinocytes produce CCL20 after stimulation with TNF-α or IL-17 but not with IFN-γ.

The activation of immune cells by chemokines via their transmembrane G-proteins binding receptors initiates the next step, which is characterized by the formation of a tight adhesion between endothelial cells and immune cells (Figure 4.3). This is achieved by integrins expressed on immune cells and their ligands expressed on endothelial cells. Integrins consist of two different, noncovalently bound transmembrane chains (α and β). Chemokines activate the immune cells, induce the association of integrins with the cytoskeleton via the adapter molecules vinculin and talin, and change the conformation of the two chains of the integrins that then form an open binding site with an increased affinity. The integrin-dependent adhesion of immune cells to the endothelial cells causes the rapid arrest of the former under physiological blood flow. CD11a/CD18 (LFA-1; α_L:β_2) seems to be the most important integrin for skin homing. It binds to CD54 (ICAM-1) and CD102 (ICAM-2) expressed by endothelial cells. Another T-cell integrin called very late antigen (VLA)-4 (α_4:β_1), which binds to vascular cell adhesion molecule 1 (VCAM-1, CD106) expressed by endothelial cells, seems to be less important in this process. Indeed, the vast majority of intraepidermal T-cells in psoriatic skin lesions express CD11a/CD18, whereas only 58% of CD4+ and 85% of CD8+ T-cells express VLA-4. The endothelium-associated chemokines trigger the instantaneous extension of bent CD11a/CD18, which leads to an increased affinity of the CD11a/CD18–CD54 binding (see above). Although the VLA-4 affinity is not altered upon chemokine signaling, subsequent VLA-4 clustering at the leukocyte–substrate contact zone results in enhanced leukocyte avidity to CD106. Importantly, resting endothelial cells only express CD102; however, TNF-α and IFN-γ induce the expression of all these adhesion molecules.

The passage of immune cells through the endothelial wall is called diapedesis and is probably carried out by pores formed between endothelial cells (Figure 4.3). T-cells, after having reduced their speed by interaction with the endothelial selectins, their activation by chemokines, and their cessation of rolling by interaction with the endothelial integrins, crawl to interendothelial junctions. TNF-α and IFN-γ cause endothelial cells to remodel the basal membrane. The passage is also dependent on integrins and, within the integrin system, more on CD11a/CD18 than on VLA-4. A small number of peripheral T-cells also migrate into noninflamed skin (see TEM cells). This is made possible by constitutive expression of P-selectin and CD102 on resting dermal endothelial cells. Consequently, in nonlesional psoriatic skin, the number of T-cells is higher than in skin from healthy participants.

In psoriatic skin lesions, CD4+ cells are mainly present in the dermis, while CD8+ T-cells primarily home into the epidermis. The reasons for these different anatomical homing patterns may lie in the different expression of chemokine receptors (such as CXCR3; see above) and integrins on CD4+ and CD8+ T-cells. Many of the T-cell molecules that are responsible for the interaction with the extracellular matrix belong to the VLA family. Among these, VLA-1 (α_1:β_1) is the major collagen IV-binding surface receptor. Additionally, epidermal CD8+ T-cells express CD103 (α_E:β_7) that binds epidermal E-cadherin and is of great importance for the movement to the epidermis.

Other immune cells such as monocytes/macrophages, DC precursors, NK-cells, and neutrophilic granulocytes use mechanisms for skin infiltration similar to those described above for T-cells. In healthy skin, there are three populations of DCs: the Langerhans cells (CD1a+CD207+) in the epidermis that express a specific type of organelle called the Birbeck granule, as well as the immature mDCs (CD1c+CD11c+) and a small number of pDCs (CD11c–CD123+CD303+) in the dermis. Psoriatic lesional and healthy epidermis contain similar numbers of Langerhans cells that might rather suppress inflammation than induce immune response. Lesional skin additionally harbours epidermal inflammatory DCs (CD1a+CD207–) that are like Langerhans cells but do not contain Birbeck granules. In contrast to normal skin, there are so-called inflammatory mDCs (CD1c–CD11c+) in the dermis. The population of inflammatory mDCs seems to comprise a few different subpopulations including slamDCs and cells that in reality may be macrophages, as they do not express any "classical" DC marker like CD1 or CD83. These additional, "inflammatory" APCs likely derive from circulating APC precursors that migrate into the skin in response to chemotactic signals. The complement component C5a and CCL20 are apparently the most important of these chemotactic factors that attract myeloid DCs in psoriatic lesions. In contrast to mDC precursors, macrophages follow CCL2 (via CCR2).

In psoriatic lesions, the number of NK-T-cells is also increased in comparison with healthy skin. NK-T-cells are a separate line of T-cells, known for (1) their expression of NK-cell receptors (CD161 and CD94), (2) their extremely restricted TCR repertoire (mostly Vα24 and Vβ11), and (3) their activation by glycolipids presented via the MHC class I-like molecule CD1d that is overexpressed in psoriatic lesions. NK-T-cells can be CD4+ or CD4–/CD8– and immediately secrete IFN-γ following activation.

Approximately 5% of the cells infiltrated in the psoriatic lesions are NK-cells. However, they are often guided to the skin by other chemotactic factors and can also use other adhesion molecules. In fact, skin-derived NK-cells have been shown to express high levels of the chemokine receptors CXCR3 and CCR5, and intermediate amounts of CXCR1, CCR6, and CCR8. In line with this, prompt migration of these cells can be induced with CXCL10 and CCL5, and, to a lower extent, with CCL20 and CCL4. For homing of neutrophilic granulocytes, interaction between the integrin MAC-1 (CD11b/CD18; αM:β2), expressed by neutrophils, and CD90, expressed by endothelial cells, does play an important role.

In the end, neutrophils migrate into the *stratum corneum* and form accumulations known as Munro's microabscesses. CXCL8, CXCL1, CXCL5, and also complement factors (C5a) may also play an important role in this infiltration. Mainly TNF-α and IL-17, but also IL-22, induce the production of neutrophil-attracting chemokines (CXCL8, CXCL1, and CXCL5) in keratinocytes.

As a consequence of the infiltration, massive amounts of immune cells are found in psoriatic lesions. Interestingly, the numbers of T-cells, macrophages, and DCs are very similar in this case.

Effector phase: immune cell activation in the skin

After their migration into the skin, the immune cells are activated. Migrant DCs might be stimulated by means of self-RNA–LL37 complexes as well as by neutrophilic granulocytes and NK-cells. In the dermis and epidermis, different APC populations such as macrophages and various types of DCs activate T-cells, and vice versa (Figure 4.4). T-cells that have migrated into the epidermis may additionally be stimulated by keratinocytes. As a consequence of activation, T-cells proliferate, and psoriatic lesions demonstrate even some characteristics of lymph nodes. The activation of immune cells in the skin can be negatively influenced by resident intraepithelial and regulatory T-cells; however, they seem to be deficient in number and function.

A convincing proof for the T-cell activation occurring in psoriatic lesions is the fact that these cells carry activation phenotypes. In fact, most epidermal T-cells express HLA-DR (86%) and CD69 (59%), representing activation markers, and are CD45RA-negative (91%; i.e. have memory phenotype). T-cells

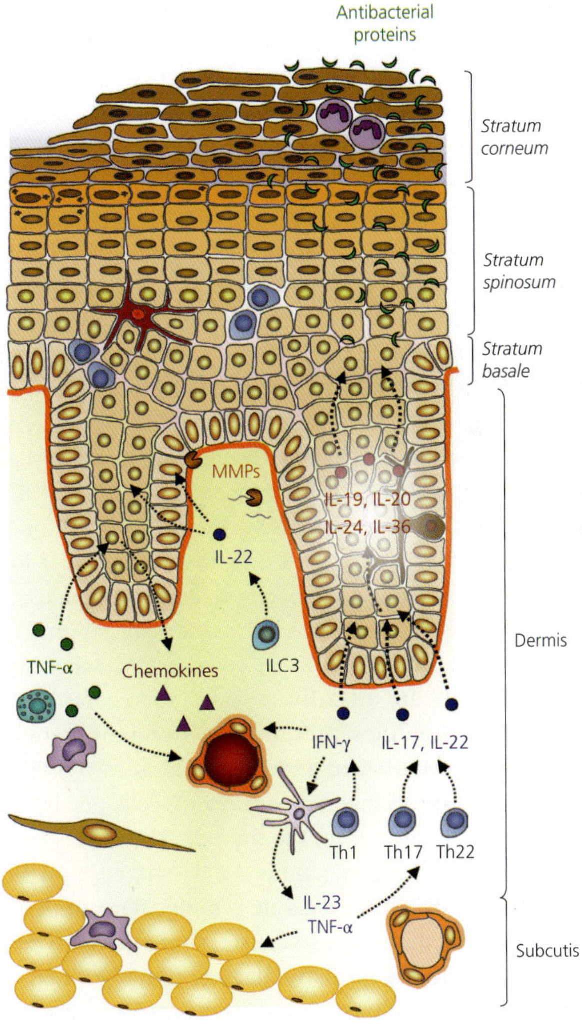

Figure 4.4 Schematic depiction of the effector phase of the psoriasis pathogenesis.

from the lesional dermis show similar characteristics except for CD69 (17%). CD69 is a surface molecule that is expressed by T-cells for only a short time after stimulation. Activated T-cells proliferate and produce cytokines. The T-cell mediators with the highest expression in psoriatic lesion and the biggest difference between nonlesional and lesional skin are IL-17A, IL-17F, and IL-22. IL-17A and IL-17F are apparently secreted by effector/memory Th17-cells. However, it was suggested recently that in psoriasis lesions, mast cells and neutrophilic granulocytes also produce IL-17. The main source of IL-22 in psoriatic lesions should be the T22- and Th1-cells. The expressions of IL-17A, IL-17F, and IL-22 are approximately 10 times higher than that of IFN-γ. Further cytokines present in psoriatic lesions include IL-26 with levels similar to IFN-γ, and IL-21, IL-13, and IL-4 with rather low levels. Interestingly, there does not seem to be any difference in IL-2 expression levels between nonlesional and lesional skin.

As far as is known, IL-22 is the only T-cell cytokine that is present in the blood of psoriasis patients at clearly detectable levels. Interestingly, the IL-22 blood levels correlate with the severity of disease.

As mentioned above, T-cells in psoriatic lesions are apparently activated by APC. The DCs from psoriatic lesions seem to be much more effective stimulators of spontaneous T-cell proliferation than blood-derived DCs or DCs from the skin of healthy individuals. HLA-DR, CD28 ligands, and LFA-1 are involved in this process. An important question for the understanding of the psoriasis pathogenesis is how monocytes/macrophages and DCs activate the migrant T-cells in the skin. We assume that in this process cytokines (in particular IL-23 and IL-6) produced by these APCs (e.g. after self-RNA–LL37 complex activation) play a dominating role. Indeed, the number of myeloid cells expressing IL-23 and the IL-23 expression levels are increased in psoriasis. In contrast to IL-23, IL-12p35 levels are not upregulated in diseased skin from psoriasis patients. Another question is which Ags are involved in the stimulation of T-cells in the skin. It is likely that some dermal CD4+ T-cells are activated by macrophages in dermal papillae that present parts of peptidoglycan, the major component of streptococcal cell wall. However, the proportions of such CD4+ T-cells and of concerned patients are currently unknown. A further attractive hypothesis regarding this topic is the concept of cross-reactivity of the T-cells that have been primarily generated, for example, against streptococcal Ags, and recognize auto-Ags in psoriatic skin. This might be possible because few auto-reactive T-cells persist in the organism despite the negative T-cell selection in the thymus. The model of cross-reactivity requires that a structure of an exogenous Ag be shared by a structure of the human molecule present in diseased tissue ("molecular mimicry"), in the case of psoriasis, the skin. Indeed, there is structural similarity between streptococcal M proteins and type I keratins, in particular keratin 17 (K17). M proteins are major streptococcal virulence factors composed of two polypeptide chains and are anchored to the bacterial cell membrane. Cutaneous K17 expression in healthy persons is missing except for the hair follicles, nail beds, sweat glands, and sebaceous glands. In psoriatic lesions, however, K17 is present in suprabasal keratinocytes. Both M proteins and K17 share the α-helical coiled-coil structure formed by hepta-peptide repeat patterns. Thus, K17 can be an auto-Ag for T-cells in psoriatic epidermis. It seems, however, that K17 plays a role in the activation of only few epidermal CD8+ T-cells. This can be deduced from the following observations: First, blood lymphocytes from HLA-Cw6-positive psoriasis patients incubated with peptides common in K17 and M protein and showing motifs predicted to bind to HLA-Cw6 produce more IFN-γ than blood lymphocytes from respective controls. HLA-Cw6 is a variant of MHC class I molecules that is associated with early-onset chronic plaque psoriasis and with psoriasis guttate. Second, the great majority of these responding cells express CD8 and CLA molecules. Third, as mentioned above, only a very small proportion of epidermal CD8+ T-cells (approximately 2–3%) recognize streptococcal Ags. These cells are apparently activated by keratinocytes. The keratinocytes constitutively express MHC I molecules complexed with peptides derived from mostly intracellularly synthesized proteins (e.g. K17). However, some scientists argue that the induced K17 expression in psoriatic skin is rather a secondary effect caused by activated T-cells than the reason for T-cell activation. Indeed, *in vitro*, K17 expression is induced in the keratinocyte HaCat cell line by IFN-γ and IL-17A, and, to a lesser extent, by TGF-α. Interestingly, K17 seems to influence the apoptosis sensibility and chemokine production of keratinocytes and, as a downstream mediator of IFN-γ and IL-17A, could play a role in psoriasis pathogenesis.

Keratinocytes can also stimulate CD4+ T-cells. They carry MHC II molecules and CD54 after exposure to IFN-γ. Such cells are able to induce T-cell activation and proliferation by bacteria-derived superAgs (such as staphylococcal enterotoxin A and B), processes that can be partially inhibited by mAbs against LFA-1 and by mAb against MHC II, respectively. Normally these IFN-γ-treated keratinocytes are not able to support T-cell proliferation to alloantigens. This means that such cells have impaired antigen processing and presentation via MHC II and are called nonprofessional APCs.

Keratinocytes may also play a role in the activation of NK-T-cells through CD1d. CD1d is expressed by keratinocytes in normal skin at a relatively low level and confined to upper-level keratinocytes immediately beneath the lipid-rich cornified layer. In psoriatic lesions, there is an overexpression of CD1d. Keratinocytes display enhanced CD1d following exposure to IFN-γ *in vitro*. Combining CD1d-positive keratinocytes with human NK-T-cell clones results in the clustering of NK-T-cells, and, while no significant proliferation ensues, NK-T-cells become activated to produce large amounts of IFN-γ.

The activation of T-cells in the skin should be inhibited by two subpopulations of T-cells. In normal mouse skin, but also in low amounts in human skin (up to 10% of total T-cells in healthy skin), intraepithelial T-cells can be found.

The biology of these cells is poorly understood, in particular in humans. They express the γδ TCR and often show less TCR variability, in comparison with T-cells that express the αβ TCR. Furthermore, they often enter tissues such as the skin and gut without previous priming in lymph nodes. Recent studies in laboratory animals have indicated the capacity of γδ T-cells to play major roles in the maintenance of the epidermal barrier, the regulation of cutaneous inflammation, and the protection against cutaneous neoplasms. The second subpopulation of T-cells that can inhibit Th17-, Th22-, and Th1-cells, are the regulatory T-cells. However, these cells seem to be both quantitatively and functionally deficient in psoriasis lesions in the ability to suppress the activation of other T-cells.

Besides T-cells, other skin-migrated immune cells are activated. NK-cells can be directly stimulated by neutrophilic granulocytes via LFA-1/CD50 and by APC-derived IL-23. The skin-infiltrating monocytes/macrophages and DCs are apparently activated by self-RNA–LL37 complexes, by IFN-γ produced by T-, NK-T-, and NK-cells, and possibly by heat-shock protein produced by keratinocytes. These cells then may begin to produce TNF-α, IL-1β, IL-6, IL-23, and IL-27. Macrophages in the papillary dermis are probably the main source of TNF-α. Interestingly, despite elevated IL-1β levels in psoriatic lesions the biological activity of IL-1 is not enhanced in diseased skin on the strength of increased IL-1RA expression.

Effector phase: tissue-cell response

The most striking signs of tissue-cell response in psoriatic lesions are the profoundly changed epidermis and the extension of the blood vessels in the upper dermis. Keratinocytes are apparently activated during the initiation of psoriatic lesions mainly by mediators produced by Th1-cells (IFN-γ, IL-22) as well as Th17- and Th22-cells (IL-17, IL-26, IL-22; Figure 4.2 and 4.4). However, over time, the cytokines produced by macrophages and DCs (TNF-α, IL-6, IL-24), and lastly by stromal cells in the dermis [keratinocyte growth factor (KGF), insulin-like growth factor 1, and fibroblast growth factor 10 (FGF-10)] might become increasingly important. Activated keratinocytes secrete chemokines (e.g. CXCL8, CCL20, CXCL9) and show enhanced CD56, CD1d, MHC I, and MHC II expression that together strengthen the influx of immune cells in the lesions and facilitate the immune cell activation, respectively. Furthermore, they produce numerous mediators such as IL-19, IL-20, TGF-α, and nerve growth factor (NGF) that activate stromal cells in the dermis and, in autocrine self-amplifying loops, add to their own activation. Importantly, the stimulation of keratinocytes by the cytokine mix present in psoriatic lesions leads to (1) increased proliferation of these cells, (2) alteration of their maturation, and (3) elevated production of antibacterial proteins. The strongly enhanced presence of antibacterial proteins ensures that despite the troubled integrity of the epidermis, cutaneous infections are not common in psoriasis. Furthermore, the mediators of activated immune cells and tissue cells induce angiogenesis.

The considerably elevated keratinocyte proliferation in psoriatic lesions is caused by an increase in the interfollicular epidermal stem cells number and by an approximately fivefold shortening of their cell-cycle duration and leads to the characteristic thickening of epidermis (*acanthosis*). Until today, the mediator(s) responsible for this fast proliferation could not be identified. We know that activated APCs release factors that increase the keratinocyte proliferation. The formidable improvement of diseased skin as a consequence of therapeutic neutralization of TNF-α strongly suggests that this cytokine plays an important role in keratinocyte hyper-proliferation in psoriatic skin. However, many studies have shown that TNF-α does not increase the division of these cells *in vitro*, and thereby the profound *in vivo* effects have to be indirect. The strong inhibitory impact of type I IFNs that are secreted by pDCs on the keratinocyte proliferation suggests that these mediators do not play an important role in visible epidermis changes. At this point, it should be noted that a discrepancy between the presence of IFN-α in psoriatic lesions and the increased proliferation of keratinocytes does not necessarily exist. First, the expression of type I IFNs seems to be limited to the first time of the lesional development, and second, the psoriatic keratinocytes show extenuated signaling in the type I IFNs pathway compared with normal keratinocytes. However, type I IFNs can play a role in the early stages of the effector phase by: (1) increasing the immigration of immune cells into the skin (by induction of numerous chemokines in keratinocytes such as CCL2, CXCL2, CXCL9, CXCL10, and CXCL11), (2) activating monocytes, macrophages, DCs and endothelial cells, and (3) upregulating MHC class I, MHC class II, CD1d, and CD54 in keratinocytes. Besides APCs, activated T-cells release mediators that increase keratinocyte proliferation. Interestingly, the neutralization of IFN-γ in T-cell supernatants partially diminishes their stimulatory potency. Because IFN-γ by itself inhibits the keratinocyte proliferation, this must mean that IFN-γ amplifies the effects of other T-cell cytokine(s). Furthermore, other T-cell mediators (IL-6, IL-17, IL-22, IL-26) have only minimal if any pro-proliferative effects on keratinocytes.

In addition to mediators from T-cells and APCs, there are at least two mediators from tissue cells that could be jointly responsible for the keratinocyte hyper-proliferation in psoriatic lesions: TGF-α and NGF. TGF-α messenger RNA and protein are much more abundant in lesional psoriatic epidermis than in normal-appearing skin of psoriatic patients or in epidermis from healthy people. TGF-α binds to the epidermal growth factor (EGF) receptor, stimulates proliferation of keratinocytes, and accelerates epidermal regeneration. NGF can increase the proliferation of keratinocytes through high-affinity NGF receptors (trk). NFG levels are also strongly elevated in lesional compared with nonlesional skin. However, the trk expression is downregulated in keratinocytes of nonlesional and lesional skin in patients with psoriasis.

The keratinocyte proliferation in diseased skin is also apparently affected by micro-RNAs as interregulators. Micro-RNAs are approximately 22-nucleotide-long noncoding, single-stranded RNAs that mediate posttranscriptional silencing of specific target messenger RNA. In the last months, a few micro-RNAs have been described whose expression is altered in psoriatic lesions in comparison with healthy skin and that regulate the keratinocyte proliferation.

The alteration of keratinocyte differentiation contributes to acanthosis and additionally leads to hyperkeratosis, parakeratosis, and hypogranularity. In normal skin, the way of keratinocytes from the basal layer to the cornified layer takes approximately 28 days. This process is shortened in psoriatic lesions to approximately 5–7 days. The last steps of the keratinocyte differentiation process include a particular apoptotic process that results in the formation of the mechanically resistant cornified layer (terminal differentiation). Briefly, it includes: (1) the dissolution of the nucleus and other cell organelles, (2) the formation of the so-called cornified envelope by irreversible cross-linking of structural proteins by transglutaminases, and (3) the formation of intercorneocyte junctions, the corneodesmosomes, which are finally degraded by special proteases enabling the physiological desquamation (for a detailed description, see Chapter 3). Keratinocytes in psoriasis lesions show a massively inhibited and disrupted differentiation. In contrast to the hyperproliferation, the mediators that are very likely to be responsible for the altered keratinocyte maturation in psoriasis lesions have been identified in recent years; these include IL-22, IL-20, and IL-24. Importantly, a few cytokines such as TNF-α, IFN-γ, and IL-17 amplify many effects of these mediators by enhancing the expression of their transmembrane receptors (e.g. TNF-α, IFN-γ) or by influencing their signal transduction (e.g. IFN-γ). In contrast to IL-22, which in psoriasis lesions might be produced by T22- and Th1-cells, IL-20 and IL-24 are expressed in the epidermis above the dermal papillae and in monocytes/macrophages in the dermal infiltrate, respectively. Importantly, IL-22, IL-20, and IL-24 affect exclusively tissue cells, but not immune cells. IL-22 mediates its effects though a receptor complex, which is composed of IL-22R1 and IL-10R2. IL-20 and IL-24 can affect keratinocytes via two different receptor complexes (IL-20R1/IL-20R2 and IL-22R1/IL-20R2). It seems that the receptor chain IL-22R1 is responsible for the psoriasis-relevant effects of these three mediators. In the skin, IL-22R1 is preferentially expressed by keratinocytes and only to a minimum extent by fibroblasts, but not by resting or activated immune cells. Thus, keratinocytes are the most important targets of these cytokines, which in these cells regulate four functions: (1) the terminal differentiation, (2) their expression of antibacterial proteins, (3) their migration, and (4) their chemokine production.

First, IL-22, IL-20, and IL-24 inhibit the expression of proteins that are crucially involved in the differentiation of keratinocytes: profilaggrin, K1, K10, calmodulin-like-5, keratinocyte differentiation-associated protein (KDAP), cornified envelope protein 1B, desmocollin-1, and kallikrein 7. Importantly, reducing the levels of these proteins, IL-22, IL-20, and IL-24 affects all steps in the differentiation and leads to the appearance of corneocytes with remaining nuclei that are not continuously exfoliated because of alterations in the corneodesmosomal degradation.

Second, in keratinocytes, IL-22R1 ligands induce the production of diverse antibacterial proteins, including β-defensins 2 (BD2), BD3, S100A7 (psoriasin), S100A8, and S100A9. BD2 is especially effective in killing Gram-negative bacteria, whereas BD3 also destroys Gram-positive bacteria. S100A7 act against *Escherichia coli,* and S100A8/A9 inhibits Gram-negative and Gram-positive bacteria, and some fungi. Because of the different specificities and the different mechanisms of action, the collection of induced antibacterial proteins has a high potency in the antimicrobial defense of the skin. Importantly, besides IL-22, IL-20, and IL-24, IL-17 also induces such antibacterial proteins in keratinocytes and amplifies the action of the other mediators.

Third, IL-22, IL-20, and IL-24 enhance the migration of keratinocytes. The IL-22R1 ligand-induced, elevated expression of the extracellular matrix-degrading enzymes, called matrix metalloproteinase (MMP)1 and MMP3, might be involved in this action. MMP1 and MMP3 are inducible, secreted, zinc-dependent, neutral endopeptidases, and their expressions are upregulated in psoriatic lesions. MMP1 cleaves fibrillar type I collagen and is required to initiate keratinocyte migration in the tissue. MMP3, a protease with a wide range of substrate specificities, degrades old multicellular actin networks, thereby apparently also playing a role in the cutaneous immune-cell infiltration.

Fourth, IL-22R1 ligands induce the expression of neutrophilic granulocyte-attracting chemokines in keratinocytes (CXCL1, CXCL2, CXCL5, CXCL8).

Fifth, IL-22 provokes mechanisms that may enhance its own action, in the sense of a positive feedback regulation. An example is the induction of STAT3, which is the major transcription factor activated upon IL-22 receptor signaling and is essential for the IL-22 effects. Interestingly, mice that transgenically express a constitutively active STAT3 variant in keratinocytes, develop psoriasis-like skin alterations. Moreover, IL-22 induces the production of IL-20 in keratinocytes, which demonstrates IL-22-like effects on keratinocytes (see above).

Other characteristics of psoriatic lesions include the dilation and increased length of upper dermal blood vessels. Factors of the complement system and TNF-α might be responsible for the dilation. The strengthened angiogenesis, which is responsible for the strong vessel extension in diseased skin, is probably dependent on vascular endothelial growth factor (VEGF) and angioprotein 2. VEGF is an endothelial cell mitogen that also enhances microvascular permeability. In psoriatic lesions, VEGF levels are elevated, and the VEGF receptors kdr and flt-1 are overexpressed by papillary dermal microvascular endothelial cells. The levels of angiopoietin 1, angiopoietin 2, and their receptor (Tie2) are also increased in diseased skin compared with uninvolved psoriatic and healthy skin. Angiopoietin 1 is expressed by stromal cells in the highly vascularized papillary dermis.

Angiopoietin 2 is expressed by endothelial cells in the neighborhood of the proliferating epidermis that also abundantly expresses VEGF. VEGF elevates angiopoietin 2 and Tie2 expression in dermal microvascular endothelial cell cultures. Angiopoietin 1 induces Tie2 signaling as a receptor activator and maintains blood-vessel formation, whereas angiopoietin 2 destabilizes vessels by blocking Tie2 signaling as an antagonist of angiopoietin 1. Angiopoietin 2 then acts with VEGF to initiate angiogenesis. Interestingly, a transgenic overexpression of VEGF in keratinocytes in mice provokes the appearance of psoriasis-like skin alterations in these animals. In line with that, inhibition of angiogenesis alleviates psoriasis-like skin alterations in mouse models. In addition to keratinocytes and stromal cells of the dermis, macrophages could also play a certain role in angiogenesis. Due to the release of proteases, growth factors [basic fibroblast growth factor (bFGF), GM-CSF, TGF-α, IGF-I, PDGF, VEGF], and other cytokines, activated macrophages have the capability to influence each phase of the angiogenic process. In contrast to macrophages, it appears that T-cells do not have a profound positive impact on the angiogenesis. Even so, all IFNs dose- and time-dependently inhibit the proliferation of endothelial cells *in vitro*.

Further reading

Gerdes, S., Rostami-Yazdi, M. and Mrowietz, U. (2011) Adipokines and psoriasis. *Experimental Dermatology*, **20**(2), 81–87.

Guttman-Yassky, E., Lowes, M.A., Fuentes-Duculan, J. *et al.* (2007) Major differences in inflammatory dendritic cells and their products distinguish atopic dermatitis from psoriasis. *Journal of Allergy and Clinical Immunology*, **119**, 1210–1217.

Male, D., Brostoff, J., Roth, D.B. and Roitt, I. (2006) *Immunology*, 7th edition. Mosby, Philadelphia, PA.

Murphy, K.M. and Stockinger, B. (2010) Effector T cell plasticity: flexibility in the face of changing circumstances. *Nature Immunology*, **11**(8), 674–680.

Nestle, F.O., Di Meglio, P., Qin, J.Z. and Nickoloff, B.J. (2009) Skin immune sentinels in health and disease. *Nature Reviews Immunology*, **9**(10), 679–691.

Sabat, R., Philipp, S., Höflich, C. *et al.* (2007) Immunopathogenesis of psoriasis. *Experimental Dermatology*, **16**(10), 779–798.

Schön, M.P. (2008) Animal models of psoriasis: a critical appraisal. *Experimental Dermatology*, **17**(8), 703–712.

Wolk, K., Haugen, H.S., Xu, W. *et al.* (2009) IL-22 and IL-20 are key mediators of the epidermal alterations in psoriasis while IL-17 and IFN-gamma are not. *Journal of Molecular Medicine*, **87**(5), 523–536.

Wolk, K., Witte, K., Witte, E. et al. (2013) IL-29 is produced by T(H)17 cells and mediates the cutaneous antiviral competence in psoriasis. *Science Translational Medicine*, **5**(204), 204ra129.

CHAPTER 5

Genetics of psoriasis

Ellen Witte and Robert Sabat
Psoriasis Research and Treatment Center, Department of Dermatology and Allergy/Institute of Medical Immunology, University Hospital Charité, Berlin, Germany

Analyses of psoriasis incidence in monozygotic and dizygotic twins have provided convincing evidence for an important role of genetic factors in the etiology of psoriasis in the second half of the last century. Indeed, if one monozygotic twin suffers from psoriasis, there is approximately a 70% probability that the other will be affected, too. However, there is only a 20% probability for dizygotic twins. Furthermore, the disease tends to be similar with respect to age at onset, distribution pattern, course, and severity in concordant monozygotic twins, a situation that has not been observed in dizygotic twins. Importantly, the fact that concordance is substantially lower than 100% also underlines the environmental component in disease development.

Further hints for a role of genetic factors in psoriasis etiology were provided by familial transmission studies. In fact, the risk of a child falling ill is about 20% if one parent has psoriasis, and about 65% if both parents are affected. Interestingly, patients with a positive family history are often affected before their 40th year of life and suffer from a generalized form with an irregular course and frequent relapses. However, only about 33% of psoriasis patients have a positive family history, which again underlines the role of the environmental component in disease development.

Twin studies, pedigree studies, and recurrence-risk analysis support a multifactorial model of inheritance of psoriasis-susceptibility genes. Family-based approaches, in particular on the basis of scanning analyses using microsatellite markers for identifying allele sharing among affected relatives, have led to the description of nine psoriasis susceptibility (PSORS) loci: PSORS1 on chromosome 6p21, PSORS2 on 17q25, PSORS3 on 4q34, PSORS4 on 1q21, PSORS5 on 3q21, PSORS6 on 19p13, PSORS7 on 1p32, PSORS8 on 16q12, and PSORS9 on 4q31. Whereas linkage to, and candidate genes in, PSORS1 have been confirmed by many independent studies and also by genome-wide association studies described later in this chapter, confirmation and identification of susceptibility genes for other loci need to continue.

Psoriasis: Diagnosis and Management, First Edition. Edited by Wolfram Sterry, Robert Sabat, and Sandra Philipp.

Currently, PSORS1 unambiguously constitutes a major psoriasis-risk region. It is located within the human HLA-complex that comprises genes that have also been associated with other autoimmune diseases such as rheumatoid arthritis and inflammatory bowel disease. Although, since the 1970s, PSORS1 has been the subject of many investigations, the question of which candidate genes confer a risk for psoriasis remains to be answered. This is especially due to extensive linkage disequilibrium of genes within PSORS1. Nevertheless, the strongest association of genes located to PSORS1 with psoriasis have been described for the HLA class I alleles. In fact, certain HLA-haplotypes to some extent overrepresented in psoriasis individuals are encoded in this susceptibility locus, including HLA-Cw6 as the most popular and with the strongest disease association, but also HLA-Cw7, HLA-B13, HLA-B17, HLA-B37, HLA-B39, HLA-B57, HLA-Bw5, HLA-DR4 and HLA-DR7. However, the HLA-C region is one of the few of those identified by linkage and association studies that could be confirmed with genome-wide association studies. Interestingly, besides others, Henseler and Christophers have reported an increased frequency of HLA-Cw6 among early-onset but not late-onset-type psoriasis. The contributions of HLA-Cw6 to psoriasis pathogenesis in allele carriers might exist in the following facts: (1) the HLA-Cw6 binds the ALEEAN motif-containing peptides from both streptococcal M6 and K17; and (2) the HLA-Cw6–K17 peptide complex has a similar structure in the TCR binding surface area to that of the HLA-Cw6–M protein peptide complex. Thus, CD8+ T-cells that have been generated against this streptococcal Ag after migration into the epidermis are activated by keratinocytes, presenting K17 peptides on their MHC I molecules. Besides the individual HLA-alleles, further reported candidate genes mapping to PSORS1 include the keratinocyte proteins HCR/CCHCR1 (coiled-coil α-helical rod protein), and corneodesmosin (CDSN), which were suggested to have a functional relevance for psoriasis pathogenesis. Indeed, expression of both CCHCR1 and CDSN is increased in lesional compared with non-lesional psoriatic skin. The risk variant HCR*WWCC of CCHCR1 displays a shortened protein that may contribute to the epidermal alterations in psoriasis. In fact, keratinocyte-specific overexpression of the HCR*WWCC risk allele in contrast to the non-risk-allele led to psoriasis-typical overexpression of keratins 6, 16, and 17 in the mice. CDSN constitutes a corneodesmosomal protein with supraspinous expression, which is cleaved during physiological desquamation by proteases, a process that, as motioned in Chapters 3 and 4, is disturbed in psoriatic keratinocytes leading to aberrant scaling. The functional relevance for the allelic risk variant CDSN*5 may lie in its increased mRNA stability, elevated protein production, and hindered desquamation.

Candidate psoriasis risk genes mapped to PSORS2 include SLC9A3R1 (solute-carrier family 9 isoform 3 regulator 1), NAT9 (*N*-acetyltransferase 9), and regulatory associated protein of mTOR (RAPTOR), a protein regulating cell growth and survival via interaction with and regulation of the activity of mTOR. Additionally, regarding SLC9A3R1 and NAT9, a disease-associated single nucleotide polymorphism (SNP) in a putative runt-related transcription factor 1 (RUNX1) binding site between those two genes was reported. This disease-associated SNP could lead to defective regulation of SLC9A3R1 and NAT9 expression. Nevertheless, SLC9A3R1 and NAT9 constitute a haplotype of rather low disease association strength. Whereas the function of SLC9A3R1 may lie in the regulation of membrane dynamics important for assembly of the immunological synapse and consequently T-cell activation, NAT9 is a protein of as-yet unknown function. The third putative candidate gene of PSORS2, RAPTOR, is a signal sensing scaffold component of the rapamycin-sensitive mTORC1 complex and functions to regulate the activation of the central cell proliferation regulating protein mTOR. RAPTOR gene variants associated with psoriasis do not affect the protein-coding region but may rather play a role in transcriptional regulation. Concordantly, RAPTOR seems to be highly expressed in both lesional and non-lesional psoriatic skin.

PSORS4, another genomic region implicated early in the genetic predisposition of psoriasis, spans a region of approximately 2 Mb and contains clusters of about 45 genes of the epidermal differentiation complex (EDC) that encode, for example, loricrin, involucrin, filaggrin, trichohyalin, small S100 calcium-binding proteins, late cornified envelope (LCE) proteins, and small proline-rich proteins (SPRR). EDC proteins are crucial for the development of the epidermis and strongly involved in the normal keratinocyte differentiation (for more details, see Chapter 3). The last step of this process is the terminal differentiation of keratinocytes, which includes the dissolution of the nucleus and other organelles, the aggregation of keratin intermediate filaments to macrofibrils, and the formation of the cornified envelope, which together result in the formation of a mechanical and physical barrier built by corneocytes and lamellar sheets of characteristic lipids. Recently, the association between a deletion of the LCE3B and LCE3C genes and psoriasis has been identified and subsequently confirmed as a risk factor for psoriasis by studies with large patient cohorts. The association of EDC and psoriasis susceptibility is in line with our current understanding of the psoriasis pathogenesis. Indeed, the keratinocyte differentiation, in particular the terminal differentiation, is strongly inhibited in psoriatic epidermis and the reason for acanthosis, parakeratosis, hypogranularity, and hyperkeratosis. Interestingly, PSORS4 also contains genes encoding the peptidoglycan recognition proteins PGLYRP3 and PGLYRP4. Polymorphisms of these genes have been reported to be associated with psoriasis. This can be interpreted as a sign for the role of streptococcal wall components in psoriasis pathogenesis (e.g. in CD4+ T-cell activation).

Besides PSORS1, PSORS2, and PSORS4, limited information was gained with PSORS5 and PSORS7. A putative PSORS5 was first reported by studies in a Swedish family cohort. The gene of SLC12A8 (solute-carrier family 12 isoform 8), a potassium/chloride transporter, was described as the first candidate gene of this region. Nevertheless, in subsequent studies with German and northern European patients, the association of SLC12A8 with psoriasis was either very weak or not confirmed. Cystatin A has gained attention as a putative candidate risk gene located in the PSORS5 region. Cystatin A is a cysteine protease inhibitor that can inhibit the cathepsins B, H, L, and S. Furthermore, this protein is one of the precursor proteins of the cornified cell envelope in keratinocytes. Thus, the possible alterations of expression and/or function of Cystatin A in respective psoriasis patients can influence (1) the degradation of Ag, therewith the kind of presenting peptides, and thereby the specificity of developing effector T-cells, as well as (2) the terminal differentiation and skin barrier function.

Finally, regarding PSORS7, attention has focused on PTPN22 (protein tyrosine phosphatase nonreceptor type 22), a protein playing a role in the regulation of T-cell activation as a candidate psoriasis risk gene, but consistent results regarding the different alleles and possible disease-related consequences are still lacking.

Interestingly, some of these aforementioned psoriasis susceptibility loci overlap with those of other chronic-inflammatory diseases. Apart from the aforementioned involvement of the genomic region at chromosome 6p21 (PSORS1), the region at 19p13 (PSORS6) is associated, besides other diseases, with rheumatoid arthritis and inflammatory bowel disease as well. Candidate risk genes of 19p13 include ICAM1 (intercellular adhesion molecule 1) and Tyk2 (Tyrosine kinase 2). Moreover, the psoriasis-associated loci at chromosomes 17q25 (PSORS2), 1q21 (PSORS4), and 3q21 (PSORS5) were reported to overlap with susceptibility loci for atopic dermatitis.

The results generated by means of the genome-wide association study technique provide accumulating evidence that inheritance mainly concerns certain immunological pathways and might strengthen these during the development of psoriasis through gene variations of the involved molecules (Figure 5.1). In fact, the psoriasis-associated genetic regions include those related to the MHC I pathway (HLA-C, ERAP1), the IL-23 pathway (IL-23p19, IL-12p40, IL-23R, Tyk2), T-cell activation (IL-2, IL-21), the NFκB pathway (TNFAIP3, TNIP1, Rel, NFKBIA), the interferon pathways (IL-28R1, Tyk2), and the innate immunity (copy-number variation in HBDs, ZNF313/RNF114, IFIH1). Furthermore, the inheritance can also affect the terminal differentiation of keratinocytes (deletion of LCE3B/C) and inhibit the Th2 pathway (IL-4, IL-13). Interestingly, the most highly significant associations are SNPs in the MHC I *HLA-Cw*0602* allele. Hence, the genome-wide association study results are consistent with very early findings regarding PSORS1 and HLA-Cw6. The polymorphism of the IL-19 and IL-20 genes, previously described in many different studies, has not yet been reported in any genome-wide association studies.

The genome-wide association studies also demonstrate that psoriasis genetics are complex, the underlying alleles are not rare but relatively common in the population, and single genes contribute very little to disease risk. Furthermore, they show an overlap between psoriasis loci and those identified for other chronic immune-mediated disorders such as Crohn's disease (IL-12p40, IL-23R,

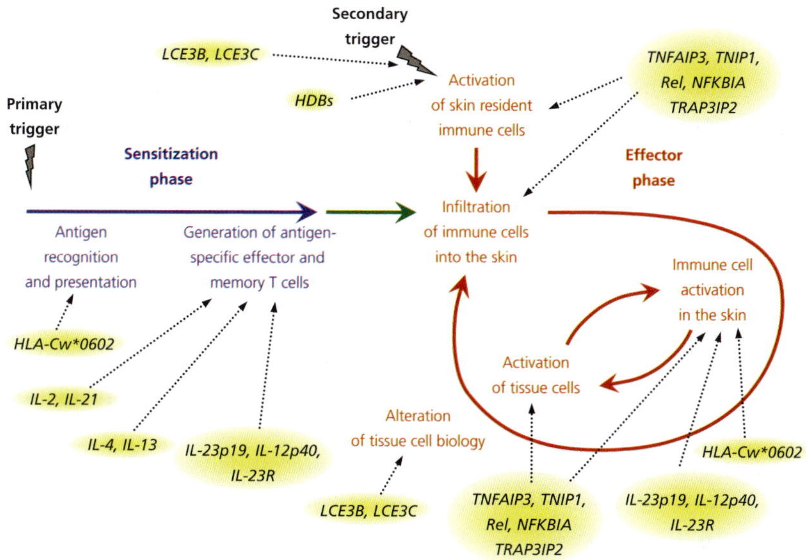

Figure 5.1 Genes associated with psoriasis susceptibility and potential role of their products during the psoriasis pathogenesis.

IL-2, IL-21) and rheumatoid arthritis (TNFAIP3, IL-2, IL-21). However, the possible functional consequences of putative risk variants are currently not known for most of the respective genes, and further investigations are needed.

Interestingly, genome-wide association studies have revealed an association between an SNP in the IL-13 promoter and psoriasis. The allele that is protective for psoriasis but is associated with risk for asthma binds the transcription factor YY1 and enhances the IL-13 production. The reason for the protective effects of the elevated IL-13 levels and therewith of this SNP for psoriasis susceptibility might be the inhibitory impacts of Th2 cytokines on Th17-cell development.

The observation that many genes of the IL-23 pathway are linked to psoriasis is in line with the view that this pathway is essential for effector function of Th17- and T22-cells, which are substantially involved in the pathogenesis of this disease (see Chapter 4). Interestingly, there are disease-associated SNPs not only for both subunits forming the IL-23 cytokine (p19 and p40) but also for the signaling receptor chain IL-23R. Whereas the relevance and possible functional consequences for allelic p40 and p19 in psoriasis have not yet been studied, there is evidence for impaired function of the putative protective IL-23R variant. Indeed, the *in vitro* generated effector Th17-cells carrying the R381Q IL-23R variant (A allele) produce less IL-17A compared with cells carrying the more common G allele. Moreover, there is also an allelic impact further downstream the IL-23 pathway through consequences arising from the identified polymorphism in TRAF3IP2 (TRAF3 interacting protein). TRAP3IP2 encodes the signaling adapter protein Act1 (NFκB activator 1 protein), which is an important component of the IL-17 signaling cascade. By binding of IL-17 to its receptor complex, Act1 is recruited to the conserved cytoplasmatic SEF/IL-17 receptor (SEFIR) domain of IL-17RA which enables the association of the TNFR-associated factor TRAF6 to the TRAF-binding domains of Act1 and subsequently activation of NFκB and mitogen-activated protein (MAP) kinase pathways. Therefore, Act1 plays an important role for IL-17 mediated immune responses. Moreover, Act1 is also a negative regulator of humoral immunity by inhibiting CD40- and B cell-activating factor of TNF family (BAFF) receptor signaling. However, functional studies of the underlying molecular mechanism have shown that the Act1 risk variant D10N has lost its ability to interact with TRAF6 through its defective folding by the hsp90 chaperone. Nevertheless, Act1-deficient mice show spontaneous skin inflammation. The reason for this interesting phenotype is the dysregulation of T-cell function in these mice associated with overproduction of IL-22 and the influence of this cytokine on skin tissue cells. Interestingly, the D10N Act1 risk variant is even more significantly associated with psoriasis arthritis than with psoriasis vulgaris, suggesting the involvement of IL-17 and NFκB pathways in both diseases.

These are very good examples of how genetic studies support our understanding of the psoriasis pathogenesis. However, there are also several mechanistic discoveries due that would enhance our currently limited understanding of the functional consequences of many players of the psoriasis-associated genetics.

Further reading

Bowcock, A.M. and Krueger, J.G. (2005) Getting under the skin: the immunogenetics of psoriasis. *Nature Reviews Immunology*, **5**, 699–711.

Elder, J.T., Bruce, A.T., Gudjonsson, J.E. *et al.* (2010) Molecular dissection of psoriasis: integrating genetics and biology. *Journal of Investigative Dermatology*, **130**, 1213–1226.

Li, Y. and Begovich, A.B. (2009) Unraveling the genetics of complex diseases: susceptibility genes for rheumatoid arthritis and psoriasis. *Seminars in Immunology*, **21**, 318–327.

Roberson, E.D. and Bowcock, A.M. (2010) Psoriasis genetics: breaking the barrier. *Trends in Genetics*, **26**, 415–423.

PART III

Clinical features/diagnostic procedure

CHAPTER 6
Plaque psoriasis

Wolfram Sterry
Department of Dermatology and Allergy, University Hospital Charité, Berlin, Germany

Plaque psoriasis

Elevated, red, and scaling lesions are the hallmark of psoriasis. Such large elevated areas are described in dermatological terminology as plaques. In contrast to many other inflammatory lesions, psoriatic plaques have well-defined borders, may be surprisingly stable, and occasionally persist without any change over months and even years.

The typical plaque is elevated 2–3 mm above the skin surface, is scaly, and shows a reddish and very sharply demarcated border (Figure 6.1). The color may vary, depending on skin type and localization of the lesions. A bright reddish color will be seen in acute forms, for example those induced by irritation, UV light, or trauma (Figure 6.2a). Older lesions may have a darker reddish coloration, sometimes with a brownish hue (Figure 6.2b). In seborrheic areas, a yellowish color may develop (see also Figure 6.9b). In persons with skin type I or II, light red and often salmon pink are typical presentations, whereas in colored skin, such as type V or IV, the red color may clinically be completely missing (Figure 6.2c). A special phenomenon occurs in certain patients during treatment with anthralin or tar products, when a whitish rim occurs in the periphery of the lesions that does not

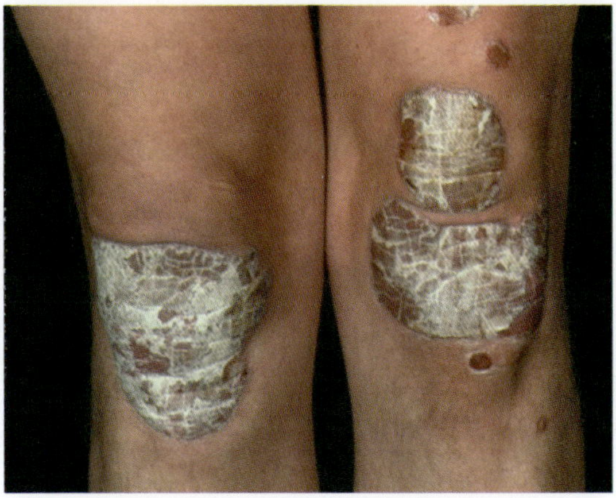

Figure 6.1 Plaque psoriasis with sharply demarcated borders, covered by silvery scales.

Psoriasis: Diagnosis and Management, First Edition. Edited by Wolfram Sterry, Robert Sabat, and Sandra Philipp.

take up any external colors; this is associated with good treatment response and named Woronow's ring, after its first describer (Figure 6.2d).

If untreated, large silvery scales containing small black dots representing inclusions of erythrocytes within the scales cover the surface (Figure 6.2e). The scales are large and often several centimeters in diameter, and their silvery, sometimes asbestos-like appearance together with their large size is unique among all erythemato-squamous skin diseases.

The scales normally are rather adherent and can be detached from the skin surface by means of a wooden spade. When scratching vigorously on the surface of a psoriatic plaque, the shiny appearance of the scales changes, and the surface suddenly becomes opaque. This phenomenon has always been compared with scratching on the surface of a candle, which initially appears quite shiny and after scratching loses its translucency. This is called the candle-wax phenomenon (Figure 6.3a). If the scales are removed from the surface of the plaque, a shiny

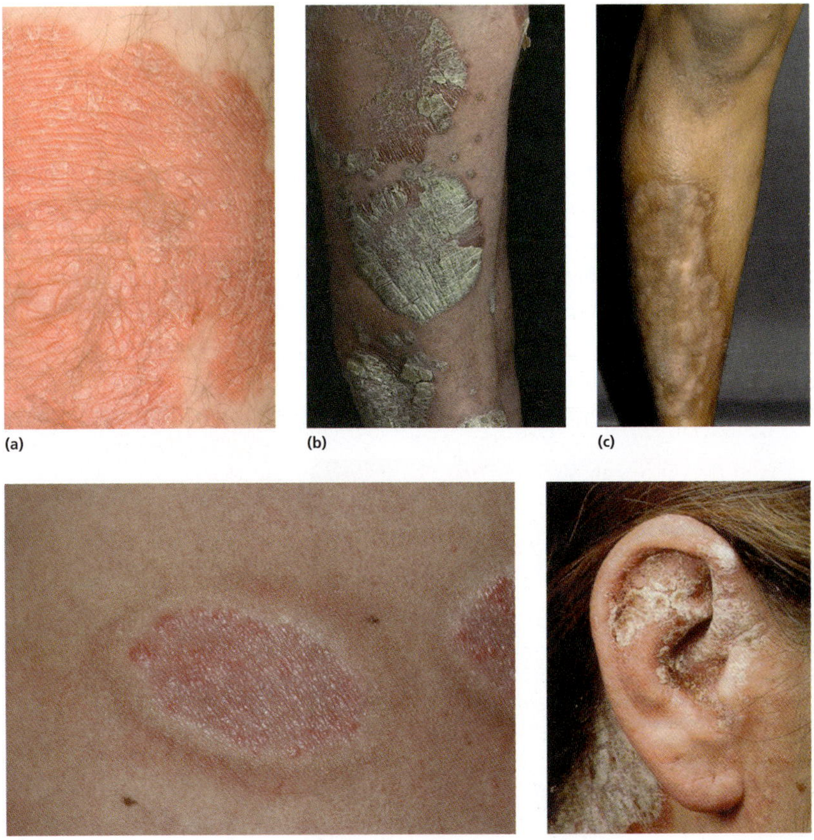

(a) (b) (c) (d) (e)

Figure 6.2 Different appearance of psoriatic plaques. (a) Psoriatic plaque with less scaling and light red color, possibly recently triggered. (b) Chronic psoriasis plaque with brownish coloration. (c) Psoriatic plaques in skin type IV: note that inflammatory signs sign as erythema are barely visible. (d) Woronow's ring during treatment, a zone that does not stain with any external color. (e) Large silvery scales, sometimes with black dots (foci of erythrocytes).

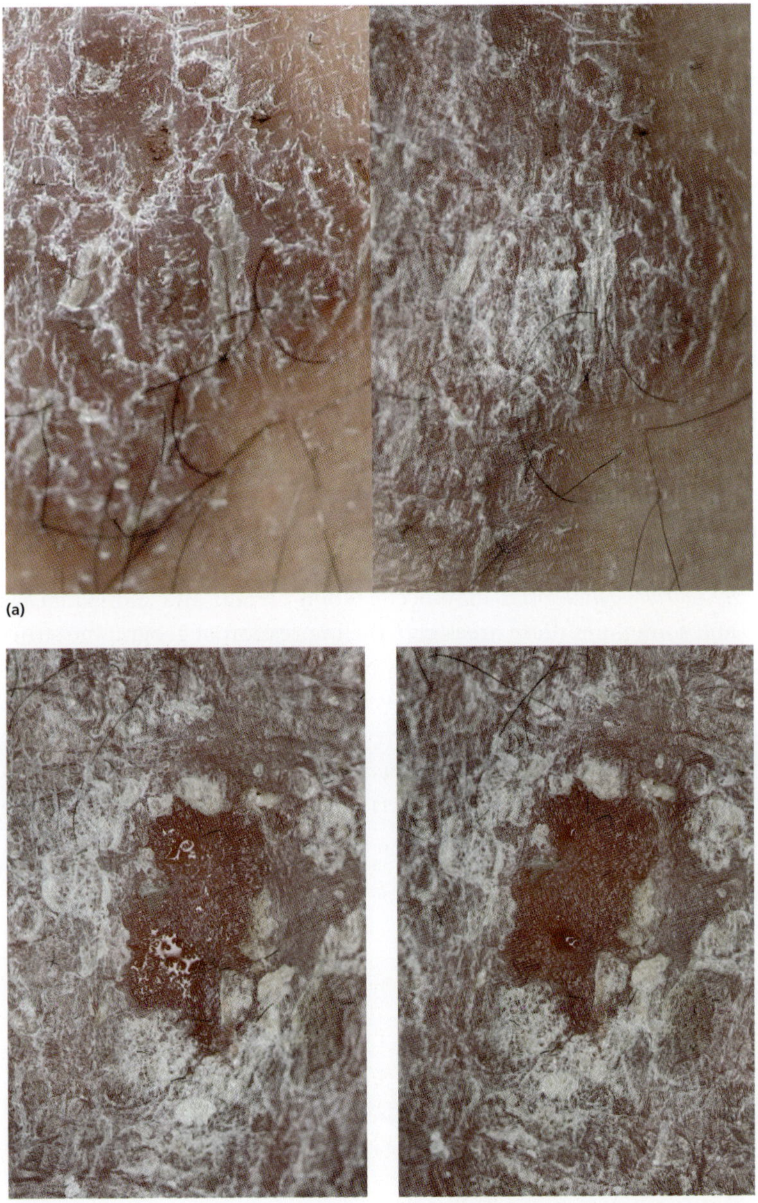

(a) (b) (c)

Figure 6.3 Characteristics of the psoriatic plaque. (a) Candle-wax phenomenon. After scratching the surface of a psoriatic plaque with a wooden spade, the horny layer loses its transparency. (b) Last cuticle. After removal of the scales, one looks at the stratum spinosum, with a glossy aspect and covered with serum droplets. (c) Auspitz phenomenon. After removal of the last cuticle, the capillary loops of the stratum papillare in the upper dermis start to bleed, causing tiny blood droplets (bloody dew).

thin membrane becomes visible, which represents the last few layers of keratinocytes of the lower *stratum spinosum* and the basal layer, just overlying the papillary body with its dilated capillaries. Consequently, this shiny membrane (also called the last cuticle) is quite red and glossy (Figure 6.3b). Scratching off the last cuticle with a wooden spade, small blood droplets appear, arising from capillaries of the papillary body. This phenomenon was first described by Heinrich Auspitz, an Austrian dermatologist, and is called Auspitz's sign (Figure 6.3c). These blood droplets are often referred to as "bloody dew." These signs can be demonstrated on all psoriatic plaques, but the demonstration is somewhat unpleasant and painful for the patient and thus not normally used for diagnostic purposes; in unclear cases, however, they prove to be very helpful.

The size of a psoriatic plaque is obviously variable, but each psoriatic plaque starts with pinpoint-sized lesions that gradually increase in size (Figure 6.4). Larger plaques may also develop by coalescence of several plaques within the same area that by continuous growth reach each other and merge into larger areas that may be up to 1 m or more in diameter (e.g. on the trunk of some patients). Typically, small and large plaques exist simultaneously.

Special morphological forms may occur when certain and individual plaques merge, and sometimes these areas give the impression of geographic structures, sometimes simulating certain countries or islands on a map. In such cases, the term *geographic psoriasis* (Figure 6.5a) has been coined. In other patients, plaques may show central healing, leaving only the active peripheral rim of a lesion; such anular lesions of the so-called *annular* or *circinate psoriasis* (Figure 6.5b) may pose specific differential diagnostic aspects and sometimes are difficult to interpret

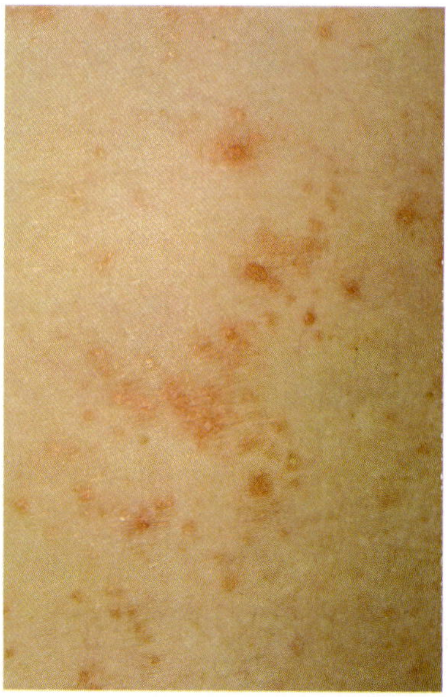

Figure 6.4 Tiny early lesions in psoriasis: pinpoint lesions.

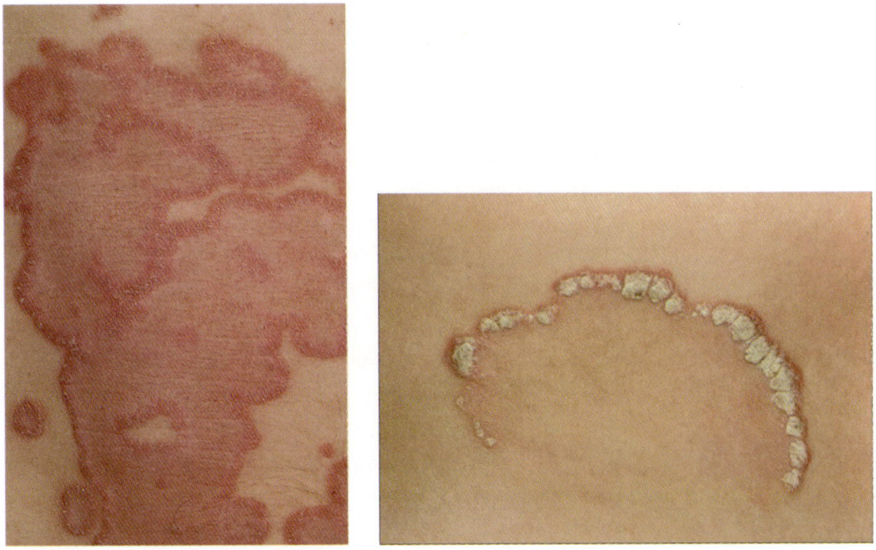

(a) (b)

Figure 6.5 (a) Geographic psoriasis (Denmark?) created by coalescence of psoriatic plaques. (b) Circinate psoriasis.

correctly for a beginner, particularly if the ring is very thin. In such instances, the presence of psoriatic lesions in other predilection sites may give a clue towards the correct diagnosis.

Cases with particularly thick scales, or those where scales are soaked with serum forming irregular horny masses resemble the surface of oysters, and thus are referred to as *rupoid* or *ostraceous psoriasis* (Figure 6.6). One has to be careful to check for joint symptoms, as this appearance is frequently found in patients with reactive arthritis (Reiter's syndrome).

Patients experience many physical and psychological symptoms (see Chapter 14), and one major problem is scaling, the constant loss of large scales that are visible on clothing but also at sites were they have been sitting or sleeping. For psoriasis patients who are travelling, loss of scales can be very distressing, because in the morning numerous scales can be found in and around the bed, and patients often bring their own vacuum cleaners in order to avoid any problems with staff in hotels or other institutions. If larger areas are involved, scales also represent a major loss of protein, which can account for up to 100g per day!

The word "psora" means itching; in Modern Greek, "psora" is the word for scabies. Although itch was never regarded as a major problem in psoriasis in earlier times, recent analyses of the quality of life of patients suffering from psoriasis have revealed that itch represents a major symptom and cause of distress, and it is noteworthy that itch as a symptom has given the name to the disease!

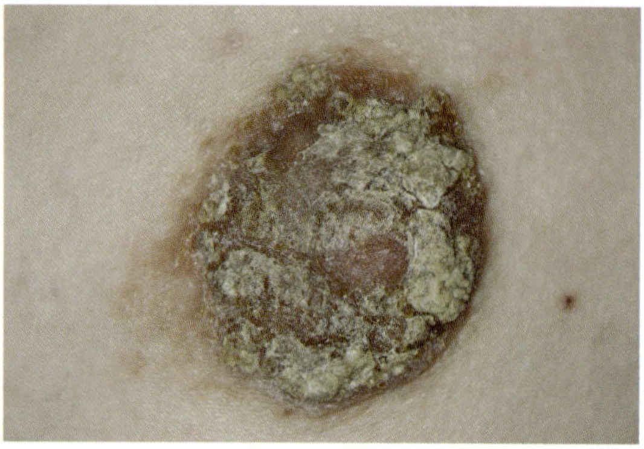

Figure 6.6 Rupoid psoriasis with large amount of serum embedded between the corneocytes.

Therefore, treatment of itch should always be considered a major part of therapy, and the treatment response should always include the relief of itching.

As scales always reflect malfunctioning keratinization, it is obvious that any shearing or mechanical stress of psoriatic plaques leads to fissures and rugae. Patients have feelings of soreness and pain in the lesions that may be severely aggravated by mechanical stress.

For the purposes of treatment, plaque psoriasis is divided into three categories: mild, moderate, and severe. Classically, mild plaque psoriasis is, as far as skin lesions are concerned, defined as plaques covering less than 10% of the body surface, and severe plaque psoriasis covering more than 10% of the body surface. Moderate psoriasis covers the poorly defined border between mild and severe psoriasis; it should be noted here that further criteria are used to define mild, moderate, and severe psoriasis, and that the percentage of body surface affected is just one of the criteria (see Chapter 14). Another important distinction is that between active (nonstable) and nonactive (stable) psoriasis. In active psoriasis, lesions increase in size and number; the tendency of the skin to react in a way consistent with the Köbner phenomenon (see below, Figure 6.14)) is more pronounced, and treatment may be more difficult. Trigger factors should be carefully excluded.

Predilection sites of plaque psoriasis include the scalp, particularly the retroauricular areas (Figure 6.7a), and the extensor sites of the extremities, in particular the elbows and knees (Figure 6.7b–c), as well as the sacroiliac region (Figure 6.7d). Sometimes small plaques, also with a high diagnostic specificity, occur in the umbilical area (Figure 6.7e) and the rima ani (Figure 6.7f). The reason for this anatomical preference of plaque psoriasis is not known.

In typical cases, psoriasis cannot be confused with any other skin diseases. However, atypical cases, such as coinciding occurrence with seborrheic dermatitis or contact dermatitis, early or irritated lesions, treated lesions, or psoriasis in atypical location (i.e. intertriginous, palmoplantar) may pose great difficulties or even make it impossible to make a correct diagnosis, even for an experienced dermatopathologist.

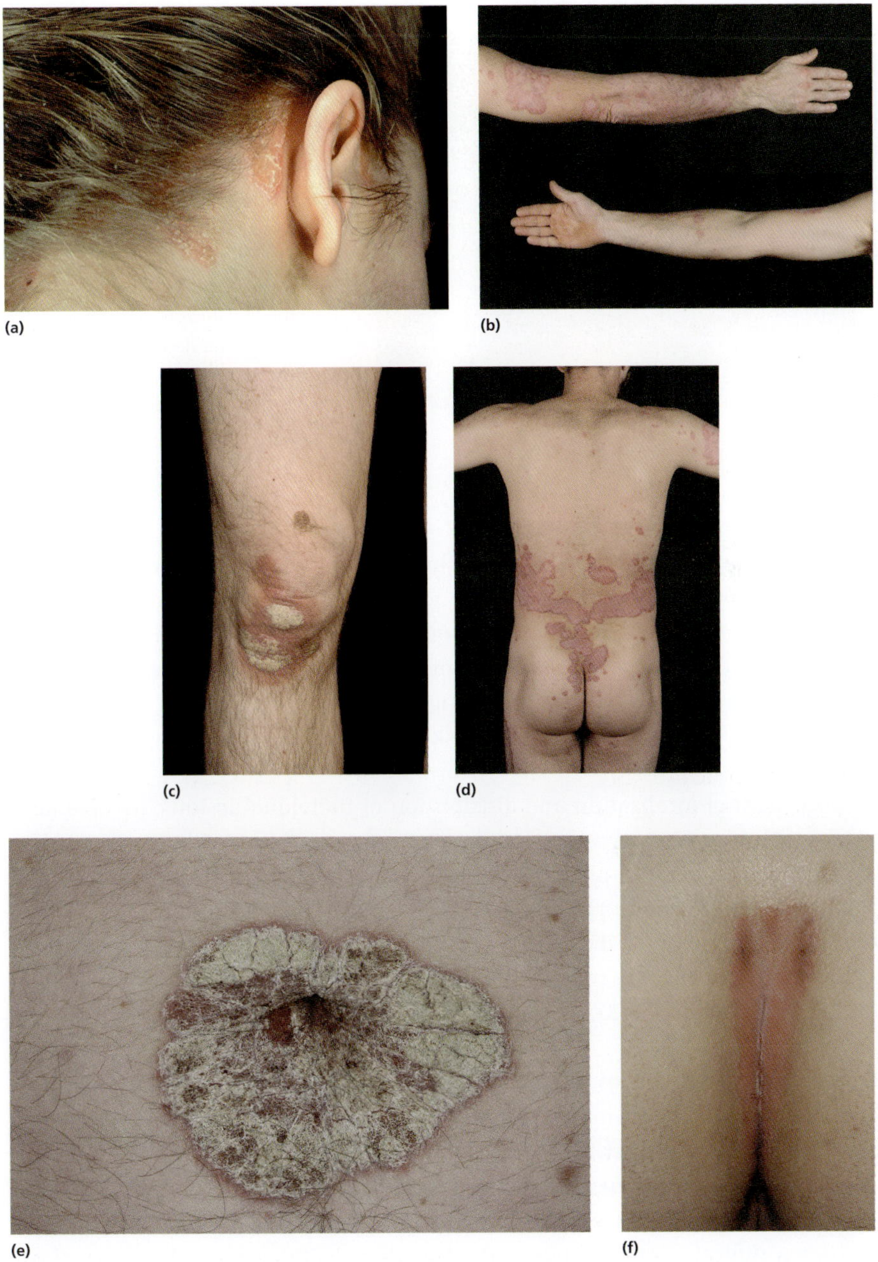

Figure 6.7 Different localization of psoriatic plaques. (a) Retroauricular plaques. (b) Lesions on the extensor sites of the arms. (c) Plaque on the extensor site of the leg. (d) Involvement of the ileosacral area. (e) Periumbilical plaque. (f) Lesion in the rima ani—note the lack of scaling.

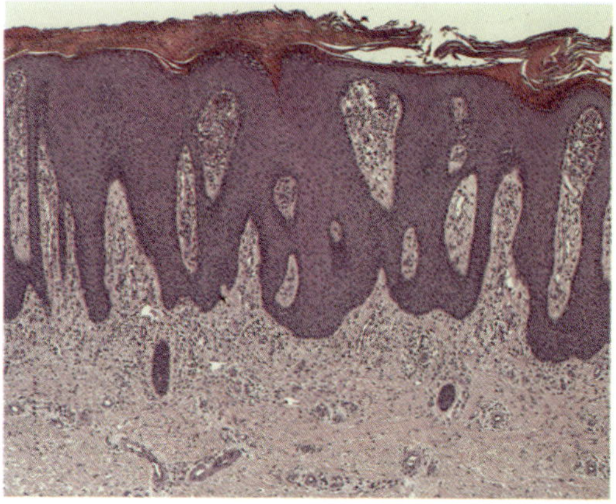

Figure 6.8 Histopathology of fully developed psoriasis, featuring hyper- and parakeratosis, acanthosis, papillomatosis, and inflammatory infiltrate.

Diagnostic approach to psoriasis

Psoriasis is diagnosed in most cases on the basis of the clinical appearance: color and morphology of the plaques, that is, a well-defined border, localization at the predilection sites, and subjective symptoms such as itch and feeling of soreness. A standardized approach to a patient with suspected psoriasis is recommended, and we routinely adhere to the following steps:

1 analysis of features of individual skin lesions: border, color, scales, and symptoms;
2 assessment of localization and distribution of individual lesions: involvement of predilection sites, symmetrical distribution, and "hidden" lesions;
3 presence of "signs of psoriasis": candle-wax phenomenon, last cuticle, and bloody dew (Auspitz's phenomenon);
4 exclusion of potential differential diagnoses: may include other investigations such as patch testing, microbial cultures, immunological investigations, and skin biopsy (Figure 6.8).

Differential diagnosis of plaque psoriasis

The following disorders may show a clinical overlap with plaque psoriasis and thus may warrant further investigation:

1 seborrheic dermatitis: particularly for scalp and facial psoriasis, it may be difficult to distinguish these from seborrheic dermatitis, especially as many patients show a clinical overlap between the two disorders (i.e. seborrhiasis) or show a history of seborrheic dermatitis with gradual transformation into unequivocal psoriasis. Typically, seborrheic dermatitis of the scalp shows medium-sized, yellowish scales, and transgression of the inflammatory border towards the nonhairy areas of the head is rarely seen (Figure 6.9a), while transgression is typical for psoriasis. In the face, seborrheic dermatitis shows small to medium-sized yellowish scales with a tendency to appear on the eyebrows, nasolabial

folds (Figure 6.9b), and, if present in males, the beard. Mycological cultures normally yield growth of the lipophilic yeast *Pityrosporum ovale* (*Malassezia furfur*).

2 tinea corporis: in immuno-competent individuals, tinea corporis is mainly caused by zoophilic dermatophytes, therefore, there is usually a brief history. Annular forms of psoriasis may mimic tinea corporis (Figure 6.9c), and mycological cultures for dermatophytes may be indicated.

3 nummular dermatitis: nummular dermatitis occurs mainly in atopic individuals and is pathogenetically based on a decreased skin barrier and staphylococcal supercolonization. Nummular dermatitis appears similar to psoriasis as erythematous and scaling plaques (Figure 6.9d), and thus sometimes needs to be distinguished from psoriasis. In almost every lesion of nummular dermatitis, one can identify features of dermatitis in the periphery, that is, papulovesicles or tiny erosions. Microbial swabs reveal high-density colonization with *Staphylococcus aureus*.

4 discoid and subacute lupus erythematosus: discoid lupus erythematosus (LE) presents with hyperkeratotic erythematous plaques (Figure 6.9e), and thus may resemble psoriatic plaques. If localized exclusively on the scalp, or in rare cases of disseminated discoid LE, clinical differential diagnosis may be difficult. However, two features clearly distinguish discoid LE from psoriasis: (i) a lack of scaling (instead, the plaques are covered with hyperkeratotic *stratum corneum*, which can be painful if one tries to remove it) and (ii) atrophy. In subacute LE and overlap collagenosis, there is a psoriasiform variant (Figure 6.9f). The history of sudden flare and triggering by UV light may help distinguish this from plaque psoriasis. In uncertain cases, an immunological workup will be necessary in order to exclude LE including blood investigations (ANA, Ro, La antibodies) as well as histology and direct immunofluorescence.

5 mycosis fungoides and pagetoid reticulosis: these two types of cutaneous T-cell lymphoma may occasionally resemble psoriasis and, in our experience, may even be mistaken by experienced dermatologists, if mycosis fungoides lesions present with large scales. In mycosis fungoides, one will always find in addition to plaques earlier lesions, that is, patch-type lesions with atrophy and sometimes fine scaling (Figure 6.9 g), particularly on the inner parts of the arms and thighs as well as on the lateral aspects of the trunk. If necessary, histology and molecular biology can be used for a clear diagnosis.

6 pityriasis rotunda: in colored skin, pityriasis rotunda may represent a clinical differential diagnosis, as the lesions are sharply demarcated and stable, as is the case in psoriasis (Figure 6.9 h). However, the degree of scaling is mild, and its occurrence is mainly confined to Africa, which may serve as a diagnostic clue.

Early pinpoint lesions of psoriasis may be confused with dermatitis, as psoriasis is usually expected to present invariably with plaques. However, psoriatic lesions may occur with numerous papules (1–2 mm in size), occasionally with follicular

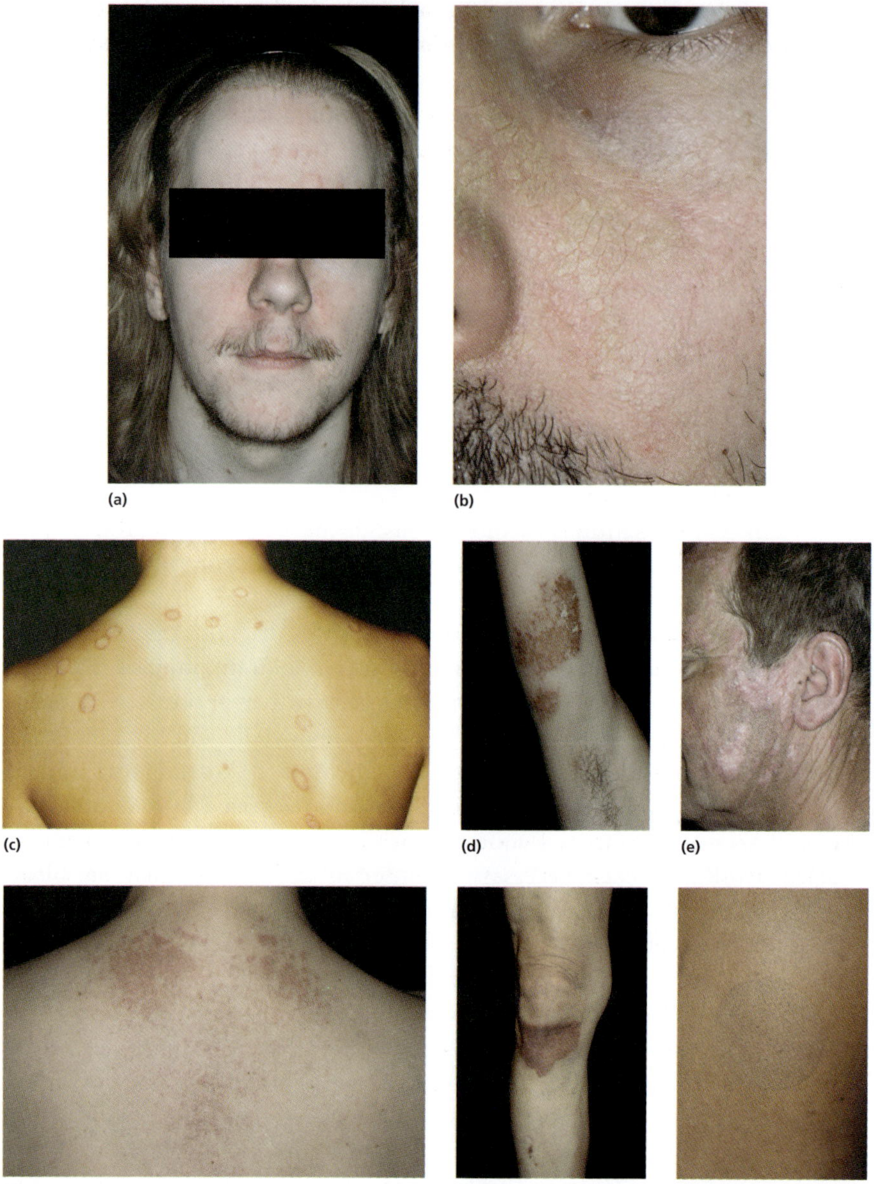

(a) (b) (c) (d) (e) (f) (g) (h)

Figure 6.9 Differential diagnosis of plaque psoriasis. (a) Seborrheic dermatitis with some overlap to psoriasis (so-called seborrhiasis). (b) Yellowish color of seborrheic dermatitis. (c) Tinea corporis resembling annular psoriasis—note the accentuated border. (d) Nummular dermatitis with papulovesicles as primary lesions at the periphery. (e) Discoid lupus erythematodes with lesions in sun-exposed areas that later will show healing with atrophy. (f) Psoriasiform lesion in overlap collagenosis. (g) Mycosis fungoides, histologically and molecular biologically proven. (h) Pityriasis rotunda.

preference. Dermatitis, however, invariably displays papulovesicles and small erosions that are lacking in psoriasis (see also Figure 6.9d). Follicular lichen planus may be occasionally hard to differentiate, but more prominent scaling, even in tiny psoriasis lesions, may serve as a clue. Histological examination is useful to differentiate between these two conditions.

In summary, although a diagnosis of psoriasis can be made in most patients on the basis of history and clinical investigation, the differential diagnosis of plaque psoriasis is broad. The diagnostic workup may require in selected cases fungal cultures, bacterial swabs, histology, direct immunofluorescence, and serological examination as well as molecular biology.

Plaque psoriasis in special localizations

Scalp psoriasis

The area most frequently affected by psoriasis is the scalp. In general terms, the lesions are similar to those occurring on the free skin of the body, but they are more difficult to visualize and examine because they are covered by the hair of the scalp. On the scalp, psoriatic lesions predominantly occur within areas of hair growth, meaning that bald areas in males or females with androgenetic alopecia or other types of alopecia are rarely affected. Characteristically, however, the psoriatic lesion may transgress the border between hairy and nonhairy areas by more than 1 cm (Figure 6.10a). The psoriatic plaques show the same type of silvery large scaling as on the free body surface, sometimes having a yellowish hue. The area most frequently affected on the scalp is the retroauricular area (see Figure 6.7a), followed by the temples. The area affected may vary from small minute papules or plaques to the entire scalp (Figure 6.10b) possibly resulting in partial or even complete hair loss due to the inflammation (Figure 6.10c). Scarring hair loss virtually never occurs.

As scalp psoriasis may cause disturbing itch, secondary problems due to scratching are frequently seen, most often indicated by bloody crusts covering the psoriatic plaques. For patients, one of the most disturbing symptoms of scalp psoriasis is the frequent production of scales, which are different from those in ordinary dandruff because of their size and color, but also sometimes because of the large number. This makes it impossible for some patients to wear dark suits, since the shoulders and back can be covered with silvery scales in a short time.

Scalp psoriasis often plays an important diagnostic role in patients with minimal psoriasis, where one is looking for clear signs of psoriasis. A careful inspection of the scalp, in particular the retroauricular area, is always helpful in confirming or excluding the diagnosis of psoriasis.

Differential diagnosis of scalp psoriasis includes all other erythematous–squamous inflammatory skin disorders affecting the scalp.

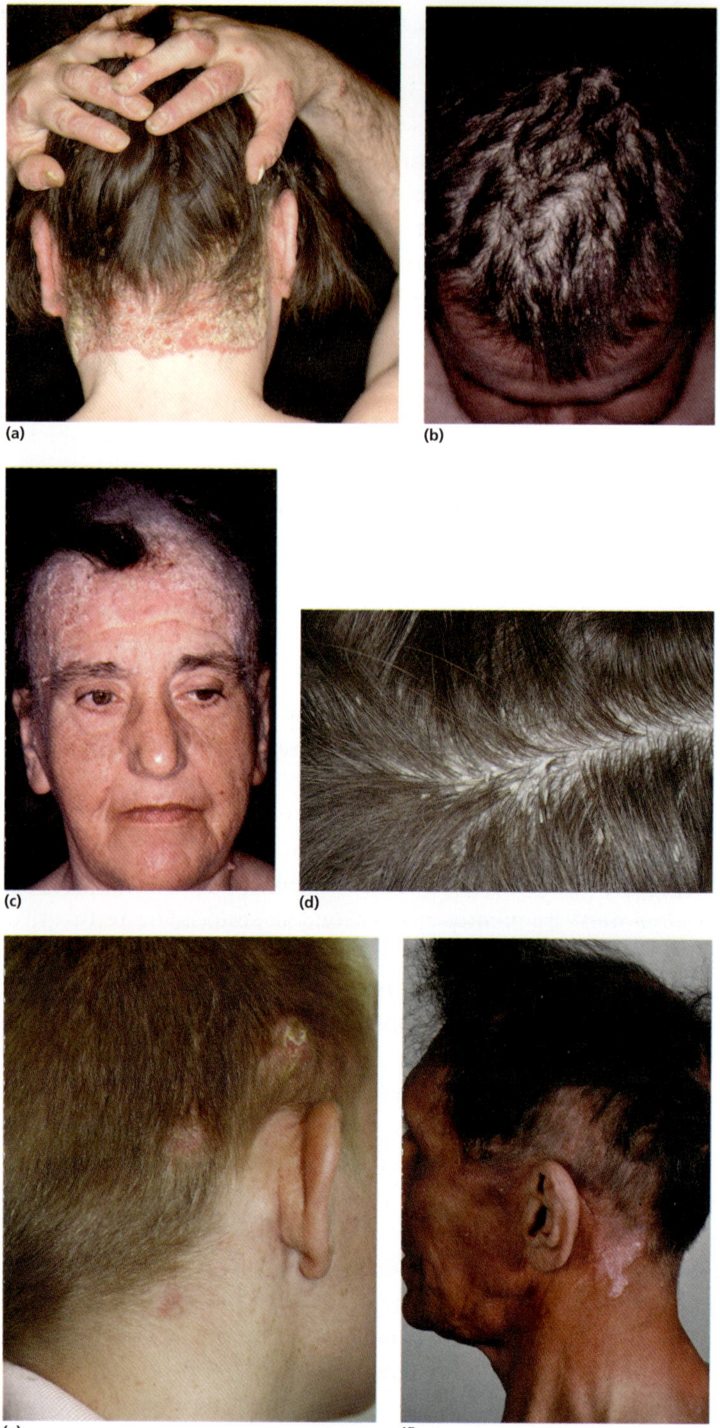

Figure 6.10 (a) Scalp psoriasis transgressing the border between hairy and nonhairy scalp. (b) Extensive scalp involvement. (c) Hair loss in extensive psoriatic scalp involvement. (d) Chronic scalp dermatitis causing tinea amiantacea. (e) Tinea capitis in a wrestler caused by *Trichophyton tonsurans*. (f) Scalp involvement of discoid lupus erythematosus with scarring.

1 Most frequently, scalp psoriasis has to be distinguished from seborrheic dermatitis. Seborrheic dermatitis results from an immune reaction against microbial hyper-colonization, particularly due to pityrosporon species. In contrast to psoriasis, seborrheic dermatitis is characterized by small to medium-sized scales, often greasy or yellowish color, is confined to areas covered by hair, and typically does not transgress to areas not covered by hair (see Figure 6.9a). It is important to stress that some patients present with seborrheic dermatitis and may develop psoriasis months or years later. This means that seborrheic dermatitis may be one of the first symptoms of psoriasis or that both disorders are triggered by common mechanisms. For patients in whom it is difficult to distinguish clearly between seborrheic dermatitis and psoriasis, the term "seborrhiasis" is used. One should avoid this term in clinical practice as often as possible, but some patients will still accept this diagnosis, as they show features of both seborrheic dermatitis and psoriasis,so that one cannot distinguish between the two disorders.
2 Regular dermatitis of the scalp, whether allergic or toxic, may be another differential diagnosis for scalp psoriasis. The scaling in scalp dermatitis is normally fine, and itching is a common complaint. On careful examination, small papulovesicles can be seen on the edges of diseased skin, a hallmark of any dermatitis. In some patients, dermatitis persists and becomes chronic; in those individuals, scaling and hyperkeratosis are the leading features, and scales may be as thick as 1–2 cm and cover the scalp like roof tiles. This condition is called "tinea amiantacea" (Figure 6.10d).
3 Tinea caused by dermatophytes represents another differential diagnosis of scalp psoriasis (Figure 6.10e). Clues to the diagnosis of tinea are broken hairs (in endothrix dermatophyte infections) or the involvement of parts of the hair channel in the infection, leading to complete hair loss and quite often purulent discharge. Zoophilic dermatophytes are the main cause of such inflammatory forms of tinea capitis.
4 Discoid lupus erythematodes may also cause reddish plaques, but the predominant feature is not scaling with hyperkeratosis but healing with scar formation. Scar formation is virtually absent in psoriasis and is thus a valuable clue for differentiation from discoid lupus erythematodes (Figure 6.10f).

Histological examination of scalp psoriasis is rarely carried out, as the diagnostic features of psoriasis are much more clearly displayed on lesions of the free skin. However, mycological cultures may be helpful in diagnosing seborrheic dermatitis (*Pityrosporum* species will grow) or tinea capitis (dermatophytes will grow). The histological diagnosis of discoid lupus erythematodes of the scalp is normally clear cut, as all classical histopathological features of discoid lupus erythematodes are present on the scalp as well as hyperkeratosis with follicular accentuation, atrophy of the epidermis, macular degeneration of the basal layer, and a lymphocytic infiltrate, which is located below the epidermis and around the hair follicles. Later, scarring will be a dominant feature together with epidermal atrophy. In immunofluorescence, deposits of IgM and IgG may be seen at the epidermal junction, and the basement membrane zone is thickened in PAS stains.

Intertriginous psoriasis

Intertriginous psoriasis is defined as psoriasis involving the intertriginous areas. Although there are many intertriginous areas in the body, the frequency of the involvement differs substantially. The locations most frequently affected are the anal fold, followed by the umbilical area, the submammary regions in obese females, and the abdominal folds in obese patients of both sexes. The involvement of the inguinal area by psoriasis also occurs quite frequently, whereas the axillae are less frequently involved.

Intertriginous psoriasis is discussed here as a separate manifestation of plaque psoriasis because the intertriginous location causes a change in morphology (Figure 6.11a–c). Frank scaling, particularly silvery-white scales, will not occur in intertriginous areas. Instead, the thickened *stratum corneum* appears macerated, that is, hydrated with a somewhat waxy and shiny aspect. The areas are red, well demarcated, and often painful. In the anal fold, fissures may complicate the clinical picture and add additionally to the burden of disease.

Intertriginous psoriasis is regarded as being triggered by microbial colonization of these areas. However, frank colonization with bacteria or candida species is not seen. Intertriginous psoriasis may be of value also when one has to establish the diagnosis in patients with only mild skin involvement. Particularly helpful is the inspection of the umbilicus and the anal fold, but as outlined above, one has to be well aware of the clinical presentation of intertriginous psoriasis in order to make the right diagnosis and not to misdiagnose these manifestations as candida infection or intertriginous dermatitis.

Histology of intertriginous psoriasis is not particularly helpful, as the classical hallmarks of psoriasis are only partially present. Hyperkeratosis is only discretely present, so the histologist is left with acanthosis and papillomatosis along with a strong inflammatory infiltrate containing numerous neutrophils.

Differential diagnosis of intertriginous psoriasis includes several disorders that have to be excluded carefully. The most important and most difficult disorder is candida infection.

1 The clinical presentation of candida infection may be quite similar to intertriginous psoriasis; however, in the peripheral zones of candida intertrigo, one will see minute satellite areas and some pustules also (Figure 6.11d). Satellite areas are rarely seen in intertriginous psoriasis. Furthermore, in candida infection biological cultures will demonstrate abundant growth of candida species.
2 Intertriginous dermatitis occurs as a result of the irritating effects of sweat, exogenous pigment, and occlusion phenomena. It is a form of dermatitis, typically displays papulovesicles in the periphery, and is almost exclusively associated with itching as well as pain, especially if erosions have developed.
3 Langerhans cell histiocytosis (LCH) is a rare, but quite important, differential diagnosis that can develop in intertriginous areas. The primary lesions of LCH

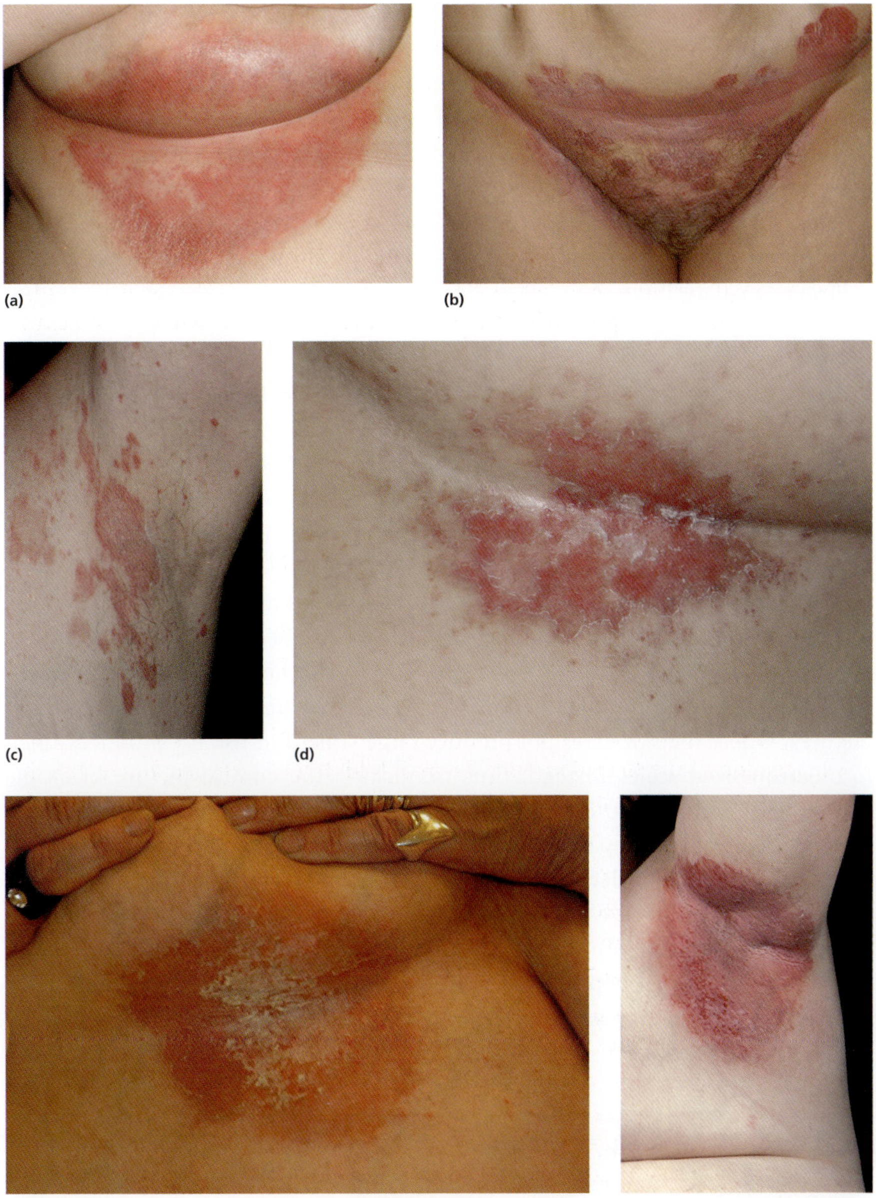

(a) (b) (c) (d) (e) (f)

Figure 6.11 (a) Submammary psoriasis. (b) Psoriasis in the genital and inguinal skin as well as the abdominal fold. (c) Axillary involvement. (d) Submammary candida infection with small peripheral satellite lesions, as well as fine scaling borders. (e) Langerhans cell histiocytosis. (f) Hailey–Hailey's disease with erosions, fine fissures, and macerated epidermis.

are reddish-brownish papules, which may be erosive or covered with crusts (Figure 6.11e). These lesions may coalesce and give rise to larger, painful, crusted areas. Histology will show the presence of dendritic cells and eosinophils;

special stains for Langerhans cells such as CD1a, Langerin, and others will help in demonstrating the presence of numerous atypical Langerhans cells.

4 Hailey–Hailey's disease also occurs in axillae and groins due to the hereditary insufficiency of the desmosomal connection between keratinocytes. It manifests almost exclusively in axillae and groins, and only rarely in other intertriginous areas. The surface is covered with fine fissures that form a reticular pattern (Figure 6.11f). The areas are painful and superinfected with Gram-negative bacteria. Diagnosis is established by histology, showing acantholysis due to desmosomal dysfunction.

Inverse psoriasis

Inverse psoriasis describes a phenotype that involves the flexural areas rather than the extensor parts of the extremities (Figure 6.12). Some authors regard inverse psoriasis to be somewhat broader and see an overlap between flexural psoriasis and intertriginous psoriasis. The latter has been discussed above in detail. Here, we will just discuss those patients showing involvement of the large flexures of arms and legs.

The reason for distinguishing flexural psoriasis from other forms of plaque psoriasis is the somewhat different clinical appearance and, therefore, other differential diagnoses that need to be excluded, predominantly atopic dermatitis.

Some patients present with psoriatic plaques occurring only on the elbow flexures, where the skin does not produce large scales but usually produces small to medium-sized scales instead, thus mimicking the clinical picture of atopic dermatitis. Careful examination will reveal sharply demarcated borders of the plaques, whereas typical papulovesicles are present in the periphery of the flexural inflammation in atopic dermatitis presenting the hallmarks of dermatitis. Clinical history will normally reveal further atopic stigmata, and distinction between the two diseases does not pose too much of a problem. The histology is that of typical plaque psoriasis (see Chapter 3), but lesions may be less acanthotic, and hyper-parakeratosis may be present to a lesser extent than in regular plaque psoriasis.

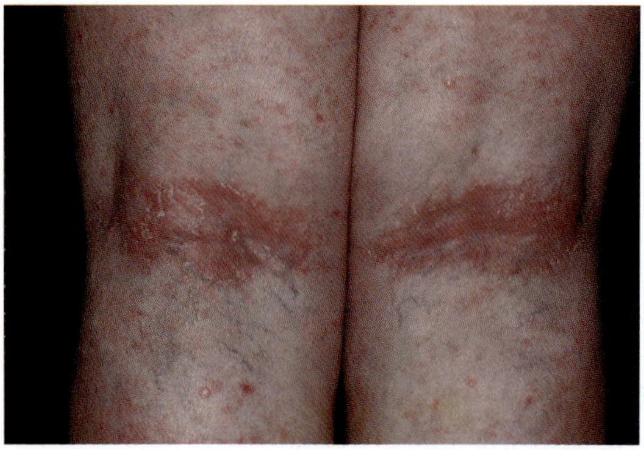

Figure 6.12 Inverse psoriasis.

Palmoplantar psoriasis

Here, we will cover psoriasis of the back of hands and feet as well as palmoplantar psoriasis sensu stricto. Psoriasis can involve both the volar and plantar aspects of the hands and feet. The extensor surfaces of hands and feet more or less present with an identical clinical appearance compared with other parts of the free skin (Figure 6.13a). The psychological distress caused by involvement of the back of the hand, however, is much higher than by lesions normally covered by clothing. Many private and professional situations are severely limited, and patients experience negative reactions from clients, friends, and even family members: Selling meat in a butcher's shop or presenting a precious necklace as a jeweller, for example, is virtually impossible.

A special situation of psoriasis of the extensor sites of hand and feet occurs when lesions affect the periungual areas. Periungual involvement is almost invariably associated with psoriasis of the nails, which in turn is often observed in patients with psoriatic arthritis of the distal interphalangeal joints. This complex situation displaying psoriatic inflammation simultaneously in the skin, the nail matrix, and the underlying enthesis (the insertion area of the extensor tendons into the bone) and joints is both highly disturbing and difficult to treat as well.

Psoriasis of the palms and soles is both diagnostically and therapeutically challenging, and involvement of the palms and soles may result from expanding plaques from the lower arms and legs (Figure 6.13b). In this context, diagnosis is easily made and equates with that of other typical psoriatic lesions elsewhere on the patient's skin. If lesions on the palms and soles are the only manifestations, however, diagnosis may become very difficult.

Palms and soles may be affected entirely or present with islets of psoriatic lesions. This latter feature may require discrimination from secondary syphilis (Figure 6.13d). Scaling is not a prominent feature of palmoplantar psoriasis. Mechanical stress may cause pain and fissures, and itching is another frequent complaint. Daily routine activities may be difficult to perform because contact with dirt, heat and cold, chemicals, or mechanical shear forces will cause pain and often worsening of the lesions. If the histology shows all the typical features of psoriasis (see Chapter 3), diagnosis is easy, but when irritated and eczema-like, things become more complicated. In patients with chronic hand or foot dermatitis that have a genetic background for psoriasis, histologic features of chronic dermatitis (acanthosis, parakeratosis, mononuclear infiltrate in the upper dermis) and psoriasis (papillomatosis, distorted blood vessels in the papillae) may be present.

Psoriasis of the palms is particularly stressful due to impairments in the sense of touch, a capacity that cannot be overestimated for daily activities such as analysis of the environment and communication.

Differential diagnosis includes other diseases with erythema and scaling. The most frequent clinical problem is distinguishing between palmoplantar psoriasis and *chronic hand and foot dermatitis*. Careful examination of the entire integument may reveal other psoriatic lesions and will support diagnosis of palmoplantar

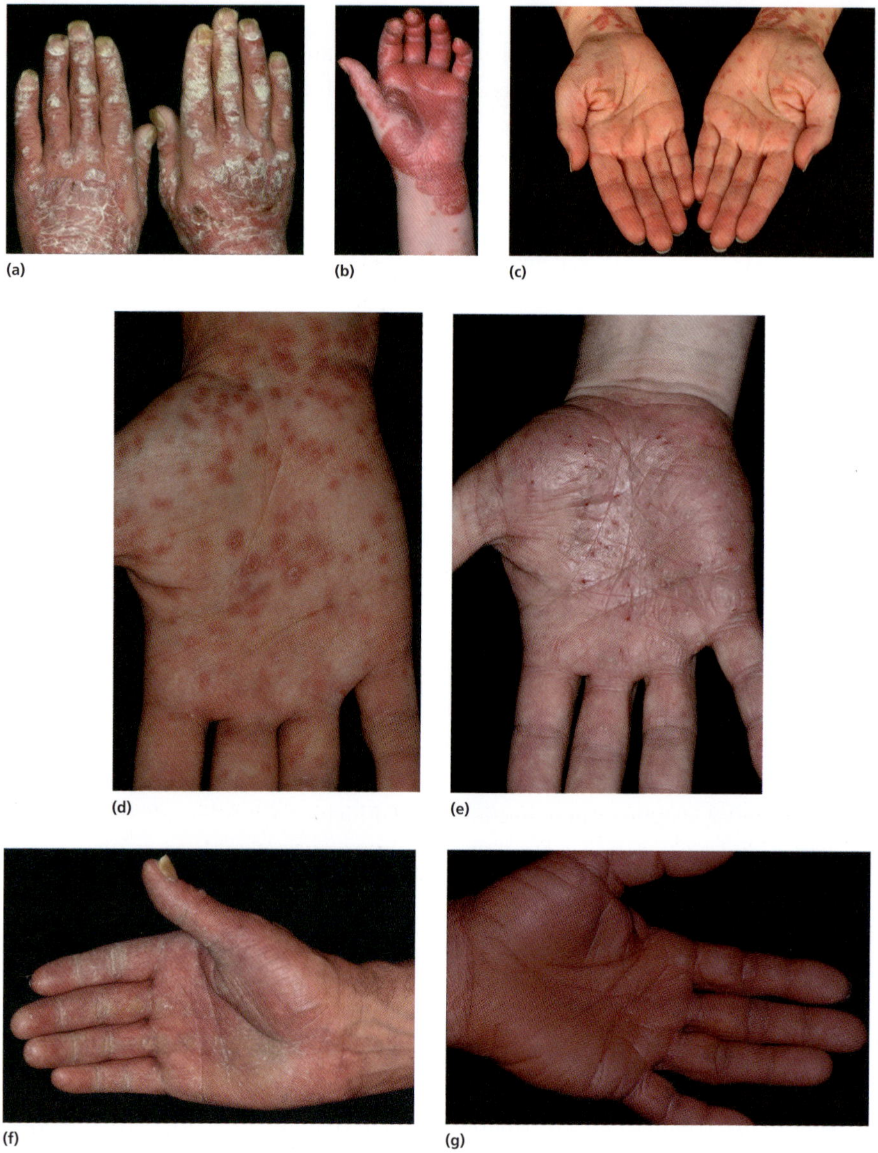

Figure 6.13 Palmoplantar psoriasis and its differential diagnosis. (a) Psoriasis of the back of hands and fingers, together with nail psoriasis. (b) Palmar psoriasis extending to the forearm. (c) Small maculopapular psoriatic lesions in the palm. (d) Maculopapular lesions in secondary syphilis. (e) Subacute hand dermatitis with small erosions having evolved from papulovesicles. (f) Tinea manuum due to *Trichophyton rubrum* infection. (g) Palmar keratoderma in pityriasis rubra pilaris with typical salmon color.

psoriasis. Even in the most chronic cases, hand and foot dermatitis will show acute or subacute lesions such as papulovesicles (Figure 6.13e), and itching may be more prominent than in psoriasis, but this is not a reliable feature. History or atopic stigmata may be present, and a detailed history of professional or private

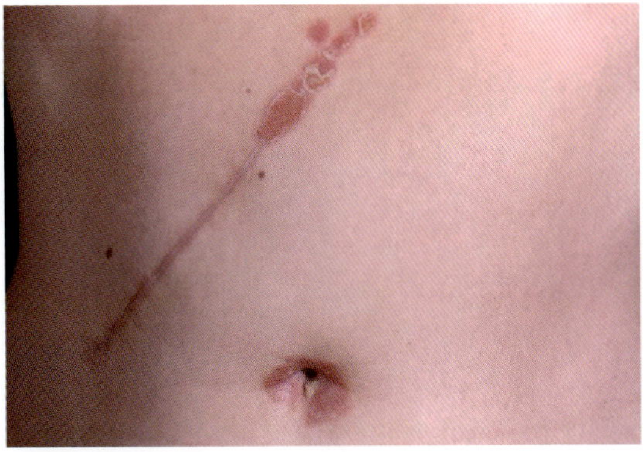

Figure 6.14 Köbner phenomenon.

exposure to allergens or toxic agents is mandatory, including patch testing if indicated. In typical cases, histology may be useful, but here the diagnosis can be made on clinical rationale alone in most cases. In patients showing clinical features of both psoriasis and eczema, one will find the features of psoriasis and eczema also in histology, which is therefore of limited value.

Tinea manuum or *tinea pedis* may resemble psoriasis, particularly if tinea shows inflammatory features (Figure 6.13f). In tinea pedis, involvement of the toenails is a valuable feature, but care should be taken not to confuse psoriatic with fungal nail involvement. Fungal cultures will help to establish the correct diagnosis.

Although rare, *Pityriasis rubra pilaris* is an important differential diagnosis (Figure 6.13g). Patients typically have palmoplantar keratoderma as well as reddish scaling lesions on the entire integument. A salmon-like color, islands of healthy skin, and a distinct histology with parakeratosis around the follicular orifices confirm a diagnosis of pityriasis rubra pilaris.

Köbner phenomenon

The term "Köbner phenomenon" refers to the occurrence of psoriasis in sites of trauma, mainly mechanical. One to two weeks after trauma, previously uninvolved skin will become psoriatic skin, and the shape of the psoriatic lesion will correspond to the area of the previous trauma or skin areas with altered structure. In fact, Heinrich Köbner from Berlin described a patient who was a horse dealer; one of the horses had bitten him in his upper arm, and after two weeks, the shape of the gnaw marks from the horse became visible as a psoriatic lesion. In order to develop a Köbner phenomenon, the psoriasis in a patient needs to be in a somewhat unstable state, and roughly one-quarter of all patients will develop a Köbner phenomenon when exposed to experimental traumatization.

The term "inverse Köbner phenomenon" is used for the disappearance of psoriasis within a given lesion after trauma. Psoriatic lesions in certain areas have been interpreted as being the result of a Köbner phenomenon, that is, psoriasis within a scar (Figure 6.14), and even intertriginous psoriasis and seborrhiasis have been regarded by some experts as being induced by toxic or microbial factors, and thus being examples of a Köbner phenomenon.

CHAPTER 7
Gutatte psoriasis

Wolfram Sterry and Frank Bachmann
Department of Dermatology and Allergy, University Hospital Charité, Berlin, Germany

We regard guttate psoriasis as a special manifestation of psoriasis, not as a variant of plaque psoriasis. Guttate psoriasis is the exanthematic form of psoriasis occurring mainly in children and young adults, often as the first manifestation of psoriasis. Guttate psoriasis often develops in the context of pharyngeal infection, mainly streptococcal, and T-cells specific for streptococcal antigen can be found both in the tonsillae and in the involved skin of these patients.

Patients typically present with a sudden onset of papules and small plaques covering the entire integument and measuring from a few millimeters to 1–2 cm in diameter (Figure 7.1). Involvement of the face is not unusual, and scaling may be less prominent than in plaque psoriasis (Figure 7.2). Therefore, the histological changes are not those of a fully developed psoriatic plaque but display features of developing psoriasis with histological signs of psoriasis being less pronounced (Figure 7.3). When sending such a biopsy to a dermatohistopathologist, special reference has to be made that clinical diagnosis is that of guttate psoriasis.

In addition to skin symptoms, patients may experience systemic symptoms such as fatigue or mild elevation of body temperature, which is not due to the pharyngeal infection alone but may reflect systemic immunological reactions.

Differential diagnosis includes pityriasis rosea, drug reactions, and secondary syphilis.

1 Pityriasis rosea occurs at the same age as guttate psoriasis. Patients develop a red and scaling primary lesion several centimeters in diameter, the so-called primary medallion. This does not exist in guttate psoriasis. The individual lesions of pityriasis rosea are larger, follow the orientation of the skin tension lines of the trunk and extremities, and are oval in shape (rather than the round lesions of guttate psoriasis; Figure 7.4). Furthermore, pityriasis rosea typically spares the face. Histology is helpful, if one cannot make the diagnosis by clinical examination alone, that is, without invasive measures.
2 Exanthematic drug reactions are rarely psoriasiform but may change to a psoriasiform aspect and via köbnerization into a typical psoriasis in predisposed

Psoriasis: Diagnosis and Management, First Edition. Edited by Wolfram Sterry, Robert Sabat, and Sandra Philipp.

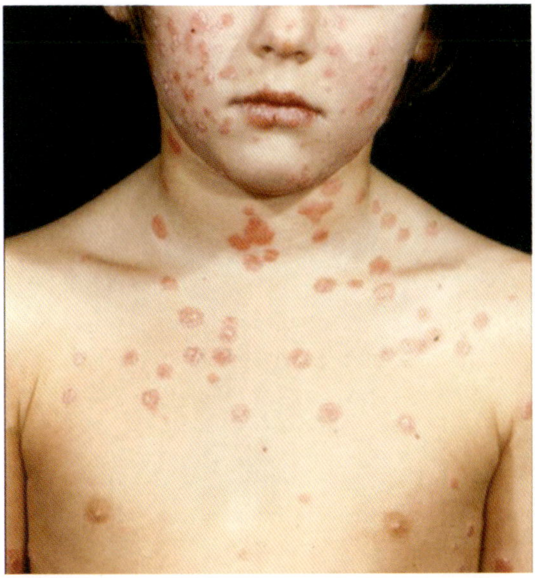

Figure 7.1 Guttate psoriasis in a boy. Note the pronounced involvement of the face.

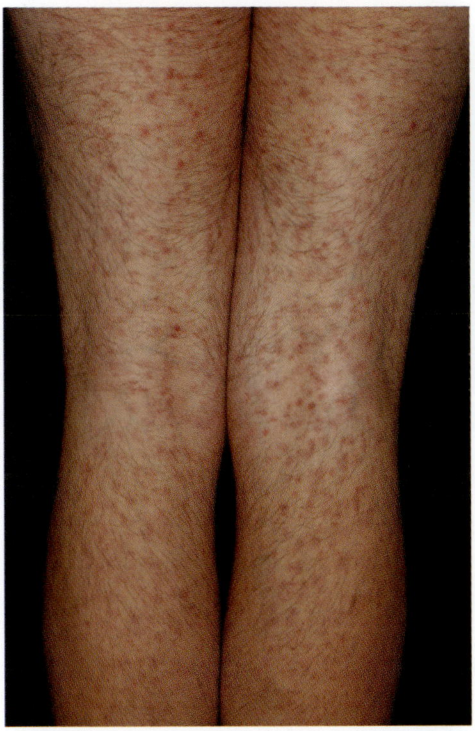

Figure 7.2 Guttate psoriasis. There is less scaling here than with plaque psoriasis.

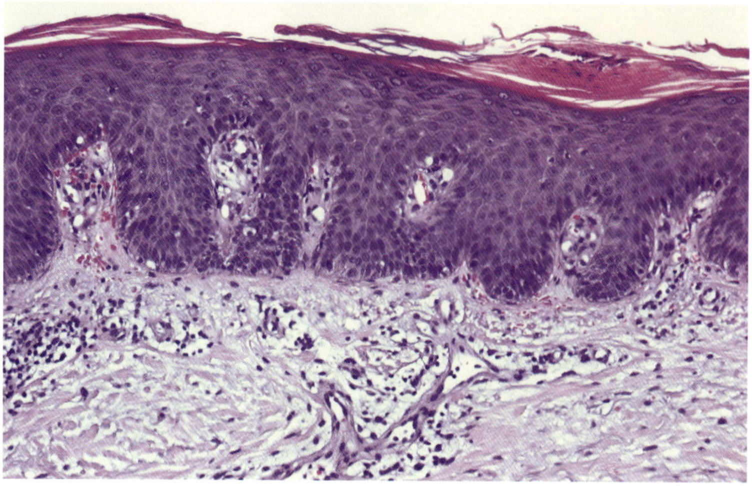

Figure 7.3 Histopathology of guttate psoriasis. All features of psoriasis are expressed but less severe than in psoriasis vulgaris.

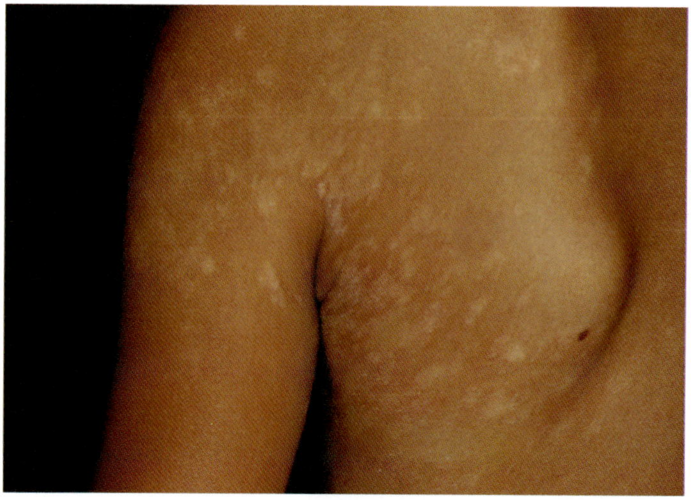

Figure 7.4 Pityriasis rosea with typical arrangement of lesions along skin tension lines.

individuals. In most cases, the medical history will establish the link between drugs and skin rashes. Classical drugs that evoke psoriasiform drug reactions are β-blockers, other antihypertensive drugs, chloroquin, and others (Table 7.1).

3 Secondary syphilis is also mainly a disease of young adults and presents with many different manifestations including psoriasiform lesions (Figure 7.5). Clues towards the correct diagnosis are other manifestations of secondary

Table 7.1 Drugs with known activity to induce psoriasiform skin lesions or to provoke psoriasis.

Drugs with causal relationship	
β-blocker • noncardioselective • cardioselective	Unknown mechanism. Hypotheses are as follows: (1) immunologic mechanisms such as impaired lymphocyte transformation, decreased IL-10 production; (2) decrease in intraepidermal cAMP through blockage of epidermal β-receptors with consequent increase in epidermal cell turnover.
Lithium	Mechanism not fully understood. Hypotheses are as follows: (1) disruption of ion-transport system leading to reduced cAMP and inositol levels, (2) dysregulation of the cyclic network, (3) stimulation of neutrophilic production by blocking the inhibitory effects of prostaglandin, (4) increase in circulating neutrophil levels and promotion of lysosomal release from leukocytes.
Synthetic antimalarials	Chemical structure similar to that of the potent transglutaminase inhibitor dansylputrescine. Transglutaminase is involved in the terminal differentiation of keratinocytes (see Chapter 3).
Nonsteroidal anti-inflammatory drugs • especially indomethacin	Influence of the arachidonic acid metabolism by inhibiting the cyclo-oxygenase or the lipoxygenase pathway.
Tetracyclines	Reduction in intracellular cAMP or by the interaction of the drug with arachidonic acid and its metabolites.
Withdrawal of corticosteroids	
Drugs with probable causal relationship but insufficient data	
ACE inhibitors	Not clearly understood. Hypotheses are as follows: (1) allergic, immune-mediated reaction, (2) pharmacological dose-dependent response.
Other cardiovascular drugs	• digoxin • clonidine • amiodarone • quanidine
Other psychotropic drugs	• benzodiazepines • fluoxetine • carbamazepine • olanzapine
Miscellaneous drugs	• terbinafine • potassium iodide • procaine • salicylate • sulfonamides • imiquimod • cimetidine • gemfibrozil
Cytokine/anticytokine therapies	
IFNs	• IFN-α2β • recombinant IFN-γ • peginterferon-α2β plus ribavirin • recombinant-DNA-derived IFN-α
TNF antagonists	Mechanism unclear.

cAMP: cyclic adenosine monophosphatase; IFN: interferon; TNF: tumor necrosis factor.

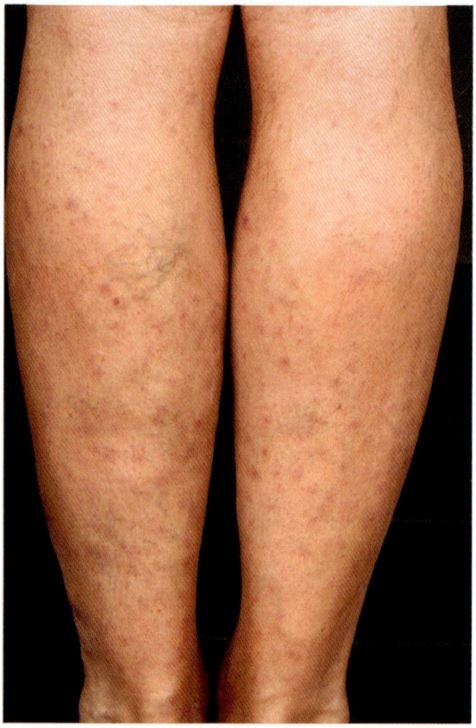

Figure 7.5 Secondary syphilis with maculopapular exanthema.

syphilis, that is, mucosal lesions, condylomata lata, and involvement of the palms and soles (syphilids). If clinical diagnosis includes secondary syphilis, specific blood tests will allow rapid clarification.

Further reading

Basavaraj, K.H., Ashok, N.M., Rashmi, R. and Praveen, T.K. (2010) The role of drugs in the induction and/or exacerbation of psoriasis. *International Journal of Dermatology*, **49**, 1351–1361.

Dika, E., Varotti, C., Bardazzi, F. and Maibach, H.I. (2006) Drug-induced psoriasis: an evidence-based overview and the introduction of psoriatic drug eruption probability score. *Cutaneous and Ocular Toxicology*, **25**, 1–11.

Diluvio, L., Vollmer, S., Besgen, P., Ellwart, J.W., Chimenti, S. and Prinz, J.C. (2006) Identical TCR beta-chain rearrangement in streptococcal angina and skin lesions of patients with psoriasis vulgaris. *Journal of Immunology*, **176**, 7104–7111.

CHAPTER 8

Erythrodermic psoriasis

Wolfram Sterry
Department of Dermatology and Allergy, University Hospital Charité, Berlin, Germany

Psoriasis may involve the entire integument without sparing a single spot (Figure 8.1); this is called "erythrodermic psoriasis." The term "suberythrodermic psoriasis" refers to almost complete involvement of the skin. The histology of erythrodermic psoriasis does not differ substantially from plaque psoriasis, except for a sometimes lesser degree of acanthosis (thickened epidermis) and papillomatosis (elongated rate ridges).

The reason why this clinical situation is regarded separately is that generalized inflammation of the entire skin has severe acute effects on the whole body. To understand the impact of erythrodermic psoriasis, try to recall your last severe sunburn where the cutaneous inflammation caused fever, chills, and malaise. While the sunburn-related symptoms subside after 24 h, psoriasis keeps on going for weeks, months, or even years. As a consequence, a catabolic metabolic situation is generated owing to protein loss via the epidermis (up to 100 g of protein per day in form of scales), intestinal malabsorption, and higher energy demand because of an increased demand of blood supply to the dilated blood vessels in the skin resulting in a stressful situation for the cardiovascular system as well. Thus, erythrodermic psoriasis, like any other kind of erythroderma, represents a dermatological emergency requiring immediate treatment.

Erythroderma may be due to a number of distinct skin disorders, and a clear diagnosis must be made before any specific treatment is initiated. Except for psoriasis, the most frequent causes of acquired erythroderma are generalized eczema (both allergic contact dermatitis and atopic dermatitis), pityriasis rubra pilaris, red man syndrome (an idiopathic erythroderma of elderly males), and Sézary syndrome (a distinct type of cutaneous T-cell lymphoma). A careful patient workup is required to establish the correct diagnosis, and so the reader is referred to textbooks of dermatology for further details. The diagnostic procedures required include the following:

1 Clinical examination: Clues for the presence of psoriasis such as psoriatic nail changes, splinter hemorrhages, pitting, or oil drops as well as psoriatic arthritis.

Psoriasis: Diagnosis and Management, First Edition. Edited by Wolfram Sterry, Robert Sabat, and Sandra Philipp.

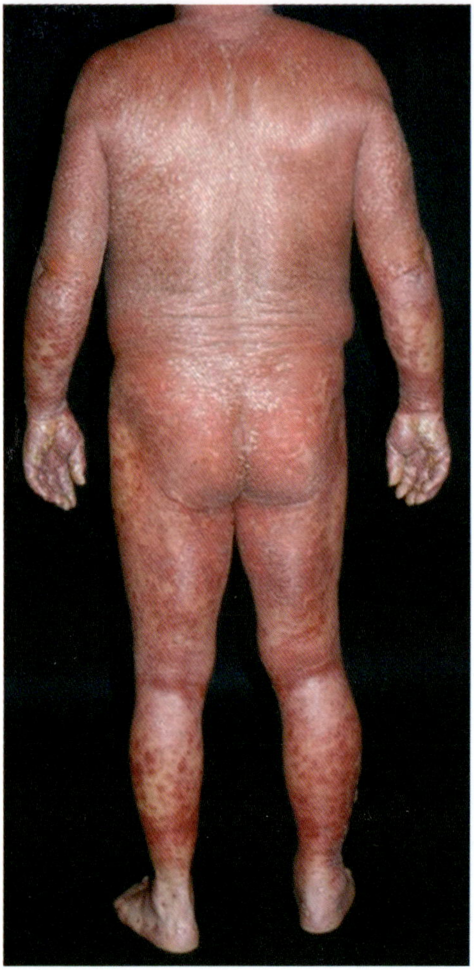

Figure 8.1 Erythrodermic psoriasis.

Presence of so-called nappes claires, spared areas of 1–2 cm, which typically occur in pityriasis rubra pilaris and Sézary syndrome. History of psoriasis, allergy, or atopy.

2 Blood examinations, particularly blood smears for presence of Sézary cells (lymphocytes with highly convoluted nuclei) and molecular biological analysis for demonstration of a dominant T-cell clone; total IgE as a hint for allergic or atopic eczema.

3 Histological and molecular biological investigations to look for specific changes in one of the potential diseases, and search for the presence of a dominant T-cell clone by T-cell-receptor rearrangement analysis in the skin, which would be suggestive of Sézary syndrome.

For a differential diagnosis of erythroderma, the reader is referred to reviews on this topic (Sterry and Steinhoff, 2012).

Further reading

Sterry, W. and Steinhoff, M. (2012) Erythroderma. In: J.L. Bologna, J.L. Jorizzo and J.V. Schaffer (eds). *Textbook of Dermatology,* 3rd edition. Mosby, Philadelphia, PA.

CHAPTER 9
Pustular psoriasis

Sandra Philipp
Psoriasis Research and Treatment Center, Department of Dermatology and Allergy/Institute of Medical Immunology, University Hospital Charité, Berlin, Germany

The term "pustular psoriasis" comprises several subtypes: (1) generalized pustular psoriasis Zumbusch type (GPP), (2) erythema anulare centrifugum-like psoriasis with and without pustulation (EACP), (3) psoriasis vulgaris with pustulation (psoriasis cum pustulatione), (4) palmo-plantar pustular psoriasis (Königsbeck-Barber), (5) acrodermatits continua suppurativa Hallopeau and (6) generalized pustular psoriasis of pregnancy (GPPP), also known as impetigo herpetiformis.

Pustular psoriasis is much rarer than psoriasis vulgaris. In surveys in Japan, the percentage of pustular variants in patients with psoriasis has been reported as 0.6–0.9% for generalized pustular psoriasis and 0.15–0.5% for localized pustular psoriasis. Further epidemiological studies in Japan and France estimated the prevalence of GPP between 7.46/million, and 1.76/million respectively, the incidence to be at least 0.64/million.

Generalized pustular psoriasis (GPP)

GPP (Figure 9.1) has been named after Leo Ritter von Zumbusch, who first described this disease in 1910. It is regarded as one of the most severe types of psoriasis with potentially life-threatening complications. However, in contrast to psoriasis vulgaris, there is no association of GPP with the typical psoriasis susceptibility loci or HLA-Cw6.

A possible pathogenic role of IL-8, tumor necrosis factor alpha (TNF-α), and IL-36 is suggested. IL-8 is an important chemokine that induces migration of neutrophils into the epidermis, and TNF-α as a potent proinflammatory mediator may be responsible for the highly inflammatory reaction in GPP. IL-36 is a novel IL-1-related cytokine that potently induces many chemokines in keratinocytes.

In GPP, inflammation is more pronounced than in plaque psoriasis. Yet, besides the increased number of neutrophils in GPP, no further significant differences in mechanism of neutrophil infiltration have been detected. Therefore, Iizuka *et al.* (2003) have suggested that the HLA distinction might

Psoriasis: Diagnosis and Management, First Edition. Edited by Wolfram Sterry, Robert Sabat, and Sandra Philipp.

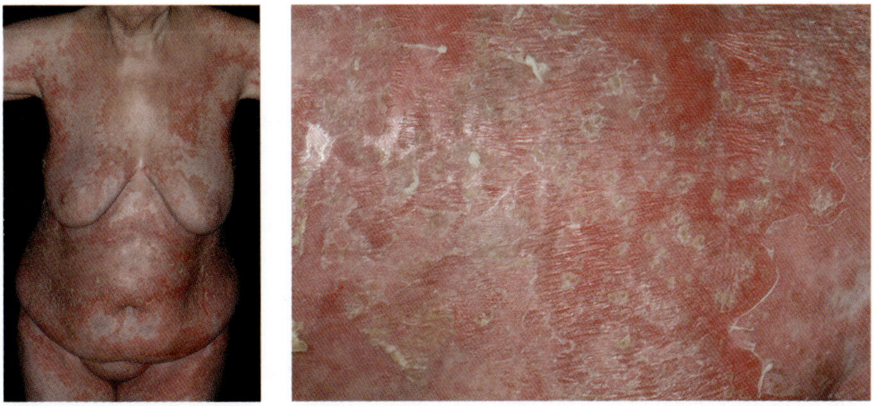

(a) (b)

Figure 9.1 (a) Generalized pustular psoriasis. (b) Generalized pustular psoriasis with erosions after shedding of dried pustules.

simply correspond to a distinct predisposition of acute neutrophilic inflammation between the two subgroups. Additionally, multiple trigger factors of GPP have been reported:

- dental- or upper-respiratory-tract infections, especially group A streptococcal infections; vaccinations;
- physical, chemical, and mechanical triggers: for example, solar irradiation or irritating topical substances;
- hypocalcemia;
- pregnancy, hormonal changes, oral contraceptives, withdrawal of corticosteroids;
- emotional stress;
- numerous medications, for example, lithium, beta blocker, and antimalaria medications, ACE inhibitors such as ramipril or topical indomethacin.

Clinical picture

Characteristic is the sudden onset of a diffuse erythema with fast-developing disseminated pinhead-sized sterile pustules (Figure 9.1a). The pustules often appear within a few hours but can persist over several days. Frequently, the pustules coalesce, thus forming large lakes of pus.

When the pustules rupture and dry out, the skin sheds off, resulting in large erosions (Figure 9.1b) that may become superinfected. The course of disease often includes multiple bursts. While existing lesions show desquamation, a new eruption of pustules may occur. Widespread confluence of the disseminated lesions can finally lead to complete erythroderma. The face is usually not affected; however, nails, palms, and soles can be afflicted. Though not frequently present, geographic tongue or pustules can be found as sign for mucosal involvement. General lymphadenopathy is common. Additionally, most patients also suffer from systemic symptoms such as fever, general malaise, and/or arthralgia.

Laboratory analyses often reveal marked leukocytosis, increased erythrocyte sedimentation rate, and eventually hypocalcemia. Recently, further extracutaneous manifestations such as liver involvement have been reported. Patients showed increased transaminases, alkaline phosphatase, and gammaglutamyl transferase, or jaundice. Evidence for biliary involvement related to neutrophilic cholangitis was found. Moreover, possible complications such as infections, electrolyte imbalance, or hypocalcemia have to be considered. A French survey reported complications and death in 17% and 2% of the cases respectively.

Diagnostic procedure

The characteristic clinical symptoms, including generalized lymphadenopathy may lead to a diagnosis. The medical history should include drug intake and family history of psoriasis.

Laboratory analyses frequently show a decisive leukocytosis, increased erythrocyte sedimentation rate, CRP, as well as raised transaminases. Hypocalcemia is not rare. If a streptococcal infection triggered the exacerbation, an increased ASL titer could be found.

The histological picture shows the characteristic spongiform pustules of Kogoj (=groups of neutrophils in the *stratum spinosum*) and the typical epidermal changes of psoriasis such as hyper- and parakeratosis, or elongation of the rete ridges.

One of the most important differential diagnoses is acute generalized exanthemateous pustulosis (drug-induced, e.g. antibiotics; frequently more acute course of fever and pustules, histology: single necrotic cells in epidermis, eosinophils, dermal vasculitis).

Topic of interest—GPP and glucocorticoids

GPP may be induced in patients with psoriasis vulgaris by tapering or withdrawal of systemic glucocorticoids, especially when patients have been subjected to a dosage greater than a Cushing dose for a prolonged period (>1 week). These patients often experience a more severe course of the disease and seem to have a higher risk for potential complications such as cardiovascular failure or infections. Furthermore, these exacerbations often respond inadequately to traditional systemic treatments. Therefore, systemic glucocorticoids (in higher dosages) should be used with great caution in patients with psoriasis and avoided whenever possible.

Generalized pustular psoriasis of pregnancy (GPPP)/ Impetigo herpetiformis (IH)

GPPP has been accepted widely to be a variant of annular pustular psoriasis occurring in pregnancy. As the disease may be potentially harmful to mother and child, early recognition and timely treatment are important in order to avoid complications. A more detailed description of psoriasis in different life situations can be found in Chapter 13.

Annular psoriasis [erythema annulare centrifugum-type (EACP)]

This was first reported by Lapiere in 1959, and later Huriez and Degos introduced the term EACP. This is a rare variant of psoriasis that may occur spontaneously in patients without a history of psoriasis or may develop in patients with plaque-type psoriasis as well as pustular psoriasis.

Clinical picture

Annular psoriasis is characterized by erythemateous macules or discrete plaques in ring form or showing a serpiginous pattern (Figure 9.2a). The margin of the lesions is covered with multiple pustules and/or colerette-like scales (scales located at the margin with their free edge directed into the center). Frequently, the course of disease includes several acute eruptions followed by rapid remissions within a few days or weeks, though some lesions also may persist for several months. In the long term, recurrent exacerbations for a number of years are possible.

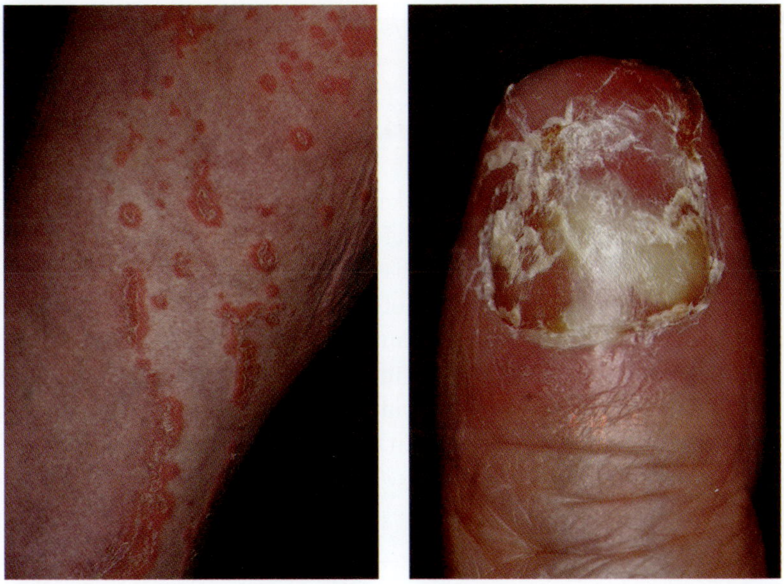

(a) (b)

Figure 9.2 (a) Annular psoriasis with collarette-like scales. (b) Acrodermatitis continua suppurativa, showing peri- and subungal confluent pustules on erythemateous base and almost complete destruction of the nail plate.

Diagnostic procedure

The characteristic annular or ring form of lesions either with or without pustules and colarette-like scales is often sufficient for the diagnosis, especially if the lesions evolve from pre-existing plaques, yet in unclear cases, a histologic examination may be warranted. Munroe microabscesses (group of subcorneal neutrophils) as well as spongiform pustules (Kogoj) are frequently seen, and the acanthosis is usually discrete. In some cases, immunofluorescence may be helpful to exclude blistering diseases.

Differential diagnoses include annular or gyrate erythemas, tinea corporis (mycology), different blistering diseases such as subcorneal pustular dermatosis of Sneddon–Wilkinson (histology, direct immunofluorescence), or pemphigus foeliaceus (immunofluorescence: reticular pattern of IgG, serology: IgG autoantibodies against desmoglein 1), as well as Sweet's syndrome (fever, arthralgias, leukocytosis with increased numbers of neutrophils, histology).

Psoriasis vulgaris with pustulation

The term psoriasis cum pustulatione is used if pustules develop on plaques during an acute exacerbation of a pre-existing psoriasis vulgaris, for example, triggered by infections or withdrawal of glucocorticoids. Diagnostic procedures and treatment correspond to plaque psoriasis and pustular psoriasis, respectively.

Palmoplantar pustular psoriasis (PPP)

PPP was first described in 1888 by Crocker as "dermatitis repens", but a relationship with psoriasis was not suggested before 1930. And still today, the affiliation of PPP with psoriasis is a matter of debate. PPP is not associated with PSORS1, the most common susceptibility locus of psoriasis vulgaris, but has been linked to variations of genes of the IL-20 subfamily of cytokines. Moreover, recent dermatoscopic investigations have shown involvement of the acrosyringium in the PPP vesicle formation, and in patients with PPP, an accumulation of inflammatory markers such as IL-17 has been found in the acrosyringium in combination with Langerhans cells close to the sweat duct. Therefore, a central role for the acrosyringium has been suggested.

Clinical picture

Frequently, PPP manifests in patients without a history of psoriasis, though about 20–25% present additional psoriatic plaques elsewhere on the body. Primarily, women are afflicted (9:1 female:male ratio), showing first symptoms in the fourth

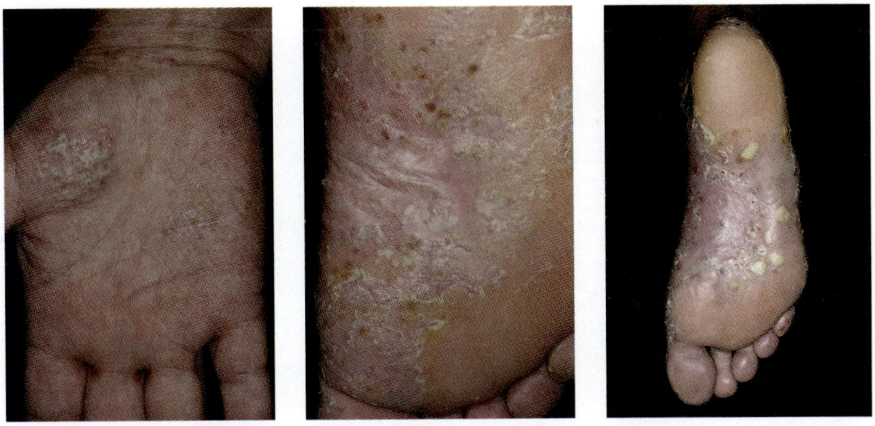

Figure 9.3 Typical clinical pictures of palmoplantar pustular psoriasis.

or fifth decade, and so an association with sex hormones might be possible. Interestingly, nearly all patients (up to 95%) are either current or previous smokers.

Initially, multiple pinhead-sized yellow pustules develop on an erythematous base. Later, one may find fresh yellow pustules side by side with older dried pustules of brown color, small erosions, crusts, and adherent fine scales on an erythematous base (Figure 9.3). Some patients present with one localized single lesion, others with complete affection of palms and soles. Typical locations on palms are thenar or hypothenar regions, whereas plantar lesions often involve the lateral or medial margin of the soles. Additional psoriatic nail affection is common. The course of disease is mainly chronic and/or shows recurrent exacerbations. Patients are often decisively impaired due to the restricted use of hands or walking.

Diagnostic procedure

Most important are the characteristic clinical symptoms, and additional affliction of the nails can be helpful to make a diagnosis. Direct microscopic examination of native preparations with potassium hydroxide and microbiological culture can be used to exclude infectious diseases.

Histologic examination may be considered in unclear cases, though differentiation between psoriasis and eczema can prove challenging, even by histology. In early phases, spongiosis and epidermal vesicles might dominate, whereas in later stages, the characteristic sterile pustules (Figure 9.4) with eosinophils and neutrophils dominate. Discrete acanthosis is common, and the papillary dermis demonstrates an inflammatory infiltrate of lymphocytes, mast cells, and eosinophils.

Most important differential diagnoses are chronic hand eczema or contact dermatitis (less explicitly demarcated lesions, exposition to irritants, and/or contact allergens) and tinea of hands or feet (skin involvement often only unilateral, positive mycology).

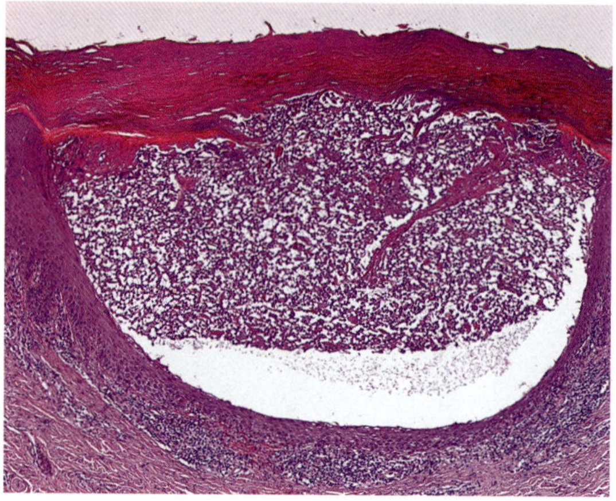

Figure 9.4 Histological picture of palmoplantar psoriasis with sterile pustules (Kogoj) as well as hyper- and parakeratosis.

Topic of interest—synovitis, acne, pustulosis, hyperostosis, and osteitis (SAPHO) syndrome

SAPHO syndrome involves osteoarticular manifestations and dermatologic diseases such as acne or palmoplantar pustulosis (neutrophilic dermatoses). Typical manifestations are osteitis and hyperostosis, most often of the anterior chest wall, such as the sternocostoclavicular joints. However, the sacroiliacal joints, upper ribs, peripheral bones, or mandibula might be involved, too. Patients complain of severe pain and swelling in these areas. Often the condition is triggered or worsened by focal infections (e.g. streptococcal throat infection). Others have suggested low-virulence pathogens, especially propionibacterium acne, as initiating factors. The course of disease is variable, but includes chronic progressive forms with recurrent flares. Nonsteroidal antirheumatics, systemic glucocorticoids, and disease-modifying antirheumatic drugs such as methotrexate show only limited efficacy. In case reports and small studies, intravenous aminobisphosphonates (pamidronate and zoledronic acid) and TNF inhibitors have been used successfully.

Topic of interest—psoriatic onycho-pachydermoperiostitis (POPP)

POPP is a recently described rare manifestation of psoriatic arthritis. The syndrome is characterized by psoriatic nail disease, arthritis of the distal interphalangeal joints, and impressively swollen distal fingers or toes (soft tissue edema). Enthesiopathy seems to play a more central role than direct affection of the periost; therefore, typical arthritis signs such as erosions are frequently missing. Psoriatic skin lesions may be present or not. So far, there is no standard treatment, though MTX and TNF inhibitors have been reported to be effective in single cases.

Acrodermatitis continua suppurativa (Hallopeau)

This disease is named after the French dermatologist, Francois Henri Hallopeau (1842–1919). Owing to its clinical picture, it has been classified as a subtype of pustular psoriasis, though this has been discussed controversially since.

Clinical picture

The disease often starts from a localized trauma or infection, frequently affecting only one or two fingers or toes. Characteristic are periungual located pustules developing on an erythematous base. When the pustules coalesce, this may lead to lakes of pus. Additional affliction of the nail bed and nail matrix frequently causes psoriatic nail changes such as pitting or oil drops, and often results in complete onychodystrophy with potential loss of the respective nail (Figure 9.2b). Usually, the lesions remain restricted to one or two digits, but rarely they can expand to the back of the hands and feet or involve additional fingers or toes. Prolonged chronic inflammation can even lead to affection of the bone resulting in osteolysis of the distal phalanx. Generally, the course of disease is chronic with recurrent pustular eruptions.

Diagnostic procedure

Characteristic clinical picture with periungual pustules and nail involvement. Infectious causes such as bacteria or fungi should be excluded by cultures of the pus. Biopsy for histologic examination might be necessary in unclear cases. The histological picture shows the typical features of pustular psoriasis, as Munro's microabscesses and pustules of Kogoj in combination with a lymphohistiocytic infiltrate. In some cases, an X-ray of the hands might be advisable to exclude affection of the bones.

Most important differential diagnoses are bacterial or fungal paronychia, allergic contact dermatitis, and dyshidrotic eczema. Nevertheless, in persistent chronic disease, a biopsy should be taken to exclude neoplasms such as spinal cell carcinoma.

Topic of interest—induction of pustular psoriasis (PP) by biologics

Although rare, new occurrences or exacerbations of psoriasis during the use of TNF inhibitors have become a well-known phenomenon. A review of 207 cases reported that 56% presented with pustular lesions. Although the pathogenic mechanism is still not clear, a change in cytokine milieu seems to be involved with an excess of interferon-α production by plasmacytoid dendritic cells in predisposed individuals. Recently, the development of pustular psoriasis has also been described in a patient with chronic plaque psoriasis after ustekinumab (anti-p40-antibody) treatment.

Further reading

Braun-Falco, O., Berthold, D. and Ruzicka, T. (1987) Psoriasis pustulosa generalisata—classification, clinical aspects and therapy. Review and experiences with 18 patients. *Hautarzt*, **38**, 509–520.

Brenner, M., Molin, S., Ruebsam, K., Weisenseel, P., Ruzicka, T. and Prinz, J.C. (2009) Generalized pustular psoriasis induced by systemic glucocorticosteroids: four cases and recommendations for treatment. *British Journal of Dermatology*, **161**, 948–970.

Christophers, E. (2008) Explaining phenotype heterogeneity in patients with psoriasis. *British Journal of Dermatology*, **158**, 437–441.

Colina, M., Govoni, M., Orzincolo, C. and Trotta, F. (2009) Clinical and radiologic evolution of synovitis, acne, pustulosis, hyperostosis, and osteitis syndrome: A single center study of a cohort of 71 subjects. *Arthritis & Rheumatism (Arthritis Care & Research)*, **61**, 813–821.

Iizuka, H., Takahashi, H. and Ishida-Yamamoto, A. (2003) Pathophysiology of generalized pustular psoriasis. *Archives of Dermatological Research*, **295**, S55–S59.

Naldi, L. and Gambini, D. (2007) The clinical spectrum of psoriasis. *Clinics in Dermatology*, **25**, 510–518.

Vocks, E., Worret, W-I. and Ring, J. (2003) Erythema annulare centrifugum-type psoriasis: a particular variant of acute-eruptive psoriasis. *Journal of the European Academy of Dermatology and Venereology*, **17**, 446–448.

CHAPTER 10

Nail psoriasis

Sandra Philipp
Psoriasis Research and Treatment Center, Department of Dermatology and Allergy/Institute of Medical Immunology, University Hospital Charité, Berlin, Germany

No recent epidemiological studies have been conducted, but the available data report the occurrence of nail affection in about 15–50% of all psoriasis patients, and in approximately 80% of patients suffering from psoriatic arthritis. The lifetime incidence of nail involvement has been estimated to be about 80–90%. Very rarely, nail lesions can present as the only clinical feature of psoriasis without skin manifestations.

The frequencies of distinct nail dystrophies associated with psoriasis vary in the literature, but the most common feature of nail psoriasis is pitting. Tham *et al.* (1988) reported a frequency of 68%, followed by onycholysis in 67%, subungal hyperkeratosis in 25%, and nail-bed discoloration in only 18%. Similarly, Zaias (1969) reported pitting as the most frequent psoriatic nail affection. However, nail-bed discoloration occurred more frequently than onycholysis or subungual hyperkeratosis.

Clinical picture and pathophysiology

The clinical symptoms of nail psoriasis are associated with the involvement of different structures of the nail (Figure 10.1) and can be divided into affection of the nail matrix and the nail bed. Nail-matrix defects comprise pits, transversal or longitudinal ridges, crumbling, leukonychia, and red spots in the lunula, and may result in onychorrhexis or complete onychodystrophy.

Pits (Figure 10.2a–b) are superficial defects within the nail plate, visible as small indentations. Involved cells in the nail matrix or proximal nail fold show an altered keratinization process (parakeratosis) that results in decreased adhesion function and thereby leads to a superficial loss of the cells, when the nail plate grows outward. If greater areas are involved, this may result in *transversal grooves or ridges* (Figure 10.2c) and long-lasting affection in *longitudinal ridges*. The whole process may end in *onychorrhexis* (longitudinal splitting of the nail). Affection of the dorsal matrix causes more superficial

Psoriasis: Diagnosis and Management, First Edition. Edited by Wolfram Sterry, Robert Sabat, and Sandra Philipp.

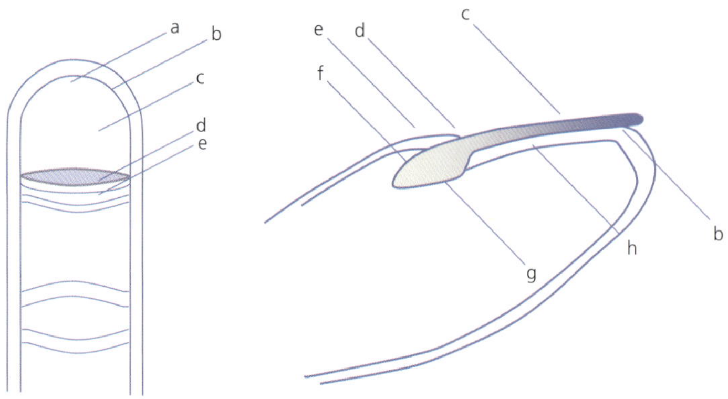

Figure 10.1 Schematic illustration of the different nail parts. (a) Free edge of the nail plate. (b) Hyponychium. (c) Nail plate. (d) Lunula. (e) Proximal nail fold. (f) Dorsal matrix. (g) Intermediate/ventral matrix. (h) Nail bed.

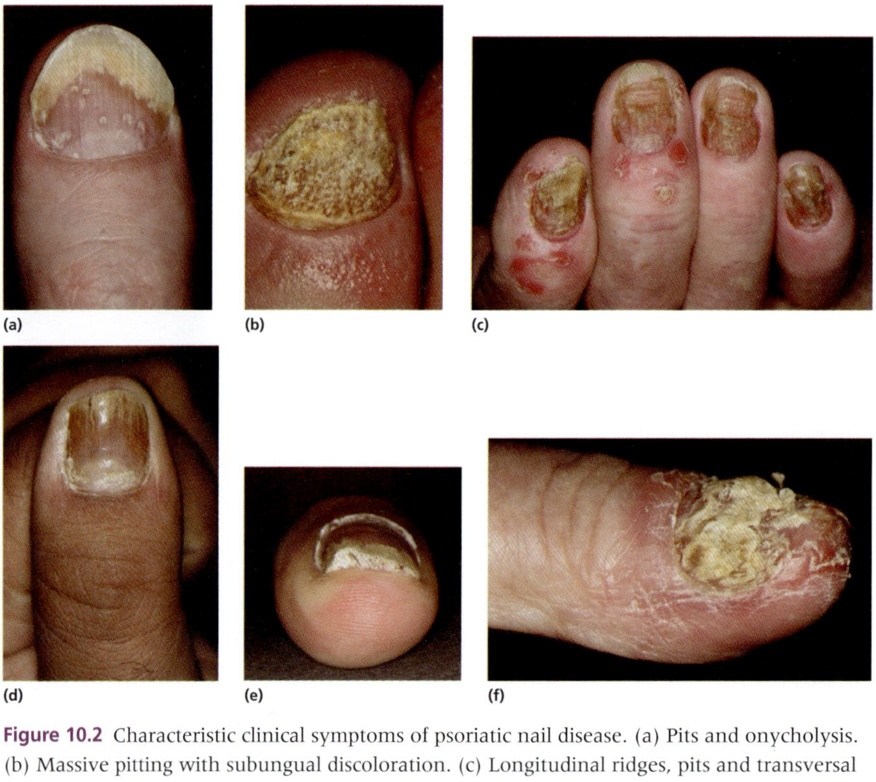

Figure 10.2 Characteristic clinical symptoms of psoriatic nail disease. (a) Pits and onycholysis. (b) Massive pitting with subungual discoloration. (c) Longitudinal ridges, pits and transversal grooves on the middle and ring fingers. (d) Nail-bed discoloration with typical "oil drops" or "salmon patches," and discrete red spots (increased transparency by thinning of nail plate). Fine splinter hemorrhages can be detected at the free nail edge. (e) Subungual hyperkeratosis with whitish crumbling material underneath the nail plate causing distal onycholysis. (f) Complete onychodystrophy of the nail.

depressions, and when additional intermediate or ventral parts are defective this leads to deeper defects with *crumbling* of the nail plate or even complete *onychodystrophy* (Figure 10.2f). If only ventral and intermediate parts of the nail matrix are impaired, the surface may stay unaffected, and the internal desquamation of the cells can either lead to a thinner nail plate with increased transparency, which results, for example, in *red spots in the lunula* arising from the gleam of capillaries in the nail bed, or cause a whitish appearance of the nail plate (leukonychia).

Affection of the nail bed includes oil-drop spots, subungual hyperkeratosis, onycholysis, and splinter hemorrhages.

Impaired keratinization of nail bed cells may lead to increased superficial desquamation of cells in the hyponychium area and thereby cause the formation of a gap between the nail plate and the nail bed, *onycholysis* (Figure 10.2a and e). When air enters the gap, the nail plate develops a whitish appearance, yet altered keratinization can also result in reduced desquamation of corneocytes with subsequent accumulation of these cells, visible as silvery-white crumbling material under the nail plate, *subungual hyperkeratosis* (Figure 10.2e). When inflammation is marked, proteinaceous exudate can change the color to gray or yellow. This process can also lead to onycholysis.

Psoriatic lesions (with acanthosis, hyper- and parakeratosis) of the nail bed appear through the nail plate as a yellowish brown discoloration and are therefore called "oil drop" spots or "salmon-colored patches" (Figure 10.2d).

Inflammatory diseases such as psoriasis seem to predispose patients to an increased fragility of dermal capillaries. The rupture of capillaries in the nail bed causes so-called *splinter hemorrhages* (Figure 10.2d), short brown to black lines, that are frequently located at the free edge of the nail plate. The linear shape can be explained by the location of these capillaries, as they follow the direction of the epidermal-dermal ridges that connect the nail plate to the nail bed.

Differential diagnoses include a broad spectrum of nail affections by other inflammatory diseases such as chronic eczema (medical or family history of atopic diseases, exposition to contact allergens or chronic irritation due to profession, less clearly demarcated skin lesions and papulovesicles), lichen planus (polygonal papules at typical locations such as the wrists or ankles, Wickham signs (reticular shaped white lines, affection of oral mucosa; Figure 10.3c), or alopecia areata (areata lesions on the scalp or other parts of the body). Onychomycosis (asymmetric affection of nails, mycology/Figure 10.3a) or trauma (medical history, leisure activities such as jogging, etc.) should also be considered. Rare diseases such as 20-nail dystrophy/trachyonychia (all nails are affected, manifestation in childhood; Figure 10.3b), or yellow nail syndrome (all nails affected, lymphedema, or respiratory diseases) could be misinterpreted as psoriasis.

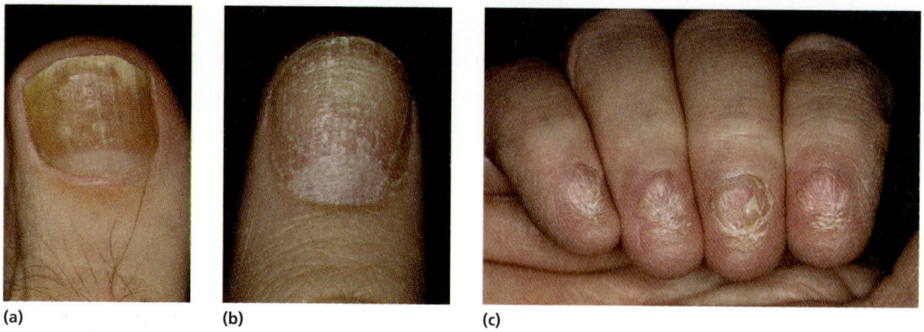

Figure 10.3 Differential diagnoses of psoriatic nail disease. (a) Onychomycosis. (b) Trachyonychia. (c) Lichen ruber.

Diagnostic procedure

In many cases, the characteristic clinical picture (e.g. pitting, salmon patch) and possible further psoriatic skin lesions on fingers or elsewhere on the body are sufficient for the correct diagnosis. If only the nails are affected, a positive family history of psoriasis may be helpful.

Infectious causes should be eliminated by examination of native preparations or by microbiological culture. Rarely, it may be necessary to do a punch biopsy or to excise part of the nail. Since the histological changes can be demonstrated in the nail bed, the biopsy does not have to include the matrix. The histological picture of nail psoriasis corresponds to the characteristic skin alterations including hyper- and parakeratosis, acanthosis as well as dilated and elongated capillaries, and the inflammatory infiltrate.

Burden of disease

Psoriatic nail affection has been associated not only with joint affliction, but also with more severe skin disease, including both the extent of skin involvement and a longer disease duration. About 90% of patients are troubled by the condition, owing to the permanent visibility of the affected nails, which causes psychological distress, feelings of embarrassment, and therefore a significant impairment of quality of life. Often patients try to conceal their hands or feet, and about half of patients complain about pain and/or functional disability, for example, with handling small objects, resulting in problems with daily activities in housekeeping or at work.

Topic of interest—close connection of nail, enthesis, and joint in psoriatic arthritis (Figure 10.4)

In patients with psoriatic nail disease, affection of the distal interphalangeal (DIP) joints is quite frequent. High-resolution MRI techniques and histological investigations have increased our knowledge about the close relationship

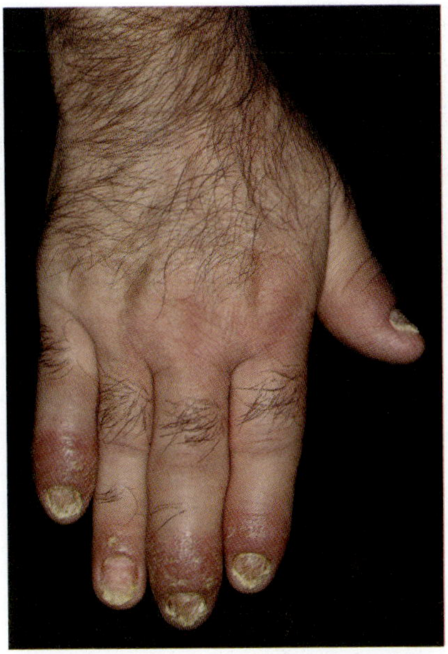

Figure 10.4 Co-occurrence of psoriatic arthritis (swollen joints), skin lesions, and nail affection.

between nail, enthesis (insertion site of tendons and ligaments), and bone by a network of enthesis fibres connected to the periosteum. Perienthesal bone edema in MRI is a typical sign of early psoriatic arthritis in the DIP joints.

It has been suggested that the entheseal inflammation may even be the starting point of the inflammation in psoriatic arthritis. The process might be induced by microdamage caused by mechanical stress in the enthesis attachment sites, in analogy with the Koebner phenomenon of the skin, with subsequent production of local tissue factors. Consequently, the inflammation may spread to the adjacent bones and nails. McGonagle (2009) hypothesized that local factors might cause a primary innate immune response at sites predisposed to disease that is independent of adaptive immunity and results in a chronic autoinflammatory reaction.

Further reading

Baran, R. (2010) The burden of nail psoriasis: An introduction. *Dermatology*, **221** (Supplement 1), 1–5.

Jiaravuthisan, M.M., Sasseville, D., Vender, R.B., Murphy, F. and Muhn, C.Y. (2007) Psoriasis of the nail: Anatomy, pathology, clinical presentation, and a review of the literature on therapy. *Journal of the American Academy of Dermatology*, **57**, 1–27.

McGonagle D. (2009) Enthesitis: An autoinflammatory lesion linking nail and joint involvement in psoriatic disease. *Journal of the European Academy of Dermatology and Venereology*, **23**(Supplement 1), 9–13.

Tham, S.N., Lim, J.J., Tay, S.H. *et al.* (1988) Clinical observations on nail changes in psoriasis. *Annals Academy of Medicine Singapore*, **17**, 482–485.

Zaias, N. (1969) Psoriasis of the nail. *Archives of Dermatology*, **99**, 576–579.

CHAPTER 11

Psoriatic arthritis

Marina Backhaus

Department of Rheumatology and Clinical Immunology, Charité-Universitätsmedizin Berlin, Berlin, Germany

Psoriatic arthritis (PsA) is an inflammatory, seronegative arthritis associated with psoriasis and has been classified to the group of seronegative spondyloarthritis along with reactive arthritis, arthritis associated with chronic inflammatory bowel disease, and spondylitis ankylosans.

Epidemiology

The exact prevalance is unknown. According to recent data, approximately 20–30% of psoriasis patients develop psoriatic arthritis, and the gender frequencies for men and women are equal. Interestingly, there is no correlation between the severity of skin manifestations and the appearance of psoriatic arthritis. Skin lesions appear in almost 70–80% of patients before the appearance of joint symptoms. In approximately 10–15% of patients, the skin and joint symptoms appear at the same time, and importantly, almost 10–15% of patients present with joint involvement before the skin symptoms appear, which may therefore complicate the correct diagnosis

Clinical picture

The clinical picture is variable. Naturally, one should look for psoriatic skin and nail symptoms, since they precede joint involvement in the majority of patients. This includes, for example, discrete affection of the scalp (e.g. retroauricular location, external ear canal) and of the buttocks (anal fold) and genital region. The musculoskeletal involvement may present in different ways. Although swelling and pain of peripheral or proximal joints represent important aspects of psoriatic arthritis, additional frequent symptoms include painful inflammation of tendon sheaths (tenosynovitis) or entheses (enthesiopathy/ enthesitis). Characteristically, PsA can involve several or all joints of a finger or toe (dactylitis). Moreover, affection of the spinal column is not rare, as in

Psoriasis: Diagnosis and Management, First Edition. Edited by Wolfram Sterry, Robert Sabat, and Sandra Philipp.

sacroiliitis, for example. Typically, there is stiffness of the joints in the morning or lower back pain that can be ameliorated by movement. Conversely, patients suffering from degenerative joint diseases often feel improvements in symptoms when resting or solely by changing position.

Peripheral arthritis in PsA

In PsA, affected joints can be inflamed with subsequent pain, swelling, and stiffness. The early disease course often starts with oligoarthritis, that is, the involvement of four or fewer peripheral joints, and may become polyarticular as more joints are involved over time. In comparison with rheumatoid arthritis, PsA is an asymmetrical arthritis with inflammation of the distal joints (DIP) or all joints of one digit (dactylitis). A polyarticular joint involvement such as rheumatoid arthritis is also possible and manifests in almost 20% of cases with PsA.

Dactylitis

Dactylitis, also called "sausage digit," is a typical clinical sign of PsA. Dactylitis includes both synovitis of the joints and tenosynovitis, especially of the flexor tendons. Chronic lymphedema in addition to tenosynovitis has also been discussed as a potential cause for chronic dactylitis, which is not so painful or red. Dactylitis affects both fingers and toes, whereas toes are more often involved than fingers. The presence of dactylitis has a predictive value for the development of destructive joint disease because patients with dactylitis develop erosive joint disease more often than patients without dactylitis.

Tenosynovitis

Tenosynovitis or tendinitis is quite frequent in patients with PsA. Inflammation of the flexor tendons of the fingers, as well as the extensor carpi ulnaris tendon, which is also often involved in rheumatoid arthritis, is typical in patients with PsA. Also, tendinitis of the Achilles tendon and fasciitis of the plantar fascia are commonly seen in PsA. Clinical symptoms include swelling and pain of the affected tendon but also may present as a burning sensation of the sole. Tendinitis is often associated with tendon nodules and responsible for disabilities and functional limitations.

Enthesitis

Inflammation of the tendon insertion into the bone is called enthesitis and is an additional characteristic feature in PsA. Enthesitis may occur at any tendon insertion site. The most frequently affected entheses are the plantar fascia, the insertion area of the Achilles tendon at the calcaneus bone, and the insertion tendons at the knee, shoulder, and pelvic bones. Enthesitis alone in the presence of psoriasis may be sufficient for a diagnosis of PsA. Also, the Classification for Psoriatic Arthritis (CASPAR) criteria deem enthesitis together with three other features to be sufficient to classify a patient with PsA (see Table 11.1).

Table 11.1 Classification of psoriatic arthritis.

Classification according to Moll and Wright (1976)

I. Distal joint involvement (DIP joints) in about 5% of PsA patients
II. Arthritis mutilans, a severe destructive pattern of arthritis in nearly 5% of PsA patients
III. Symmetrical polyarthritis like rheumatoid arthritis in 20% of PsA patients
IV. Asymmetrical oligoarthritis, affecting four or fewer joints, observed in nearly 70% of PsA patients
V. Arthritis with spinal involvement (spondyloarthritis), sacroiliitis, spondylodiscitis, and association with HLA-B27 in nearly 10% of PsA patients

CAPSAR criteria (classification of psoriatic arthritis; Taylor *et al.* 2006)

Inflammatory articular disease (joint, spine, or enthesal) with 3 or more items of the following:

1. Evidence of psoriasis (one of a, b, c)
   (a) Current psoriasis, that is, psoriatic skin or scalp disease present today as judged by a rheumatologist or dermatologist
   (b) Personal history of psoriasis that may be obtained from psoriasis patient, family doctor, dermatologist, rheumatologist, or other qualified healthcare provider
   (c) Family history of psoriasis in a first- or second-degree relative according to patient report
2. Psoriatic nail dystrophy: typical psoriatic nail dystrophy including onycholysis, pitting, and hyperkeratosis observed on current physical examination
3 A negative test for rheumatoid factor by any method except latex but preferably by ELISA or nephelometry, according to the local laboratory reference range
4. Dactylitis (one of a,b)
   (a) Current swelling of entire digit
   (b) History of dactylitis recorded by a rheumatologist
5. Radiological evidence

Ill-defined ossification near joint margins (but excluding juxta-articular new osteophyte formation) on plane X-rays of hand or feet bone formation

Data from Taylor *et al.* (2006).

Table 11.2 Clinical characteristics of psoriatic arthritis and rheumatoid arthritis.

	Psoriatic arthritis	Rheumatoid arthritis
Psoriasis	+	–
Nail dystrophy	+	–
Symmetrical	+	++
Asymmetrical	++	+
Enthesitis	+	–
Dactylitis	+	–

The typical signs of PsA are as follows:

- arthritis (swelling and tenderness) >3 joints;
  - 70% involvement of peripheral joints;
  - 60% oligoarticular;
  - 30% monoarticular in the beginning;
  - 10% polyarticular primary;

Table 11.3 Laboratory and X-ray of psoriatic arthritis and rheumatoid arthritis.

	Psoriatic arthritis	Rheumatoid arthritis
Rheumatoid factor	–	+
Erosions	+	++
Sacroiliitis	+	–
Osteoporosis, near the joint	+/–	++
Periostal proliferations	+	–

- involvement of finger- and toe joints;
- dactylitis (affections of all three joint levels of finger or toe);
- joint involvements of both, large and smaller joints, mostly asymmetrically;
- asymmetrical mono- or oligoarthritis;
- sternocostal- and jaw joints are more often involved compared with other arthritic diseases;
- enthesitis: Achilles tendon at the calcaneal bone, plantar fasciitis, musculoskeletal insertions at the pelvis, patella and clavicle; high association with spondylitis;
- bursitis, tenosynovitis, synchondritis (symphysis, sternum);
- heel pain;
- deep lower-back pain in the early morning;
- psoriatic skin or nail symptoms or positive family history of psoriasis;
- negativity of rheumatoid factor or anti-CCP and absence of rheumatoid nodules;
- X-ray: coexistent erosive-destructive changes and periostal proliferation (protuberance), periostitis, acroosteolysis, and ankylosis.

Psoriatic spondyloarthritis

Spinal involvement includes both inflammation of sacroiliac joint and spinal joints in PsA patients. The distribution of arthritis in PsA is asymmetrical, which means, for example, that involvement of the sacroiliac joint may present as affection of only one sacroiliac joint or of both with different degrees on plain radiographs. Patients with spinal involvement due to PsA often do not suffer from such severe pain or spinal limitation as patients with idiopathic ankylosing spondylitis. Fewer patients with psoriatic spondyloarthritis present with grade 4 sacroiliitis and they have fewer syndesmophytes than patients with ankylosing spondylitis.

Arthritis mutilans

Arthritis mutilans, a very destructive form of arthritis, is defined by the number of one to five or more completely destroyed joints (in X-ray) per patient. Arthritis mutilans has not been identified as an isolated arthritis group. It can occur in association with any group of distal joint disease, oligoarthritis, polyarthritis alone, or in combination with spinal involvement, as well as isolated spinal disease. In a cohort of 705 PsA patients at the University of Toronto PsA Clinic, 19.5% suffered from arthritis mutilans with one completely destroyed joint, and 8.2% presented with five or more completely destroyed joints.

One should not forget to consider additional symptoms besides the typical skin, nail, or joint manifestations. Patients may not complain about these symptoms when visiting their dermatologist, as they do not associate these signs with their skin or joint complaints.

Extradermal and extra-articular manifestations

Eye involvement, especially iritis, is an extra-articular feature often seen in spondyloarthritis (SpA) patients and is also frequently found in patients with PsA, in approximately 5–18% of cases. Uveitis is not rare, but is less common in PsA than in other patients with SpA. Bowel involvement may occur in PsA but usually manifests as nonspecific colitis. Cardiac involvement has been reported in PsA patients, including dilatation of the aortic arch. In addition, PsA patients have a higher risk for cardiovascular diseases related to the metabolic abnormalities associated with PsA, including hyperlipidemia, hyperuricemia, and lifestyle factors such as obesity and smoking.

Clinical classification of PsA

Multiple clinical subsets reflect variable clinical patterns such as distal joint affection, arthritis mutilans (destructive arthritis), oligoarthritis (up to four joints), polyarthritis resembling rheumatoid arthritis without positivity for rheumatoid factor, and spondylitis. There is an association with human leukocyte antigen (HLA)-B27 and spinal involvement, as well as other extra-articular features seen in patients with PsA.

In 1973, Moll and Wright identified five subsets of PsA, and more recently new classification criteria have been suggested, the CASPAR criteria (see Table 11.1).

Diagnostic procedures

Typical clinical signs include pain, tenderness, and/or swelling of joints, either single joints such as the knee or shoulder or multiple joints with frequent involvement of the finger or toes. In contrast to rheumatoid arthritis, distribution of involved joints is commonly asymmetrical. Affection of the tendons (e.g. Achilles tendon) may present as tenderness or swelling and manifest as palpable nodules.

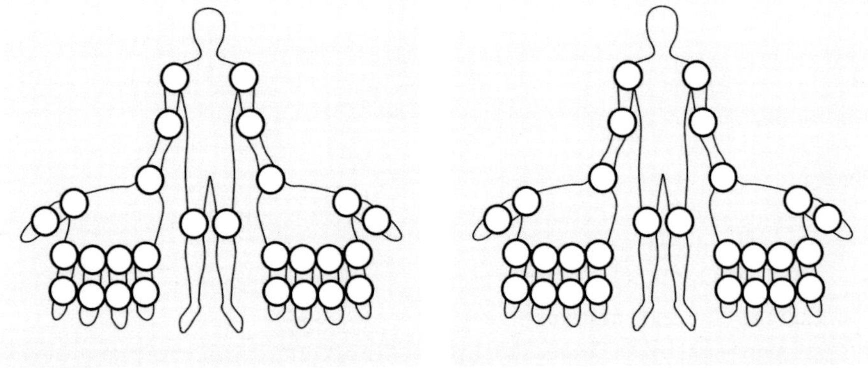

(a) (b)

Figure 11.1 Joint count: (a) tender joints; (b) swollen joints.

One should explicitly ask about morning stiffness and document the duration in minutes to hours as well as for lower back pain, especially if symptoms occur in the early morning. In addition, it may be helpful to ask the patients what ameliorates the pain. Improvement by movements speaks in favor of an inflammatory component of the joint disease.

To document the involvement of the joints in the course of the disease one may use different methods. A simple method is to ask the patients about the joint pain using a visual analog scale ranging from 0 to 10, with 10 signifying very severe pain. The use of so-called joint counts might be more precise, albeit time-consuming and requiring specific training. This means examination of the joints by palpation to detect tenderness and swelling, and documenting each result separately for swelling and tenderness (see Figure 11.1).

Laboratory findings

Unspecific inflammatory parameters include C-reactive protein and erythrocyte sedimentation rate, though in contrast to patients suffering from rheumatoid arthritis, both are often in the normal range in PsA patients. Interestingly, the level of IgA is often increased (15–35%), albeit unspecific.

The HLA-B27 marker is positive in 15% of patients with peripheral joint manifestation, and in 50% with spinal involvement in comparison with 8% in healthy volunteers.

Autoantibodies such as rheumatoid factor and anti-CCP antibodies are negative in the majority of cases. However, some patients suffering from PsA may present with low titers of rheumatoid factor (up to 10–15%) or more rarely with anti-CCP antibodies.

Imaging

Imaging techniques are useful for the documentation of the joint involvement and for detecting destructive joint disease.

X-ray

Plane radiographs are a standard diagnostic procedure and should be applied in two perpendicular planes:

- peripheral joints: wrists, hands, forefoot and other symptomatic joints depending on the clinical symptoms;
- spine/pelvis: sacroiliac joints, and eventually of cervical spine, as atlanto-axial subluxation is not rare.

Typical changes in X-rays include:

- signs of both erosive-destructive changes and periostal proliferation (protuberance; Figure 11.2);
- periostitis;
- acroosteolysis;
- ankylosis;
- pencil-in-cup phenomenon;
- asymmetrical sacroiliitis;
- asymmetrical syndesmophytes.

MR imaging

MRI allows early detection of inflammatory soft tissue and bone lesions. It is especially helpful to detect

- sacroiliitis;
- spondylitis;
- spondylodiscitis.

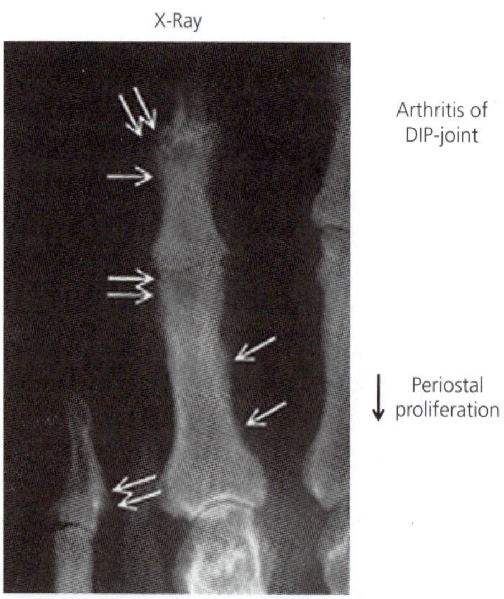

Figure 11.2 Typical radiological findings.

Bone scan (scintigraphy)

This might be used in special indications, for example:

- to detect subclinical arthritis (sternoclavicular joint, sacroiliac joint, spondylitis);
- to assess joint involvement/distribution, helpful if patients complain about pain in several changing locations;
- to detect locations of enthesitis.

Sonography

Musculoskeletal sonography allows the early detection of inflammatory soft tissue and bone processes as synovitis, joint effusion, tenosynovitis, tendinitis, enthesitis, bursitis, and superficially located bone erosions (Figure 11.3).

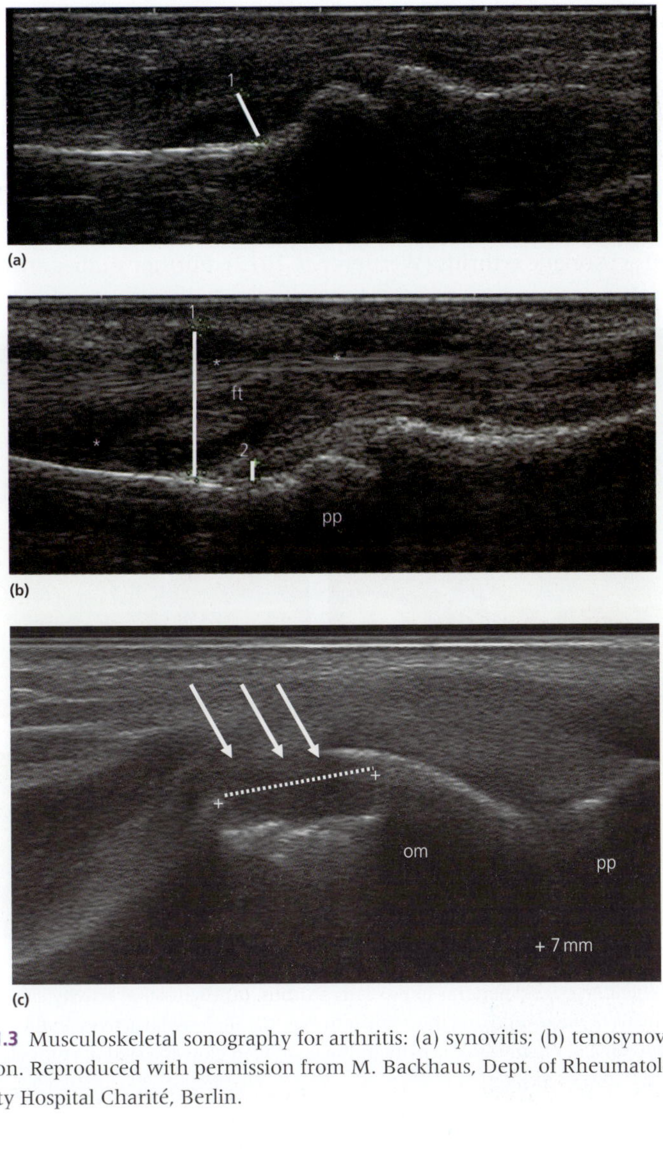

Figure 11.3 Musculoskeletal sonography for arthritis: (a) synovitis; (b) tenosynovitis; (c) erosion. Reproduced with permission from M. Backhaus, Dept. of Rheumatology, University Hospital Charité, Berlin.

Sonography of the abdomen may be considered, to exclude the differential diagnosis of paraneoplastic arthritis.

Fluorescence optical imaging (Xiralite®), Rheumascan

Rheumascan is a new fluorescence optical imaging (FOI) technology for visualizing inflammation of the hands. The method measures the fluorescence of the fluorophor indocyanine green (ICG) and thereby displays active inflammatory activity in a variety of different diseases. Indocyanine green is approved in Europe as an agent for imaging diagnostics of microcirculation. In experimental models of arthritis, ICG-enhanced FOI findings corresponded to histologically proven synovities (Fischer *et al.* 2006; Meier *et al.* 2010). The feasibility of this approach in humans was tested, and an FOI system with fixed optical geometry was developed (Xiralite® system; Salvarani *et al.* 1999; Brockbank *et al.* 2005). The Xiralite® system, a new FOI technology, is a rapid and safe procedure that does not use any potentially harmful radiation. For FOI, the dye indocyanine green is made visible with dark red light. It is possible to visualize the involvement of joints and tendons with FOI but also enthesitis and periostitis in cases of dactylitis. PsA patients present a characteristic pattern of signal distribution. The morphological aspects indicate an association with the synovio-entheseal complex (Figure 11.4). FOI could be helpful in better discerning nail involvement and arthritis of DIP joints in patients with psoriasis and/or psoriatic arthritis (Werner *et al.* 2012). Further studies are ongoing.

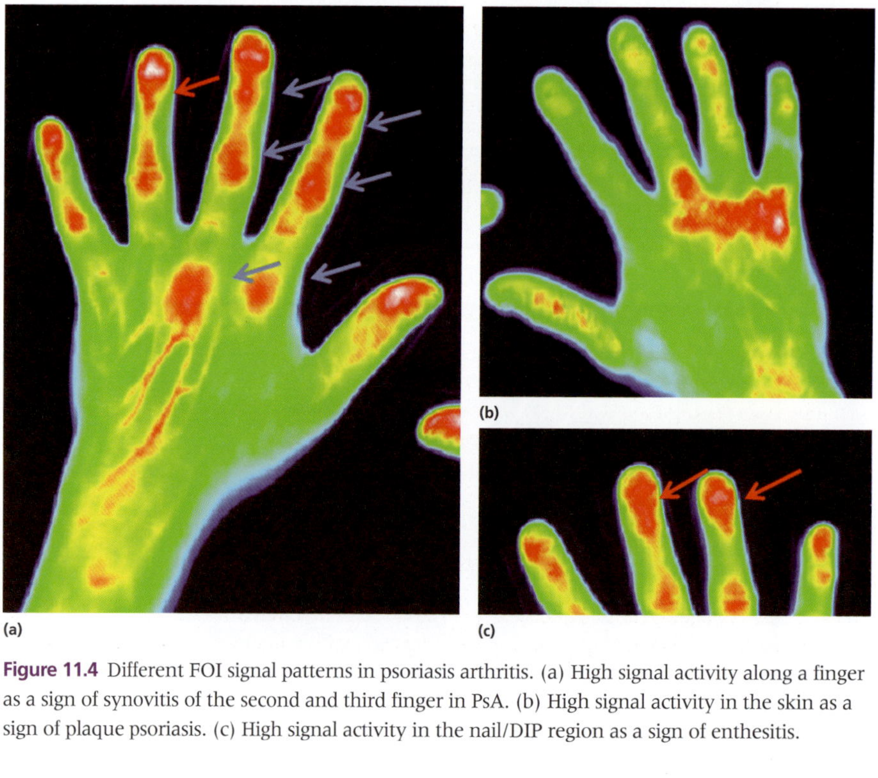

(a) (b) (c)

Figure 11.4 Different FOI signal patterns in psoriasis arthritis. (a) High signal activity along a finger as a sign of synovitis of the second and third finger in PsA. (b) High signal activity in the skin as a sign of plaque psoriasis. (c) High signal activity in the nail/DIP region as a sign of enthesitis.

Important differential diagnoses of PsA include:

- rheumatoid arthritis (see Tables 11.2 and 11.3);
- metabolical arthritis as gout;
- osteoarthritis;
- enteropathic arthritis;
- paraneoplastic syndromes, for example, bronchial-Ca, non-Hodgkin's lymphoma;
- other spondyloarthritis.

Prognosis

Thirty percent of patients with PsA present destructive arthritis followed by permanent handicaps, and 5% show arthritis mutilans with profound joint deformity. More severe courses may develop in cases of axial involvement. Definite prognostic parameters are not currently available, and in the majority of cases the disease course might be less severe compared with rheumatoid arthritis.

Further reading

Brockbank, J., Stein, M., Schentag, C.T. *et al.* (2005) Characteristics of dactylitis in psoriatic arthritis (PsA). *Annals of the Rheumatic Diseases*, **62**, 188–190.

Fischer, T. Gemeinhardt, I., Wagner, S. *et al.* (2006) Assessment of unspecific near-infrared dyes in laser-induced fluorescence imaging of experimental arthritis. *Academic Radiology*, **13**, 4–13.

Gladman, D.D. Brubacher, B., Buskila, D. *et al.* (1993) Differences in the expression of spondyloarthropathy: a comparison between ankylosing spondylitis and psoriatic arthritis. Genetic and gender effects. *Clinical and Investigative Medicine*, **16**, 1–7.

Klippel, J.H., Stone, J.H., Crofford, L.J., White, P.H. (eds) (2008) Psoriatic arthritis clinical features. In: *Primer on the Rheumatic Diseases*, 13th edition. Springer, New York.

Meier, R., Krug, C., Golovko, D. *et al.* (2010) Indocyanine green-enhanced imaging of antigen-induced arthritis with an integrated optical imaging/radiography system. *Arthritis & Rheumatism*, **62**, 2322–2327.

Peters, M.J., van der Horst-Bruinsma, I.E., Djikmans, B.A. *et al.* (2004) Cardiovascular risk profile of patients with spondyloarthropathies, particular ankylosing spondylitis and psoriatic arthritis. *Seminars in Arthritis and Rheumatism*, **34**, 585–592.

Salvarani, C., Cantini, F., Olivieri, I. *et al.* (1997) Isolated peripheral enthesitis and/or dactylitis: a subset of psoriatic arthritis. *Journal of Rheumatology*, **24**, 1106–1110.

Salvarani, C., Cantini, F., Olivieri, I. *et al.* (1999) Distal extremity swelling with pitting edema in psoriatic arthritis: evidence of 2 pathological mechanisms. *Journal of Rheumatology*, **26**, 1831–1834.

Taylor, W., Gladman, D., Helliwell, P. *et al.* CASPAR Study Group (2006) Classification criteria for psoriatic arthritis: development of new criteria from a large international study. *Arthritis & Rheumatism*, **54**, 2665–2673.

Werner, G.W., Langer, H.E., Ohrndorf, S. *et al.* (2012) Inflammation assessment in patients with arthritis using a novel in vivo fluorescence optical imaging technology. *Annals of the Rheumatic Diseases*, **71**, 504–510.

Wright, V. and Moll, J.M.H. (1976) Psoriatic arthritis. In: *Seronegative Polyarthritis*. North Holland Publishing, Amsterdam, pp. 169–223.

CHAPTER 12

Mucosal presentation of psoriasis

Georgios Kokolakis
Psoriasis Research and Treatment Center, Department of Dermatology and Allergy/Institute of Medical Immunology, University Hospital Charité, Berlin, Germany

Besides skin, joints, and entheses, psoriasis can rarely also affect mucous membranes. The underlying pathogenetic mechanism does not differ much from that involved in the evolution of cutaneous plaques. However, the anatomical structure of mucosal surfaces influences the clinical appearance of the disease. Mucosae are moist epithelia and show quite different patterns of keratinization or no keratinization at all.

The structure of transition epithelia and mucosal surfaces contributes to the presentation of psoriatic inflammation in these sites. The pattern of keratinization in the oral mucosa is characteristic where parakeratosis and absence of the granular and horny layer are considered normal. The epithelial surface is permanently moist due to saliva secretion. Similar to the vermilion border of the lips, the inner site of labia majora represents the transition from skin to mucosa, whereas the labia minora are completely mucosal. The space between the glans penis and the inner aspect of the foreskin is a closed space. The inner aspect of the foreskin is similar to the outer skin, also covered by cornifying epithelium. Thus, the area under the foreskin represents an intertriginous site; likewise, the perianal region is moist with skin surfaces typical for intertriginous areas.

Oral psoriasis can affect both the lips and the mucosal surfaces.

Several manifestations—both specific and nonspecific—in the transition zone between perioral skin, lips, and oral mucosa are distinguished:

1 Perlèche (angular cheilitis) with erythema and scaling on the mouth corners has been described in psoriasis patients.
2 Exfoliative cheilitis may accompany flares of either plaque-type or generalized pustular psoriasis.
3 Typical erythematosquamous plaques of the perioral cutaneous skin may transgress the vermilion border and consequently affect the buccal mucosa.

Unlike psoriasis plaques of the body, lesions of the oral cavity are usually temporary and migratory, and thus may vary in their presentation. Typical oral psoriasis lesion present as white annular, serpiginous, or polycyclic papules and plaques. Less frequently, erythematous patches and erosions may appear. This clinical picture is commonly known as migratory stomatitis or annulus migrans,

Psoriasis: Diagnosis and Management, First Edition. Edited by Wolfram Sterry, Robert Sabat, and Sandra Philipp.

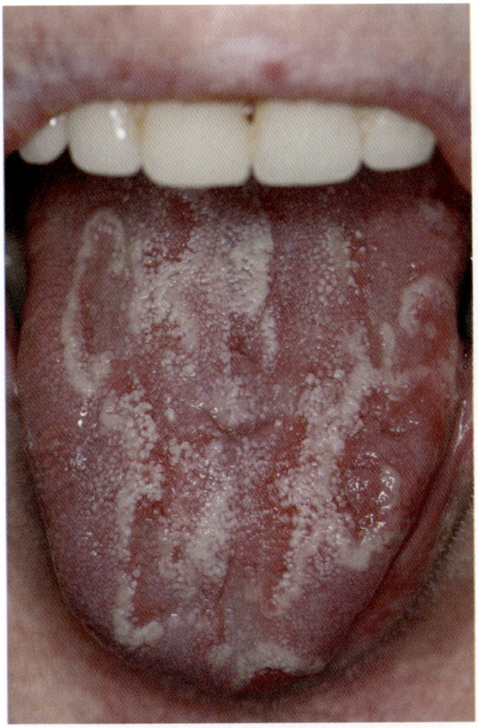

Figure 12.1 Geographic tongue.

stomatitis areata migrans or geographic stomatitis. These lesions are clinically similar to evolving plaques of geographic tongue. Geographic tongue (Figure 12.1) has been reported to occur in 5–10% of psoriasis patients. The differential diagnosis of oral psoriasis is rather broad and includes Reiter's syndrome, lichen planus, syphilis, lupus erythematosus, pemphigus and mucous membrane pemphigoid, candidiasis, leukoplakia, and trauma. Since oral lesions resolve with systemic therapies for the cutaneous disease, a special treatment is not required. In persisting cases, topical corticosteroids are the treatment of choice. Viscous lidocaine or diphenhydramine, emollient dental paste, magnesium and aluminum hydroxides, and alkaline rinses have also been recommended.

Involvement of the genitalia occurs in 29–40% of patients with psoriasis with a remarkable prominence of male patients. However, manifestation of psoriasis exclusively on genital skin occurs in only 2–5% of the psoriatic patients. Similarly, as in the skin, genital psoriasis can be triggered by local trauma, injury, or infections (Köbner phenomenon; see Chapter 6). Urine, faeces, tight-fitting clothes, and sexual intercourse may also act as triggers. Psoriasis of the genitalia is clinically presented as asymptomatic or slightly irritating, thin, erythematous, well-demarcated plaques usually lacking the typical scaling because of maceration or involvement of noncornifying epithelia.

The clinical appearance of vulvar psoriasis can vary from silver-scaly patches limited to the outer parts of the labia majora to moist grayish plaques or glossy

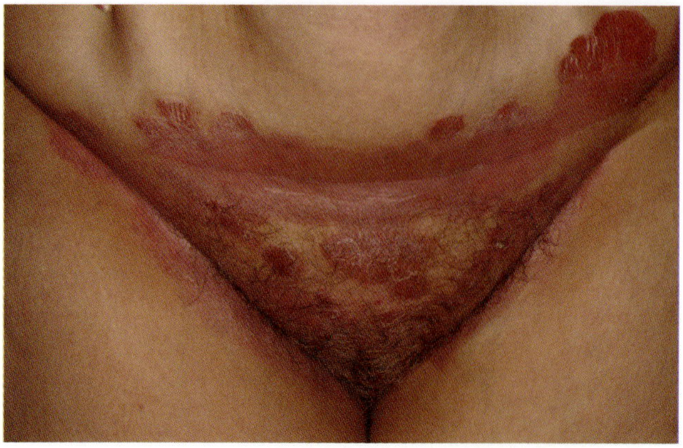

Figure 12.2 Psoriasis of intertriginous areas and external female genitalia.

red plaques without desquamation within the skin folds (Figure 12.2). The distribution pattern of genital psoriasis in female patients is usually symmetrical.

In male patients, scrotal and penile skin as well as the glans penis can be affected by psoriasis. In uncircumcised patients, nonscaling psoriasis plaques are usually identified under the prepuce and on the proximal glans. In circumcised male patients, however, the reddish lesions usually appear on the glans and corona. Besides plaque-type psoriasis, in very rare cases the pustular form of the disease can also affect the male genital skin. It can present either as localized plaque or—in the context of generalized pustular psoriasis—on an erythematous base. The most common differential diagnoses of genital psoriasis include diverse forms of dermatitis, dermatophytosis or candidiasis, squamous cell carcinoma and its variants, secondary or tertiary syphilis, lichen planus, and lichen simplex chronicus. Weak or moderate corticosteroids and vitamin D analogs either as monotherapy or as combined, coal-tar products, immunomodulators, antibiotics, or antimycotics in case of infections are recommended for the treatment of genital psoriasis. In severe cases, systemic treatment is needed (see also Chapter 17).

Ocular involvement in psoriasis patients occurs, although epidemiologic data are missing, based on expert opinion in about 10%. Each compartment of the eye from the eyelids to the lens can be affected. Besides the typical psoriasis plaques, even pustular in some cases, a red swollen sometimes crusted and flaky lid with scales covering the lashes is the most common manifestation. Regarding the conjunctiva, a chronic nonspecific conjunctivitis with or without eyelid margin lesions can present in psoriasis patients. Demarcated, yellowish-red plaques on the palpebral conjunctiva or xerotic areas on the bulbar conjunctiva can appear. Corneal complications in psoriasis are rare and rather secondary to eyelid or conjunctival involvement. They mainly include xerosis and trichiasis with punctuate epithelial keratitis and lesions with superficial or deep opacities, stromal infiltrates, neovascularization, erosions, scarring, and even stromal necrosis. Another serious ophthalmic complication of psoriasis

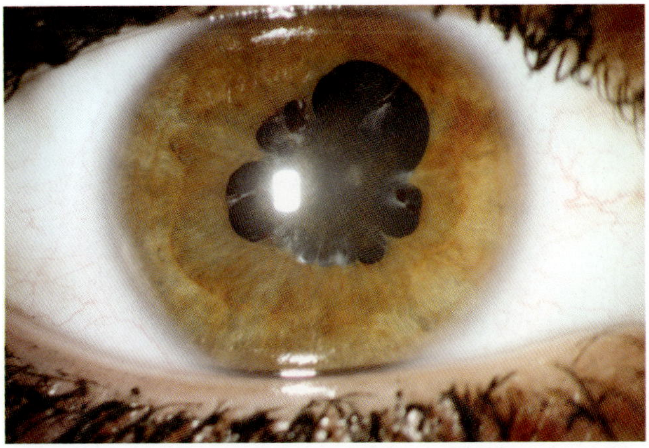

Figure 12.3 Uveitis in a psoriatic arthritis patient. Courtesy of Professor Pleyer, Dept. of Opthalmology, Charité University Medicine, Berlin

is uveitis (Figure 12.3). Involvement of the lens, with cataract as the main complication, is basically regarded as an incidental finding, and together they are usually associated with the treatment of psoriasis, including photochemotherapy and corticosteroids, rather than with the disease itself. For the treatment of ophthalmic involvement in psoriasis, besides systemic therapy and surgical interventions in severe cases, the application of lubricating or antibiotic eye drops, corticosteroids, and cytostatic or immunosuppressive agents is recommended. Close cooperation with experienced ophthalmologists in inflammatory ocular disease is also recommended.

Further reading

Braun-Falco, O., Burgdorf, W.H.C., Plewig, G., Wolff, H.H. and Landthaler, M. (2009) *Braun-Falco's Dermatology*, 3rd edition. Springer, Berlin.

Bruce, A.J. and Rogers, R.S., 3rd. (2003) Oral psoriasis. *Dermatologic Clinics*, **21**, 99–104.

Meeuwis, K.A., de Hullu, J.A., Massuger, L.F., van de Kerkhof, P.C. and van Rossum, M.M. (2011) Genital psoriasis: A systematic literature review on this hidden skin disease. *Acta Dermato-Venereologica*, **91**, 5–11.

Rehal, B., Modjtahedi, B.S., Morse, L.S., Schwab, I.R. and Maibach, H.I. (2011) Ocular psoriasis. *Journal of the American Academy of Dermatology*, **65**, 1202–1212.

CHAPTER 13
Psoriasis in different life situations

Sandra Philipp
Psoriasis Research and Treatment Center, Department of Dermatology and Allergy/Institute of Medical Immunology, University Hospital Charité, Berlin, Germany

Psoriasis in children

Psoriasis in children is quite common. About 30–45% of all patients suffering from psoriasis experience the first symptoms of the disease already in childhood or adolescence, and recent data have revealed a prevalence for psoriasis of 0.71% in children younger than 18, with almost linear increasing rates from 0.12% at the age of 1 year to 1.2% at the age of 18.

In accordance with the genetic background of psoriasis, children are at a higher risk of developing psoriasis if relatives are affected. Individuals with parental involvement showed a prevalence of the disease in 14% compared with 3% in children without parental psoriasis.

The impact of the disease on the children should not be underestimated. The quality of life is significantly impaired, and some feel embarrassed or isolated by the disease. A small recent study revealed that 65% of the affected children experienced stigmatization, though most suffered only from mild psoriasis. The majority also reported physical symptoms such as itching (71%) and 43% even fatigue. These data indicate the negative effect on physical, emotional, and social well-being of the affected children.

In addition, juvenile psoriasis has been associated with obesity, hyperlipidemia, hypertension, diabetes mellitus, and further chronic inflammatory diseases such as rheumatoid arthritis and Crohn's disease. The rate of comorbidities in children and adolescents (<20 years) with psoriasis has been found to be twice as high as that in subjects without psoriasis. Therefore, in children with severe psoriasis, respective monitoring, including measurement of waist circumference, blood pressure, or blood lipids should be considered in infancy, and individual counseling of parents and children is demanded.

Clinical picture

Principally all clinical subtypes of psoriasis may develop in childhood, with plaque psoriasis being the most common form. However, there are some differences with respect to adults. First manifestation of disease may present

Psoriasis: Diagnosis and Management, First Edition. Edited by Wolfram Sterry, Robert Sabat, and Sandra Philipp.

in early childhood as psoriatic diaper rash. Typically sharply demarcated brightly erythematous lesions are located in the genital and/or perianal region, frequently expanding to the inguinal area. Usually, psoriatic diaper rash starts before the age of 2 years, often followed by chronic recurrent exacerbations. Many affected children develop characteristic psoriatic lesions later in their lives elsewhere on the body.

The most important differential diagnoses comprise irritant diaper dermatitis and candida infections (mycology, small satellite lesions at the margin) or streptococcal dermatitis (vesicles, pustules, bacterial culture), less often erythrasma (reduced inflammation, red to brownish color; bacterial culture) or acrodermatitis enteropathica (perioral, perianal vesicles, or pustules, malabsorption, zinc level).

One of the most typical manifestations in childhood is guttate psoriasis (Figure 13.1), though the reported frequencies are quite variable, ranging from 6% to over 40%. Characteristically, guttate psoriasis starts abruptly with an exanthematous eruption of disseminated small light red flat papules and plaques with a diameter of 0.5–1.0 cm, covering the trunk, proximal parts of the extremities, the face and the scalp. Scales are mainly fine. Guttate psoriasis often occurs as a first appearance of the disease, and commonly manifests after preceding infections. Occasionally, the rash-like skin lesions resolve spontaneously after 3–4 months; though in most cases children will develop further psoriatic lesions in the subsequent years.

Guttate psoriasis might be misdiagnosed as tinea (mycology), pityriasis rosea (starting with a single "mother" lesion followed later by eruption of smaller lesions), lichen planus (Wickham sign, flat polygonal papules, typically located at the wrists, knuckles, intense pruritus, mucosal involvement) pityriasis lichenoides chronica (typical central scale, histology), or pityriasis rubra pilaris (nappes claires, follicular bound papules).

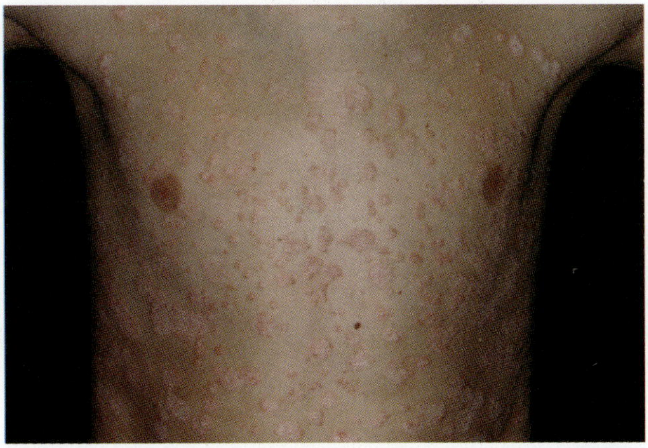

Figure 13.1 Disseminated red papules and small flat plaques on the trunk (guttate psoriasis).

Trigger factors such as infections, trauma (Köbner phenomenon), or psychological distress seem to play an important role, particularly in childhood psoriasis. Characteristic are streptococcal infections, such as sore throat, but also perianal streptococcal dermatitis. Therefore, one has to search for potential infections, such as by swabbing of pharynx, blood analysis (leukocytosis), or ASL titer. A consultation with an otorhinolaryngologist may be advisable. Rarely, the withdrawal of oral or extensively used topical corticosteroids has been reported as a possible trigger factor.

Chronic plaque psoriasis in children can appear as characteristically sharply demarcated plaques with silvery-white scales in typical locations such as the head, elbows, knee, and buttocks as in adults. However, sometimes the plaques may be thinner and less scaly, and therefore may complicate the diagnosis. In addition, pruritus seems to be more frequent in children.

With regard to plaque psoriasis, the most important differential diagnoses include nummular dermatitis (papulovesicles, crusting), tinea corporis (annular lesions, mycology), seborrhoic dermatitis, or atopic dermatitis (location, less sharply demarcated, papulovesicles).

In contrast to adults, affection of the face and inverse psoriasis with flexural or genital involvement are more frequent (Figures 13.2 and 13.3). In case of inverse psoriasis, the typical scales are missing, so lesions present as deeply red erythema with potentially painful fissures. Sometimes psoriasis may present only as vulvitis, balanitis, or perianal itchy erythema. Candida infections should be excluded (mycology, satellite lesions).

Besides the typical scaly plaques, severe scalp affection may present as tinea amiantacea, with thick adherent scales around the hair shafts dominating the clinical picture. The erythema is often only discrete, but locally restricted reversible hair loss is not rare in these cases. For differential diagnoses, tinea capitis (mycology, short cut hairs) and seborrhoic dermatitis (restriction to the area

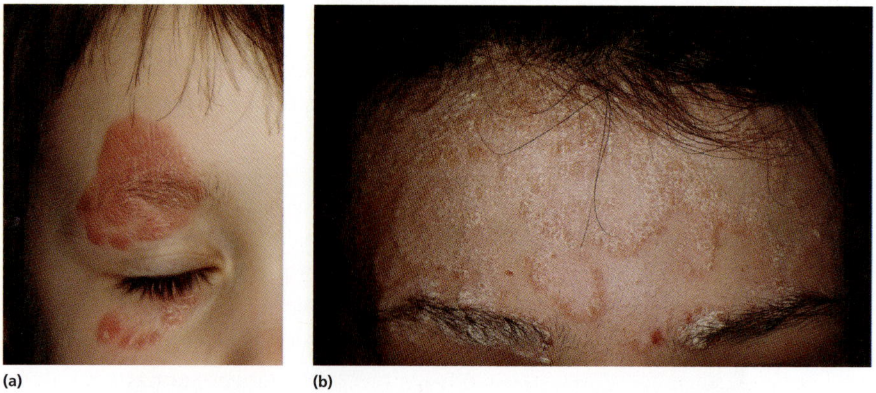

(a) (b)

Figure 13.2 (a) Characteristic erythemateous psoriasis plaques around the eye. (b) Typical scaly plaques on the forehead.

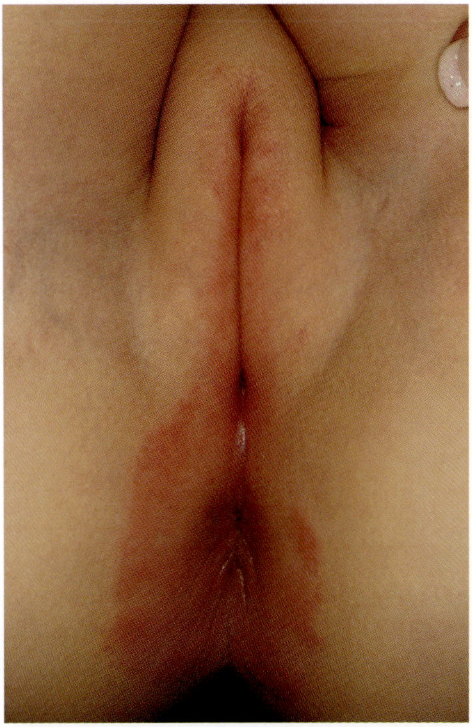

Figure 13.3 Sharply demarcated red plaques in the anogenital region, typical for inverse psoriasis.

covered with hair) have to be taken into consideration. Affliction of the scalp and face is particularly harmful for children due to the permanent visibility, and lesions in the genital area, for example, may also lead to avoidance of sports and swimming as a child tries to hide the disease.

Palms and soles may also be affected, resulting in sharply demarcated erythema, commonly showing a prominent demarcation at the wrist or lateral margins of the foot. The erythema may be covered with thick scales and include deep painful fissures.

Linear psoriasis is a rare variant of psoriasis that may occur in childhood. Characteristic is the appearance of scaly erythematous plaques following the Blaschko lines and therefore showing a linear shape. Often the skin lesions develop during the first years of life, and family history is positive. The manifestation has been explained by alterations taking place during embryogenesis leading to mosaic forms of keratinocytes with cells having lost the heterozygosity of a gene predisposing to psoriasis and thus being more susceptible to psoriasis. These cells are then distributed along the Blaschko lines. Later in life, some patients may develop typical psoriatic lesions elsewhere on the body; this has been described as "superimposed linear psoriasis." Linear psoriasis has to be distinguished from an inflammatory linear verrucous epidermal nevus (pruritus, histology, e.g. hypergranulosis, absence of involucrin).

In general, the pustular subtypes of psoriasis are rare in children, with annular psoriasis being the most frequent form. The latter often shows a highly inflammatory pattern, characteristically with erythematous lesions in ring form with margins covered with pustules and/or colarette-like scales.

There are also case reports about generalized pustular psoriasis (Zumbusch type) in children. Typical is the sudden onset of widespread deep red erythematous macules covered with numerous pinhead-sized pustules, and the majority of patients experience additional systemic symptoms such as fever, malaise, or arthralgia. Rupture of the pustules followed by shedding of the skin may result in large areas of crusting and erosions that are at risk of being superinfected. Prompt diagnosis and treatment are important to avoid potentially life-threatening complications. Possible differential diagnoses include drug-induced generalized erythemateous pustulosis, as well as staphylococcal scalded skin syndrome (histology, pharyngeal, nasal swab) or subcorneal pustulosis of Sneddon–Wilkinson (intertriginous area, histology, ELISA: IgA against desmocollin).

Manifestations of pustular psoriasis of palms and soles as well as acrodermatitis continua suppurativa are rarities in childhood. In contrast, psoriatic nail disease is quite frequent in children (Figure 13.4). It has been estimated that about 32–40% of affected children present with nail abnormalities, most often with pitting. In a recent study, pitting was found in 87% of cases, followed by onycholysis (10%), subungual hyperkeratosis (8%), and salmon patches (5%). However, splinter hemorrhages and complete onychodystrophy have been

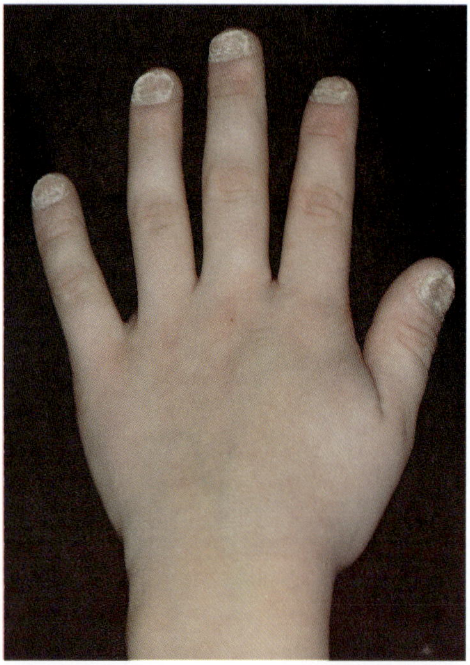

Figure 13.4 Pronounced pitting of all nails.

reported, too. Genetic disorders such as 20 nail dystrophy or trachonychia have to be considered as differential diagnosis.

Juvenile psoriatic arthritis has been classified as a subgroup of idiopathic juvenile arthritis, with an incidence in literature of 16–400/100.000. Though affection of the joints by psoriasis is not that common in children, it has been estimated that 2–11% of children or adolescents diagnosed with arthritis might suffer from psoriatic arthritis. Therefore, psoriasis is an important differential diagnosis if children complain about pain or swelling of joints. When typical skin lesions are absent, a positive family history or nail affection can be helpful. The manifestation shows two peaks, at the age of 2–4 years and 9–11 years. Interestingly, recent data suggest that patients younger than 5 years might present a distinct clinical phenotype with a female preponderance, ANA positivity, and more frequent cases of dactylitis or polyarticular affection. In contrast, psoriatic arthritis in older children shows no gender preference and, more often, enthesitis, axial involvement, and oligoarticular affection. Therapy for paediatric psoriasis is detailed in Chapter 21.

Psoriasis in pregnancy

Epidemiology and pathophysiology

Most dermatologists will have to treat pregnant women suffering from psoriasis, as the disease is not rare in women of childbearing potential. In fact, almost half of psoriasis patients are females. In addition, women frequently develop psoriasis earlier than males. The mean age of first diagnosis has been reported to be 28 years, with about two-thirds of patients developing symptoms before the age of 40. It has been estimated that in the US alone, 65,000 to 106,000 women yearly suffering from psoriasis give birth to a child, including approximately 9000–15,000 who experience moderate to severe diseases. It is well known that the course of psoriasis may be altered during pregnancy. Fortunately, 40–60% of women show an improvement of the disease, often by the late first and second trimester, but in 10–20% psoriasis becomes aggravating with the potential need for intensive therapy. In addition, more than 50% report a flare-up postpartum, though usually the symptoms appear to be no worse than before the pregnancy. Interestingly, notwithstanding improvement or worsening during the first pregnancy, similar responses can be expected in the following pregnancies. Corresponding to psoriasis of the skin, most patients (up to 80%) with psoriatic arthritis experience an improvement or even remission of joint involvement during pregnancy and a worsening after delivery (in up to 70%). However, some patients show remissions for years.

What happens during pregnancy? The maternal immune response is modulated to allow the survival of the fetus. Raised cortisol and epinephrine levels result in a decrease of IL-12 or TNF-α. Moreover, progesterone induces IL-4 and IL-5, while estrogen inhibits IL-2. These changes favor a Th2 response and reduce the proliferation rate of T-cells. Overall, the downregulation of the proinflammatory processes may at least partly explain the improvement of psoriatic symptoms in pregnancy and the aggravation postpartum. However, it is still not completely understood why psoriasis worsens in a certain group of pregnant women. It has been suggested, that the estrogen/progesterone ratio might be more important than the absolute values of the single hormones, as patients showing an improvement achieved higher levels of estrogen relative to progesterone compared with patients experiencing worsening or no change at all.

So far, psoriasis (with the exception of generalized pustular psoriasis of pregnancy) was not believed to have a negative influence on the outcome of pregnancy. Conversely, recent data have shown evidence that patients with psoriasis might have an increased risk of adverse effects in pregnancy. Cohen-Barak *et al.* (2011) reported an association of moderate to severe psoriasis with spontaneous and induced abortions, pregnancy-induced hypertensive disease, premature rupture of membranes, large-for-gestational age newborns, and macrosomia. Registry data further suggested that a potentially higher risk for adverse pregnancy outcomes in psoriasis may be due to associated comorbidities and/or lifestyle factors, as women with psoriasis were found to be more frequently obese (2.37 times), to smoke or suffer from depression, and to ingest vitamin supplements less often. However, other observations have revealed only an increased risk for low birth weight (1.4 times) in pregnant women with severe psoriasis, and no excess risk in cases of mild psoriasis. Whatever proves correct, the potential association of moderate to severe psoriasis with comorbidities of the metabolic syndrome (hypertension, diabetes), which includes women of childbearing potential, might increase the risk for adverse pregnancy outcomes. Therefore, we recommend respective counseling for the patient.

Clinical picture

Information on the incidence of clinical subtypes of psoriasis in pregnancy is rare. In comparison with all individuals suffering from psoriasis, there appears to be no significant difference in the clinical forms occurring in pregnancy, with plaque psoriasis being the most common subtype. However, there are two exceptions: first, generalized pustular psoriasis of pregnany (GPPP), a special variant of annular pustular psoriasis appearing in pregnancy, and second palmoplantar pustulosis, which seems to be very rare during pregnancy. The latter is in line with the observation that palmoplantar pustular psoriasis mostly manifests later, in the fourth and fifth decade.

GPPP/impetigo herpetiformis (IH)

GPPP, formerly known as impetigo herpetiformis, is today generally accepted to be a form of annular pustular psoriasis occurring during pregnancy. Different pathogenetic factors have been suggested, such as high progesterone levels during the last trimester of pregnancy or low calcium levels. Others have proposed that a decreased activity of skin-derived antileukoproteinase favors the development of epidermal pustules. Furthermore, it is known that hypoparathyroidism or thyroidectomy can trigger GPPP.

GPPP primarily affects women during the third trimester, although it may manifest earlier or during the postpartum period.

Typically, the first lesions appear symmetrically in the flexures and intertrigineous areas, especially in the inguinal region, later followed by distribution over the entire body, usually sparing the face, hands, and feet. Characteristically, small sterile pustules develop at the margin of erythematous macules, thereby creating ring-forms. The rupture of pustules leads to crusts and erosions that facilitate secondary infection. After the lesions have healed, residual postinflammatory hyperpigmentation is not uncommon, and the nails or mucosal affection in the form of erosions can be involved. Although the symptoms usually disappear after delivery, they can rarely persist postpartum. Recurrences of GPPP in subsequent pregnancies are common, and there are reports of exacerbations due to the use of oral contraceptives.

Besides skin lesions, the vast majority of patients experience additional systemic symptoms. Fever, chills, nausea, vomiting, diarrhea, and arthralgia are most common. Potentially harmful complications such as dehydration and tetany have to be considered. Moreover, many patients present with hypocalcemia, and with increasing severity, the risk of seizures appears to be greater. Therefore, early recognition and prompt treatment are important to minimize or avoid complications.

Maternal prognosis has improved and is quite good today. However, despite intensified treatment, placental insufficiency and electrolyte imbalance may still cause fetal complications such as fetal abnormalities, stillbirth, or neonatal death.

Diagnostic procedure

Medical history, inspection, and clinical examination

The sudden occurrence of pustules on an erythematous base in the third trimester and the characteristic begin in the intertriginous areas, especially in the inguinal region, leads to a suspicion of GPPP. As serious disease, it often requires hospitalization. Interdisciplinary gynecologic care is important.

Laboratory findings include elevated erythrocyte sedimentation rate (ESR), leukocytosis, neutrophilia, decreased serum calcium and phosphate levels, hypoalbuminemia, and iron deficiency anemia. In unclear cases a biopsy should be taken, the histological picture is comparable to generalized pustular psoriasis (see Chapter 9).

Differential diagnosis comprises the specific dermatoses of pregnancy as pemphigoid gestationis (commonly starts earlier, initially urticarial papules and plaques, direct immunofluorescence) or pruritic urticarial papules and plaques of pregnancy (PUPP, starts on abdomen, mainly in striae distensae, navel not affected). Additionally, pustular drug eruptions (drug intake), and bullous dermatoses such as subcorneal pustular dermatosis (pustules from the very beginning, direct immunofluorescence: intercellular IgA; serology: IgA antibodies against desmoglein 1+3 or desmocollin), pemphigus vulgaris (frequently oral involvement, vesicles, bullae, erosions, antibodies against desmoglein 1 or 3, direct immunofluorescence: intercellular IgG+C3), and dermatitis herpetiformis (itchy vesicular lesions, mostly located on extensor sites, direct immunofluorescence: papillar located granular IgA+C3) have to be taken into consideration.

Counseling of women with psoriasis and childbearing potential

Data are limited with respect to the influence of moderate to severe maternal psoriasis (with the exception of GPPP) on fetal development. However, the potential associated disorders such as obesity, hypertension, or diabetes might increase the risk for adverse pregnancy outcomes, and therefore respective counseling and monitoring may prove beneficial. Although the majority of patients experience improvements in symptoms, therapeutic options should be planned beforehand, especially in patients with severe disease or involvement of joints.

Furthermore, parents might be concerned about the risk of their offspring being affected by psoriasis. The concordance of psoriasis manifestations among identical twins has been reported to be 70% compared with only 20% in dizygotic twins, and therefore stresses the genetic component. The risk of children if one parent is affected has been estimated at approximately 20% and increases when both parents suffer from psoriasis to about 41–75%. If one sibling developed psoriasis while the parents are not affected, the risk of subsequent children is about 6–20%. Treatment of psoriasis in pregnancy is detailed in Chapter 22.

Psoriasis in the elderly

Currently, psoriasis belongs to the top 10 of the most frequent dermatological diseases in the elderly, and this will become increasingly important with regard to the increasing number of people aged 65 years or older in the population. Demographers estimate that the elderly will constitute up to 34% of the European population by 2050.

Clinical picture

Without age-related differences, plaque-type psoriasis is considered to be the most common clinical subtype in the elderly. Conversely, inverse or flexural forms are more frequently encountered than in the younger ones, particularly in obese or bedridden patients. Complications such as erythrodermic or generalized pustular psoriasis may prove to be especially challenging. As psoriatic arthritis shows an increased cumulative incidence with the years of existing disease, more elderly patients may suffer from additional joint involvement. However, age-related osteoarthritis or osteoporosis should be considered as a differential diagnosis.

Naturally occurring degenerative processes and external factors such as sun exposure or smoking alter the aging skin, resulting in increased vulnerability and potentially impaired skin function. In addition, the frequent dryness of the skin in the elderly may cause pruritus and thus potentially aggravate the disease (Köbner phenomenon). Therefore, consequent use of emollients is of particular importance.

Furthermore, elderly patients often present with multiple comorbidities and thus receive numerous medications such as beta blockers or ACE inhibitors, which might result in drug-induced or drug-aggravated psoriasis.

Another important aspect, particularly in elderly patients, is the current psychosocial situation and potentially existing physical or mental limitations, especially if patients are living alone. Can they care for themselves? Do they need help with daily activities or treatment? Do they understand the treatment instructions, and the potential risks? It is of upmost importance in care to have additional help by social workers or nursing services when necessary to enable optimal management of the disease.

Therapy

Limited data are available with respect to specific single treatment options in aged patients, as usually no special evaluations dedicated to elderly have been carried out.

First-line treatments for older patients with localized psoriasis are topical treatments with vitamin D analogs, glucocorticoids, and tazarotene. Yet, special caution has to be taken to avoid widespread or prolonged use of topical glucocorticoids for possible absorption and because of the already-present increased skin fragility. In addition, the use of glucocorticoids or potentially irritating substances in sensitive areas such as flexures or face should best be avoided. Possible physical restraints that prevent patients from applying topical substances, for example, on the back or head, have to be taken into account. Simple therapeutic regimens are strongly recommended, particularly in case of potential mental constraints.

Phototherapy may be the first choice for more widespread disease. However, the practicability might be restricted in patients with physical restraint due to the need for frequent visits to the doctor's surgery. Another limiting factor is the potential cumulative UV exposure in the past. Close monitoring is required with respect to an increased risk of nonmelanoma skin cancer in the elderly. UV-B (narrowband) may be favored, though topical psoralen plus ultraviolet A (PUVA) (bath-PUVA) may be used alternatively. Combinations with anthralin are quite effective but require hospitalization.

If topical treatment and UV therapy are not sufficient to control disease, systemic treatment might be considered. Careful attention should be given to the fact that aged patients are more susceptible to adverse drug reactions because of alterations of drug metabolism, in particular the reduction in the elimination capacity of the kidney. In addition, liver disorders such as fatty liver disease can make the substances more toxic to the liver. Thus, in some cases, it might be advisable to start first with lower dosages to test for tolerability, before initiating the anticipated dosage needed to achieve the respective treatment response.

Moreover, frequent comorbidities with consequent intake of multiple medications further complicate the choice of treatment owing to potential interactions (Table 13.1). Methotrexate (MTX) can be used safely in the elderly when decreased renal function is taken into consideration. If creatinine clearance (Ccl) is reduced to 80 mL/min or less, the dosage of MTX has to be adapted (Ccl = 80 mL/min → 75%, Ccl = 60 mL/min → 63% of standard dosage, <60 mL/min, no treatment). Remarkably, although many drugs can affect MTX metabolization

Table 13.1 Selected interactions of traditional systemic therapies with a focus on the elderly.

Substance	Interactions
Methotrexate	Use of NSAIDs on the day of MTX intake is best avoided (nephrotoxicity) Penicillin, sulfonamides, proton-pump inhibitors, and ciprofloxacin might increase nephrotoxicity Certain anesthetics and sulfonamides could increase the risk of myleosuppression Azathioprine, leflunomide, retinoids, and sulfasalzine may enhance hepatotoxicity Phenytoin, tetracycline, and tranquilizer may increase toxicity (impairment of binding to plasma proteins)
Cyclosporine	Aminoglykosides, NSAIDs, trimethoprim/sulfomethoxazole, H_2 antagonists, MTX can increase nephrotoxicity Ketoconazole (and other azoles), macrolide antibiotics, doxycyline, Ca-antagonists, and grapefruit juice may increase the level of Cya due to metabolism by CYP3A4 CyA can influence clearance of digoxin and colchicine To avoid myotoxicity, the dosage of statins has to be reduced if combined with CyA CyA + repaglinide may cause hypoglycemia; CyA + nifedipine increases risk of epulis CyA + medications that spare potassium (some diuretics, ACE inhibitors, ATII antagonists) may increase potassium levels CyA + other immunosuppressive medications might increase risk of infections or NHLs
Acitretin	Interactions with diabetes medications, methotrexate, and phenytoin are known. Combination with tetracycline might cause pseudotumor cerebri. Additional use of vitamin A, other retinoids or St. John's wort should be avoided
Fumaric acid esters	No drug interactions are known, but it is recommended that the long-term combined use with nephrotoxic substances such as MTX, retinoids and CyA, as well as other immunosuppressive medications, be avoided

(Table 13.1), clinically significant drug interactions are not frequent. Nevertheless, it is advisable to avoid concurrent use of nephrotoxic substances and the intake of nonsteroidal anti-inflammatory drugs (NSAIDs) at the same day of MTX application. A potential benefit of MTX may be its effect on cardiovascular disease. A retrospective study in US veterans suffering from psoriasis or rheumatoid arthritis showed a significantly reduced risk of vascular disease when treated with low to moderate cumulative doses of MTX.

Retinoids are considered a relatively safe treatment option in the elderly. However, the potential risk of elevated blood lipids should be monitored carefully and, if necessary, treated accordingly. Special caution might be warranted in patients with diabetes, as interactions with oral antidiabetic medications are possible. In addition, the dryness induced by retinoids may be a limiting factor in the elderly and requires consequent use of emollients. Moreover, potentially existing melancholy should be addressed for the possible induction of depression by retinoids.

Therapy with fumaric acid esters is generally believed to be safe and reasonable in the elderly, and the absence of interactions with other medications is advantageous. Still, combinations with potential nephrotoxic substances should be avoided. Any increase in creatinine has to be controlled carefully. If creatinine continues to rise, treatment should be stopped, and moreover, regular monitoring of differential blood counts and liver enzymes is warranted. In case of persistent leukocytopenia (<3000/μL), or lymphocytopenia (<500/μL) fumaric acid esters should be discontinued.

CyA should be used with caution in the elderly because of its potential to induce hypertension, renal dysfunction, and multiple drug interactions. Control of blood pressure and kidney function is essential. An additional examination of the glomerular filtration rate might be considered in elderly patients, especially when they are taking medications that may increase CyA levels. As CyA potentially increases the risk of non-melanoma skin cancers (NMSCs) close monitoring is recommended.

Published information on the use of the different TNF inhibitors, ustekinumab, or alefacept in the elderly as well as investigations dedicated to the elderly are rare. Yet, small studies conducted in older patients treated with etanercept (a TNF inhibitor) and alefacept (a T-cell blocker) have revealed no age-related differences with regard to safety or toxicity. Similarly, according to the manufacturer's package inserts, data deduced from clinical phase III trials have demonstrated no altered efficacy or safety profile except for a slightly increased rate of serious infections. In studies with rheumatoid arthritis patients treated with either infliximab (+MTX) or adalimumab, the frequency of serious infections was reported to be 11.3% and 3.9% in patients older than 65 years compared with 4.6% and 1.4% in patients younger than 65 years, respectively. Conversely, recent data from the British Biologic Registry have revealed no sign of an increased relative risk of infection by anti-TNF-therapy with age.

Though specific studies in patients with renal or liver impairment have not been conducted, the available data have revealed no evidence for pharmacokinetic changes, so far. Therefore, dose adjustment is not needed.

Investigations regarding concurrent use of biologics with other systemic medications are limited, though all TNF-inhibitors have been combined with MTX without the need for dose adjustment. With respect to the elderly, it might be of special interest that two small studies showed no interactions of etanercept and digoxin or warfarin. Moreover, in clinical studies with etanercept, no signs for interactions with glucocorticoids, NSAIDS, analgesics, or salicylates (with the exception of sulfasalazine) have been detected. Interestingly, the combination of etanercept with sulfasalazine led to a significant decrease in leukocytes.

Ustekinumab showed no sign of interactions with the most frequently used comedications in clinical studies such as paracetamol, ibuprofen, ASS, Metformin, Atorvastatin, and levothyroxin.

In conclusion, these data suggest a reasonably good safety profile for the use of biologics in elderly patients with psoriasis. However, all substances target the immune system, and it is well known that elderly patients already possess an increased background risk for infections due to the aging of the immune system. Therefore, respective counseling and monitoring are of upmost importance, and the vaccination status should be updated, though life vaccines are not allowed during therapy. Moreover, the incidence of certain malignancies such as NMSCs is higher in the elderly and might be additionally enhanced by the use of biologics, and so careful controls are recommended.

Further reading

Augustin, M., Glaeske, G., Radtke, M.A., Christophers, E., Reich, K. and Schäfer, I. (2010) Epidemiology and comorbidity of psoriasis in children. *British Journal of Dermatology*, **162**, 633–636.

Bandoli, G., Johnson, D.L., Jones, K.L. *et al.* (2010) Potentially modifiable risk factors for adverse pregnancy outcomes in women with psoriasis. *British Journal of Dermatology*, **163**, 334–339.

Beattie, P.E. and Lewis-Jones, M.S. (2006) A comparative study of impairment of quality of life in children with skin disease and children with other chronic diseases. *British Journal of Dermatology*, **155**, 145–151.

Benoit, S. and Hamm, H. (2007) Childhood psoriasis. *Clinics in Dermatology*, **25**, 555–562.

Cohen-Barak, E., Nachum, Z., Rozenman, D. and Ziv, M.J. (2011) Pregnancy outcomes in women with moderate-to-severe psoriasis. *Journal of the European Academy of Dermatology and Venereology*, **25**, 1041–7.

Cvitanović H., Knezević E., Kuljanac, I. and Jancić, E. (2010) Skin disease in a geriatric patients group in outpatient dermatologic clinic Karlovac, Croatia. *Collegium Antropologicum*, **34** (Supplement 2), 247–251.

de Jager, M.E.A., de Jong, E.M.G.J., Evers, A.W.M., van de Kerkhof, P.C.M. and Seyger, M.B. (2011) The burden of childhood psoriasis. *Pediatric Dermatology*, **28**, 736–737.

Dogra, S. and Kaur, I. (2010) Childhood psoriasis. *Indian Journal of Dermatology Venereology & Leprology*, **76**, 357–365.

Farage, M.A., Miller, K.W., Berardesca, E. and Maibach, H.I. (2009) Clinical implications of aging skin, cutaneous disorders in the elderly. *American Journal of Clinical Dermatology*, **10**, 73–86.

Furue, M., Yamazaki, S., Jimbow, K. *et al.* (2011) Prevalence of dermatological disorders in Japan, a nationwide, cross-sectional, seasonal, multicenter, hospital-based study. *Journal of Dermatology*, **38**, 310–320.

Galloway, J.B., Hyrich, K.L., Mercer, L.K. *et al.* (2011) Anti-TNF therapy is associated with an increased risk of serious infections in patients with rheumatoid arthritis especially in the first 6 months of treatment, updated results from the British Society for Rheumatology Biologics Register with special emphasis on risks in the elderly. *Rheumatology*, **50**, 124–131.

Grozdev, I.S., Van Voorhees, A.S., Gottlieb, A.B. *et al.* (2011) Psoriasis in the elderly: from the Medical Board of the National Psoriasis Foundation. *Journal of the American Academy of Dermatology*, **65**, 537–545.

Horn, E.J., Chambers, C.D., Menter A. and Kimball, A.B., for the International Psoriasis Council (2009) Pregnancy outcomes in psoriasis, Why do we know so little? *Journal of the American Academy of Dermatology*, **61**, e5–8.

Kanda, N. and Watanabe, S. (2005) Regulatory roles of sex hormones in cutaneous biology and immunology. *Journal of Dermatological Science*, **38**, 1–7.

Kira, M. and Katayama, I. (2010) Superimposed linear psoriasis. *Journal of Dermatology*, **37**, 1063–1065.

Marji, J.S., Marcus, R., Moennich, J. and Mackay-Wiggan, J. (2010) Use of biologic agents in pediatric psoriasis. *Journal of Drugs in Dermatology*, **9**, 975–986.

Oumeish, O.Y. and Parish, J.L. (2006) Impetigo herpetiformis. *Clinics in Dermatology*, **24**, 101–104.

Ravelli, A. and Martini, A. (2007) Juvenile idiopathic arthritis. *Lancet*, **369**, 767–778.

Raychaudhuri, S.P., Navare, T., Gross, J. and Raychaudhuri, S.K. (2003) Clinical course of psoriasis during pregnancy. *International Journal of Dermatology*, **42**, 518–520.

Rogers M. (2002) Childhood psoriasis. *Current Opinion in Pediatrics*, **14**, 404–409.

Roth M-M., Feier, V., Cristodor, P. and Moguelet P. (2009) Impetigo herpetiformis with postpartum flare-up. *Acta Dermatovenerologica Alpina, Pannonica et Adriatica*, **18**, 77–82.

Stoll, M.L., Zurakowski, D., Nigrovic, L.E., Nichols, D.P., Sundel, R.P. and Nigrovic P. (2006) Patients with juvenile psoriatic arthritis comprise two distinct populations. *Arthritis & Rheumatism*, **54**, 3564–3572, 2006

Tauscher, A.E., Fleischer, A.B. Jr, Phelps, K.C. and Feldman, S.R. (2002) Psoriasis and pregnancy. *Journal of Cutaneous Medicine and Surgery*, **6**, 561–570.

Weatherhead, S., Robson, S.C. and Reynolds, N.J. (2007) Management of psoriasis in pregnancy. *British Medical Journal*, **334**, 1218–1220.

Ya-Wen Yang, Chin-Shyan Chen, Yi-Hua Chen and Herng-Ching Lin (2011) Psoriasis and pregnancy outcomes: a nationwide population-based study. *Journal of the American Academy of Dermatology*, **64**, 71–77.

Yosipovitch, G. and Tang, M.B. (2002). Practical management of psoriasis in the elderly, epidemiology, clinical aspects, quality of life, patient education and treatment options. *Drugs & Aging*, **19**, 847–863.

PART IV

Evaluation of disease severity

CHAPTER 14

Evaluation of disease severity—clinical scores and questionnaires

Frank Bachmann

Department of Dermatology and Allergy, University Medicine Charité, Berlin, Germany

The assessment of disease severity in psoriasis patients serves different goals: (1) to assess the burden of disease as objectively as possible, (2) to determine the indication for treatment, especially systemic therapy, and (3) to evaluate treatment response and possibly the need for adjustment. There are more than 40 different clinical measures for psoriasis, most of which are poorly standardized and lack validation. Here, we will concentrate on the most relevant instruments for disease assessment.

Assessment of skin involvement

For assessment of skin involvement, three scoring systems are most commonly used: Psoriasis Area and Severity Index (PASI), Body Surface Area (BSA), and Physician's Global Assessment (PGA), here, mainly the static PGA.

The PASI was first introduced by Fredrickson and Pettersson in 1978. Since then, the PASI has been one of the most important assessment tools in clinical trials. The PASI presents a scoring system that ranges from 0 to 72 points. Here, both the severity and extent of the disease are calculated separately for four body regions: head, trunk, upper and lower extremities. PASI measures erythema, induration, and scaling on a five-point-scale ranging from 0 (no symptoms) to 4 (very severe symptoms) for each criterion. The area is assessed depending on the involvement of the specific region; 0 to 6 points are attributed: 1 = 1–9%, 2 = 10–29%, 3 = 30–49%, 4 = 50–69%, 5 = 70–89%, and 6 = 90–100%. To account for the difference in body surface involvement as a proportion of the whole integument, a factor is applied, ranging from 0.1 to 0.4 for the head, the upper extremities, the trunk, and the lower extremities (see Tables 14.A.1-3). With experience, the PASI is quick and simple.

While changes in characteristics of the plaque such as erythema, induration, and scaling are assessed on a continuous scale reflecting gradual improvement or worsening, changes in affected surface area eventually lead to a jump because of

Psoriasis: Diagnosis and Management, First Edition. Edited by Wolfram Sterry, Robert Sabat, and Sandra Philipp.

its character as a multiplicator. The difference of 9% compared with 10% (affected area) results in a doubling of the score for the affected body region. If BSA is less than 10%, changes in PASI rely solely on the changes in plaque morphology and, therefore, reduce the sensitivity to further changes in BSA, thereby possibly underestimating improvement.

Therefore, some authors feel that skin involvement needs to be emphasized more and that changes especially within the first 10% need to be assessed with a more differentiated or even logarithmic scale. Others believe that a broader differentiation in body regions may overcome that problem as well. For this reason, modified PASI scores have been introduced to correct the "improper" weighting of area scores, such as the Psoriasis Log-based Area and Severity Index (PLASI), the Psoriasis Exact Area and Severity Index (PEASI), and the Copenhagen Psoriasis Severity Index (CoPSI).

The BSA assesses the involvement of the skin regardless of the body region involved. The area involved ranges from 0 to 100% such as in erythrodermic patients. Assessment can be performed by the "rule of nine" similar to that in severely burned patients as introduced by Wallace in 1951. Assessment by palm is another quick and easy approach. The patient's palm and thumb plus proximal phalanges of the fingers are used to estimate the affected surface area. It is assumed that one palm equals 1% of the body surface. More experienced physicians might estimate the body surface involvement, using the so-called eyeball technique. Note that in most cases, and even with experienced investigators, the area is overestimated, so this should be assessed as objectively as possible.

The PGA is a five-, six-, or seven-point ordinal rating scale ranging from "clear" to "very severe" to provide a subjective overall evaluation of disease severity. Two systems exist: one is dynamic and the other static. The dynamic PGA shows improvement by comparison with baseline disease severity, while the static PGA assesses severity at a specific moment. Although BSA is not part of the PGA, physicians tend to be influenced by the extent of the disease. The *Patient's Global Assessment (PaGA)* is a similar ordinal rating scale assessed by the patient.

The *Lattice System Physician's Global Assessment (LS-PGA)* presents a global assessment of disease severity and quantifies psoriasis into eight descriptive nominal categories ranging from "clear" to "very severe." Like the PASI, it involves BSA and morphological characteristics. The LS-PGA was developed to address some of the limitations of PASI and others while maintaining their benefits.

In conclusion, the PASI enables a historical comparison between different clinical trials and remains the best-evaluated objective method to define disease severity in plaque psoriasis. Despite limitations such as its low response in mild disease, or its complexity and lack of consensus on interpretability, the PASI remains the best-studied and evaluated scoring system. Most of the measures designed to overcome these limitations could not exceed the PASI on most of the clinimetric properties. Therefore, we recommend the PASI for clinical and scientific evaluation of severity of plaque psoriasis. However, as there is no one measure that captures the whole picture, we believe that the introduction of a different measure such as PASI, BGA, or PGA best reflects the severity and impact of the plaque psoriasis.

Assessment of nail psoriasis

Nail involvement is common in plaque psoriasis and present in most patients with psoriatic arthritis. Nail psoriasis has a huge impact on quality of life. Because of the variation in nail findings, the evaluation of nail involvement severity is difficult. Rich and Scher introduced an objective, numeric, and reproducible grading system for nail psoriasis in 2003, the *Nail Psoriasis Severity Index (NAPSI)*. The NAPSI includes the extent of disease as well as the location of the defects in nail plate or nail bed. The nail is divided into four quadrants. Each quadrant is evaluated for the presence or absence of nail matrix or nail bed disease, and so 0 or 1 point is attributed, which equals a maximum of 8 points for each nail. *Nail matrix* changes comprise pitting, leukonychia, red spots in lunula, and nail-plate crumbling, while *nail bed* changes include oil drop discoloration, onycholysis, nail bed hyperkeratosis, and splinter haemorrhage. A more practical approach, however, is the assessment of an index nail. The major limitation is that NAPSI measures the absence or presence, but not severity of symptoms, for example, one pit weighs as much as five or 10 pittings in one quadrant.

Cassell *et al.* (2007) introduced a *modified NASPI (mNAPSI)* in order to address the limitation mentioned above. The authors abandoned the division of the nail into four quarters in order to address asymmetric involvement and the difficulty in precisely quantifying quadrants in many cases. Furthermore, a more quantitative aspect has been added to account for the amount or severity of the most prominent features. Here, nail pitting, crumbling, and onycholysis were scored 0 to 3, depending on the number or extent of involvement, while the other features were scored according to the original NAPSI as 0 = absence or 1 = presence of symptoms.

Yet another approach presents a three-point scale: 0 = no involvement, 1 = less than 50% of involvement, and 2 = more than 50% of involvement. This score is an objective, much less time-consuming, and easily performed scoring system. Here, we suggest using the NAPSI for an index nail for more accuracy.

Assessment of psoriasis arthritis (PsA)

Asking for joint pain is the most fundamental step in assessing joint involvement possibly associated with psoriasis. Most patients do not mention joint pain spontaneously, leaving them undiagnosed and more importantly untreated. Nightly awakening, improvement by mobilization, and morning stiffness point towards inflammatory joint pain, whereas improvement while resting is more typical for degenerative joint pain. A *joint count* of swollen and painful joints may help to recognize a pattern typical for PsA or other rheumatic disease. Joint pain upon pressure is easily assessed; swelling, on the other hand, may pose a considerable challenge in untrained physicians. Therefore, dermatologists are encouraged to focus on assessment of joint pain either to refer to a rheumatologist or to initiate further diagnostics.

The key assessment is the counting of the number of tender and swollen joints. A variable number of joints are counted, but for PsA the *Tender Joint Count (TJC)* of 68 and *Swollen Joint Count (SJC)* of 66 joints are recommended. Reduced joint counts show reduced validity because they might fail to detect joints predominately affected in PsA. Joint counts can serve as a screening tool as well as a response measure for treatment.

Additionally, TJC and SJC may be incorporated into other disease severity scoring systems such as the *American College of Rheumatology (ACR)* response criteria or the *Disease Activity Score (DAS)*.

Spine assessment

Different outcome measures exist for assessment of ankylosing spondylitis: Bath Ankylosing Spondylitis Disease Activity Index (BASDAI), Bath Ankylosing Spondylitis Function Index (BASFI), and Bath Ankylosing Spondylitis Metrology Index (BASMI). These tools are complex and more suitable for clinical trials. Moreover, especially in elderly patients, it is difficult to differentiate between pain from inflammatory and degenerative spine disease. For clinical practice, duration of morning stiffness, spinal pain, and nocturnal pain might be sufficient.

Assessment of enthesitis

Enthesitis is frequently present in PsA and is characterized by inflammation at the sites of the tendon, ligament, and joint capsule insertion into bone. Insertions of the Achilles' tendon and plantar fascia to the calcaneus, ligamentous insertions, and insertions into the pelvis and to the bones of the thorax and spine are commonly affected. Two enthesitis measures have been developed: the *Mander Enthesitis Index (MEI)* and the *Maastricht Ankylosing Spondylitis Enthesis Score (MASES)*.

Assessment of dactylitis

Dactylitis is characterized by swelling of a whole digit and represents a combination of synovitis and inflammation of tendon and ligament insertions. The presence or absence of dactylitis before and after drug treatment may present a simple way of assessment. A more objective measure is the *Leeds Dactylitis Index*

(LDI), which compares the circumference of the affected digit to the circumference of the digit on the opposite hand or foot. A minimum difference of 10% defines dactylitis. A four-point tenderness score (Ritchie index) or a modified binary score (*LDI basic*; 0 = nontender or 1 = tender) is multiplied by the ratio of circumference.

Imaging techniques

X-ray is a routine imaging modality for following destructive changes in clinical practice in patients with arthritis. However, many studies suggest that both *ultrasound (US)* and *magnetic resonance imaging (MRI)* are more sensitive for detecting bone changes and especially inflammatory and destructive changes compared with X-ray. Therefore, MRI and US are more likely to detect early signs of psoriatic arthritis, especially before destructive changes manifest.

Today, ultrasound might become the screening tool of choice because systemic treatment is recommended before bone changes (X-ray) suggest psoriatic arthritis. Here, clinical assessment and US may lead to the diagnosis.

Visual analog scale (VAS)

VASs allow subjective burdens such as pruritus and pain to be measured rapidly. Furthermore, a rapid estimation may be assessed such as for arthritis activity. VAS helps in the decision as to whether or not to treat symptoms that cannot be assessed objectively and allows the treatment response to be estimated. However, most of these symptoms are rather fragile and are affected by the mood and psychological well-being of the patient.

Quality-of-Life (QOL) Questionnaires

Many questionnaires have been developed in order to measure the burden of disease. Most of them assess psoriasis severity, while only a few of them focus on psychometric QOL. Validated QOL questionnaires are mandatory in clinical trials and are becoming increasingly important in clinical practice as well; for example, a Dermatology Life Quality Index (DLQI) > 10 indicates the need for systemic treatment. Because of the good construct and content validity, internal consistency, reproducibility, acceptability, and responsiveness, we recommend the *Short Form 36 (SF36)* and *DLQI* (Table 14.A.4) followed by *Skindex 29* and *Psoriasis Index of Quality of Life (PSORIQOL)*. The DLQI is probably the most commonly used questionnaire followed by SF36. The DLQI and the SF36 can be completed within 5 min.

Another questionnaire for assessment of QOL is the *Health Assessment Questionnaire (HAQ)* originally developed to assess disability in rheumatoid arthritis. The HAQ focuses on physical disability and pain, and has been used in inflammatory arthritis clinical trials including PsA.

The *Psoriatic Arthritis Screening and Evaluation (PASE) questionnaire* is a 15-item, self-administered, and easy-to-use tool designed for screening for PsA among patients with psoriasis. The *PASE* can distinguish between symptoms of PsA and osteoarthritis. However, it does not replace a rheumatologist but rather indicates if prompt referral to a rheumatologist is indicated. The PASE may also reflect treatment response. Another new screening tool is the German Psoriasis Arthritis Diagnostic questionnaire, which is still being validated at the time of writing.

Other screening tools are the *Psoriatic Arthritis Questionnaire (PAQ)* and the *Toronto Psoriatic Arthritis Screening Tool (ToPAS)*. The ToPAS was designed to screen for PsA in any population and has been broadly validated. It refers to the patient's history of skin or joint symptoms.

Further reading

1 Bronsard, V., Paul, C., Prey, S. *et al.* (2010) What are the best outcome measures for assessing quality of life in plaque type psoriasis? A systematic review of the literature. *Journal of the European Academy of Dermatology and Venereology*, **24** (Supplement 2), 17–22.

2 Cassell, S.E., Bieber, J.D., Rich, P. *et al.* (2007) The modified Nail Psoriasis Severity Index: validation of an instrument to assess psoriatic nail involvement in patients with psoriatic arthritis. *Journal of Rheumatology*, **34**, 123–129.

3 Puzenat, E., Bronsard, V., Prey, S. *et al.* (2010) What are the best outcome measures for assessing plaque psoriasis severity? A systematic review of the literature. *Journal of the European Academy of Dermatology and Venereology*, **24** (Supplement 2), 10–16.

4 Spuls, P.I., Lecluse, L.L., Poulsen, M.L., Bos, J.D., Stern, R.S. and Nijsten, T. (2010) How good are clinical severity and outcome measures for psoriasis?: quantitative evaluation in a systematic review. *Journal of Investigative Dermatology*, **130**, 933–943.

Appendix

PASI (Tables 14.A.1 14.A.2 14.A.3)

Table 14.A.1 Psoriasis Area and Severity Index.

	Head	Upper extremities	Trunk	Lower extremities
Erythema	0 1 2 3 4	0 1 2 3 4	0 1 2 3 4	0 1 2 3 4
Induration	0 1 2 3 4	0 1 2 3 4	0 1 2 3 4	0 1 2 3 4
Desquamation	0 1 2 3 4	0 1 2 3 4	0 1 2 3 4	0 1 2 3 4
Sum				
Area %	0 1 2 3 4 5 6	0 1 2 3 4 5 6	0 1 2 3 4 5 6	0 1 2 3 4 5 6
Factor	0.1	0.2	0.3	0.4
Sum × area × factor				
			PASI:	

The scoring system for the signs of the disease (erythema, induration, and scaling) is as follows: 0 = none, 1 = slight, 2 = moderate, 3 = severe, 4 = very severe.

Table 14.A.2 Scores for the signs of psoriasis.

	Erythema	Induration	Scaling
1 = slight	Light red	0.25 mm	Mainly fine scale, some of lesion covered
2 = moderate	Red, but not deep red	0.50 mm	Coarser, thin scale, most of lesion covered
3 = severe	Deep red	1.00 mm	Coarse, thick scale, most lesion covered, rough
4 = very severe	Very deep to dusky red	1.25 mm	Very thick scale, all of lesion covered, very rough

Table 14.A.3 Area score based on body surface area.

Assign the score according to the percentage of surface covered by plaques in each region:	Please note:
0 = no involvement	(1) The neck is considered part of the head
1 = 1–9% involvement	(2) The axillae and groin are part of the trunk
2 = 10–29% involvement	(3) The buttocks are part of the lower extremities
3 = 30–49% involvement	
4 = 50–69% involvement	
5 = 70–89% involvement	
6 = 90–100% involvement	

The PASI formula is: $\text{PASI} = \{0.1 \times [(E_H + I_H + S_H) \times A_H]\} + \{0.2 \times [(E_U + I_U + S_U) \times A_U]\} + \{0.3 \times [(E_T + I_T + S_T) \times A_T]\} + \{0.4 \times [(E_L + I_L + S_L) \times A_L]\}$.

Physician's Global Assessment (PGA)—static 5-point scale

Overall lesions will be graded for induration, erythema, and scaling based on the scales below. The sum of the three scales will be divided by 3 to obtain a final PGA score.

Induration (I):

0 = no evidence of plaque elevation
1 = minimal plaque elevation = 0.25 mm
2 = mild plaque elevation = 0.5 mm
3 = moderate plaque elevation = 0.75 mm
4 = marked plaque elevation = 1 mm
5 = severe plaque elevation = 1.25 mm

Erythema (E):

0 = no evidence of erythema; hyperpigmentation may be present
1 = faint erythema
2 = light red coloration

3 = moderate red coloration
4 = bright red coloration
5 = dusky to deep red coloration
Scaling (*S*):
0 = no evidence of scaling
1 = minimal; occasional fine scale over less than 5% of the lesion
2 = mild; fine scale dominates
3 = moderate; coarse scale dominates
4 = marked; thick, nontenacious scale dominates
5 = severe; very thick tenacious scale dominates
Add $I+E+S=$______ / 3 = ______ (total average)

PGA based on above total average:
0 = cleared, except for residual discoloration
1 = minimal; majority of lesions have individual scores $I+E+S$ / 3 that average 1
2 = mild; majority of lesions have individual scores $I+E+S$ / 3 that average 2
3 = moderate; majority of lesions have individual scores $I+E+S$ / 3 that average 3
4 = marked; majority of lesions have individual scores $I+E+S$ / 3 that average 4
5 = severe; majority of lesions have individual scores $I+E+S$ / 3 that average 5
Scores should be rounded to the nearest whole number; for example, if total ≤ 1.49, score = 1, if total ≥ 1.5, score = 2.

BSA

Palm method

Patient's palm to PIP joints and thumb equals 1% of body surface. The sum of the number of palms is the BSA.
head and neck = 10% (10 palms)
upper extremities = 20% (20 palms)
trunk (axillae and groin) = 30% (30 palms)
lower extremities (buttocks) = 40% (40 palms)
total BSA score = 100% (100 palms)
Note:

- If there are many small lesions, try to put several together to make one patient palm.
- If central clearing is present, include edges only without areas that have cleared.

Documentation

BSA: ________%

Palm method according to the body areas: 1 palm in the head and neck area corresponds to 10% of this area. Similarly, 1 palm corresponds to 5% of the upper extremities region, 3.3% of the trunk area, and 2.5% of the lower extremities.

DLQI (Table 14.A.4)

Table 14.A.4 Dermatology Life Quality Index. Each question is scored on a 4-point Likert scale: Not at all/Not relevant = 0, A little = 1, A lot = 2 and Very much = 3. Scores of individual items (0–3) are added to yield a total score (0–30); higher scores mean greater impairment of patient's QoL.

Over the last week, how itchy, sore, painful, or stinging has your skin been?	Very much O A lot O A little O Not at all O
Over the last week, how embarrassed or self-conscious have you been because of your skin?	Very much O A lot O A little O Not at all O
Over the last week, how much has your skin interfered with you going shopping or looking after your home or garden?	Very much O A lot O A little O Not at all O Not relevant O
Over the last week, how much has your skin influenced the clothes you wear?	Very much O A lot O A little O Not at all O Not relevant O
Over the last week, how much has your skin affected any social or leisure activities?	Very much O A lot O A little O Not at all O Not relevant O
Over the last week, how much has your skin made it difficult for you to do any sport?	Very much O A lot O A little O Not at all O Not relevant O
Over the last week, has your skin prevented you from working or studying? If "No," over the last week how much has your skin been a problem at work or studying?	Yes O No O Not relevant O A lot O A little O Not at all O
Over the last week, how much has your skin created problems with your partner or any of your close friends or relatives?	Very much O A lot O A little O Not at all O Not relevant O
Over the last week, how much has your skin caused any sexual difficulties?	Very much O A lot O A little O Not at all O Not relevant O
Over the last week, how much of a problem has the treatment for your skin been, for example by making your home messy, or by taking up time?	Very much O A lot O A little O Not at all O Not relevant O

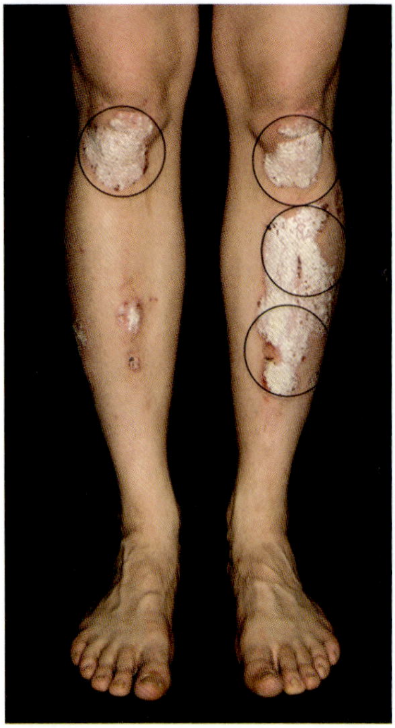

Figure 14.A.1 Assessment of BSA and disease characteristics: legs.

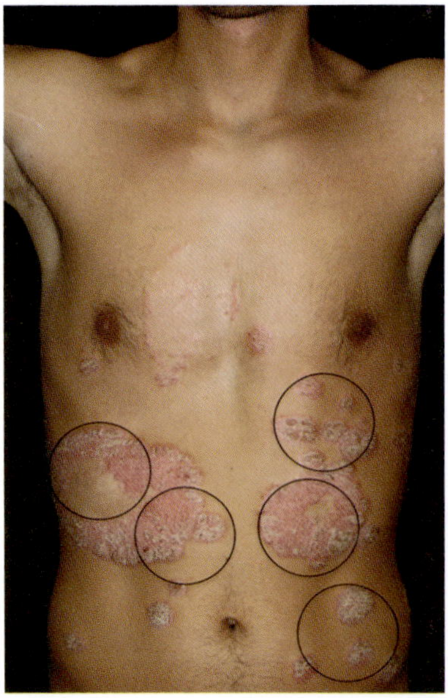

Figure 14.A.2 Assessment of BSA and disease characteristics: trunk.

Example 1 (Figure 14.A.1)

Using the palm method and adding the small lesions to the larger ones, the sum of the number of palms is 4, which means a total BSA of 4% or 10% with respect to the body region (lower extremities). If a lesion is almost completely covered by scales, erythema is difficult to assess and best seen at the scale-free rim of the plaque. Here, the erythema is deep red (3). The lesion is completely covered with thick to very thick scales with rough surfaces (4). The plaques are elevated at least 1.0 mm (3); however, induration is difficult to assess from a picture.

Example 2 (Figure 14.A.2)

In this case, some of the plaques present with central clearing, so care should be taken not to overestimate the BSA. Again, try putting several smaller plaques together to form one and to fill the central clearing. Here, the BSA is something around 5% (total BSA) or 16.5% for the trunk alone. The erythema is deep red (3), the plaques are clearly elevated (3), and the scaling is thick and covers most of the lesion (3).

PART V
Psoriasis and associated diseases

CHAPTER 15
Psoriasis and associated diseases

Steven M. Nwe and Kenneth B. Gordon
Department of Dermatology, Northwestern University, Feinberg School of Medicine, Chicago, IL, USA

While psoriasis remains a chronic inflammatory disease that is characterized most visibly through its clinical dermatological manifestations, mounting evidence suggests that it is associated with a number of systemic and psychosocial comorbidities. The same inflammatory response that precipitates the formation of psoriatic plaque lesions may also predispose individuals with psoriasis to other disease states in which chronic inflammation serves as a point of pathogenesis. Thus, in discussing the systemic implications of psoriasis, it is important not only to look at the various comorbidities of the disease, but also to inquire whether each is present as a result of psoriasis and/or treatment, or coexists with it as a possible spectrum of the same inflammatory state. The aim of this section will be to introduce the diseases associated with psoriasis as well as highlight the multidisciplinary approach that goes into what might traditionally be thought of as purely a skin disease.

Cardiovascular disease and metabolic syndrome

Cardiovascular disease continues to be the leading cause of death in the world. The increase in both global prevalence and incidence of the disease has motivated the medical community to aggressively identify those with risk factors and attempt to modify those risk factors. Evidence continues to show a link between psoriasis and risk factors contributing to cardiovascular disease and related mortality, stressing the importance of addressing these risk factors in this patient population.

Framingham risk scores (a composite measurement that predicts the absolute risk of having a major cardiovascular event at 5 and 10 years) are significantly higher in the psoriasis population when compared with patients who have other, nonpsoriasis skin disease. In addition, psoriasis patients admitted at least once to an inpatient facility show a 50% greater risk of cardiovascular mortality when compared with the general population. A retrospective cohort study reported that the risk of having a myocardial infarction was greater in patients with psoriasis. This risk was most pronounced in young patients with severe disease, further illustrating the prevalence of cardiovascular morbidity and mortality in psoriasis patients.

Psoriasis: Diagnosis and Management, First Edition. Edited by Wolfram Sterry, Robert Sabat, and Sandra Philipp.

The increased cardiovascular disease seen in psoriasis patients is multifactoral. In addition to an increased prevalence of risk factors thought to be due to the psychosocial effects of psoriasis on patient lifestyle choices (e.g. smoking) and an increased use of medications with cardiac effects (e.g. cyclosporine-related hypertension), there is a suggestion that patients with psoriasis may have an increased risk of cardiovascular disease due to interrelated inflammatory pathways. In this regard, and based on epidemiological observations, psoriasis has been suggested to be a risk factor for cardiovascular disease independent of traditional risk factors.

Atherosclerosis, the hallmark of cardiovascular disease, shares many of the same characteristics of immune-mediated diseases such as psoriasis. T-cell activation, inflammatory cytokine release, and immunologic cell interaction with the extracellular matrix are a few examples of the many histological and molecular similarities between the two disease processes. Tumour necrosis factor (TNF)-α, and its function in the propagation of the inflammatory response, also plays a very integral role in both diseases. Methotrexate, a folate analog and anti-inflammatory medication used to successfully treat psoriasis and rheumatoid arthritis, has been shown to decrease the incidence of vascular disease in those two groups, further highlighting the common thread of chronic inflammation in the pathogenesis of atherosclerosis and psoriasis.

Metabolic syndrome (also known as metabolic syndrome X) is a grouping of interrelated medical traits that, when present, indicate an increased risk of developing noninsulin-dependent diabetes mellitus and/or cardiovascular disease. Data extracted over two cycles (2003–2006) of the National Health and Nutrition Examination Survey, a cross-sectional survey of the US population aged 20–59 years, revealed that the prevalence of metabolic syndrome was 40% in patients with a self-reported history of psoriasis. This is compared with the estimated prevalence of metabolic syndrome of 15–34% in the general population.

Many variations of the concept of metabolic syndrome have existed since the 1950s, and while there are a myriad of definitions that exist today, the most commonly used are the American Heart Association/National Heart, Lung and Blood Institute's 2005 update of The National Cholesterol Education Program Adult Treatment Panel III (ATP III) definition and the International Diabetes Federation (IDF) criteria. The ATP III identified six components of the metabolic syndrome; abdominal obesity (measured by waist circumference), atherogenic dyslipidemia [demonstrated by high triglycerides and low high-density lipoprotein "good" cholesterol (HDL-C) cholesterol concentrations], elevated blood pressure, insulin resistance, a proinflammatory state (commonly manifested as an elevated C-reactive protein), and a prothrombotic state (characterized by elevated plasma plasminogen activator inhibitor and fibrinogen). Clinical diagnosis of metabolic syndrome, however, is dependent on the identification of any three or more of the risk factors listed in Table 15.1.

The IDF criterion is similar to the ATP III criteria with notable exceptions. The first exception is that fulfillment of abdominal obesity criteria is required for the

Table 15.1 ATP III Criteria for metabolic syndrome.

Abdominal obesity (waist circumference)	
Men	≥40 inches (102 cm)
Women	≥35 inches (88 cm)
Atherogenic dyslipidemia	
Triglycerides	≥150 mg/dL or drug treatment for elevated triglycerides
HDL cholesterol	< 40 mg /dL in men, <50 mg/dL in women or drug treatment for low HDL cholesterol
Blood pressure	≥130/85 mmHg or drug treatment for elevated blood pressure
Fasting glucose	≥100 mg/dL or drug treatment for elevated blood glucose

Based on ATP III Criteria, patients need to meet any three of the conditions shown in bold to be diagnosed with metabolic syndrome.

diagnosis of metabolic syndrome. The second difference is that waist-circumference cut-off values are determined by a patient's ethnic origin (e.g. Asian men ≥90 cm).

Though the concept of a metabolic syndrome helps to highlight the interplay of various risk factors, for the present purposes we will examine them separately as they relate to psoriasis.

Obesity

A key component to the metabolic syndrome is obesity. Obesity is defined as a body mass index (BMI) of 30 kg/m^2 or greater (overweight defined as a BMI of 25 kg/m^2), with the criteria for metabolic syndrome focusing on abdominal obesity measured by waist circumference. Abdominal obesity correlates with visceral organ adiposity and in particular appears to be strongly associated with insulin resistance in adipose tissue. Insulin resistance in adipose tissue leads to the release of abnormally high levels of nonesterified fatty acids in the serum and accumulation of lipids in nonadipose tissue. Additional cytokine release from adipocytes may also contribute to the vascular endothelial dysfunction and inflammation that promotes atherosclerosis.

For years, there has been recognition by clinicians of the association between obesity and psoriasis. Several European epidemiological studies confirmed the association, showing that patients with obesity had an odds of having psoriasis of 1.9 when compared with nonobese patients. Data gathered in the Utah Psoriasis Initiative confirmed that the prevalence of obesity in patients with psoriasis was almost twice that of the general population, and that psoriasis patients who were obese were more likely to have severe disease (defined in the study as more than 20% BSA involvement). The study also attempted to answer the question of whether psoriasis predisposed to obesity or vice versa. Retrospective analysis of patient-reported body size prior to onset of psoriasis seemed to suggest that psoriasis tended to precede obesity, with most patients having a normal

BMI at age 18. Seventy-one percent of patients later developed elevated BMIs at some point following a diagnosis of psoriasis.

Prospective data from the Nurses' Health Study, following 892 patients with self-reported psoriasis found a graded association between several measures of increased adiposity (waist circumference, hip circumference, waist/hip ratio, BMI) and the risk of incident psoriasis, supporting the thought that obesity may be a risk factor for psoriasis. Further support for obesity being an independent risk factor for the development of psoriasis includes several case reports of improvement of refractory psoriasis with bariatric surgery. Despite the association between psoriasis and obesity, the role of less invasive methods of weight loss such as diet and exercise in psoriasis treatment is still mostly unclear.

There are many hypothesized reasons for the interrelationship between psoriasis and obesity. The psychosocial impact of psoriasis may promote a lifestyle that lends itself to the development of obesity. Both limited cutaneous psoriasis vulgaris and psoriatic arthritis have been shown to decrease the functional status of patients, affecting mobility, energy, and sleep patterns predisposing to a more sedentary lifestyle. In addition, psoriasis-related increases in social isolation and depression, coupled with higher saturated fat and alcohol consumption, have been postulated as mechanisms for psoriasis predisposing to obesity.

Meanwhile, the recognition of obesity itself as a chronic inflammatory condition has helped implicate it as a possible risk factor for the development and/or worsening of psoriasis. TNF-α, notable for its role in recruiting T-cells to the skin and joints, and therefore serving as a critical signal in the formation of psoriatic plaques, can be released from adipose tissue. Obese patients, likely due to higher amounts of adipose tissue, have up to two and a half times higher expression of TNF-α messenger RNA when compared with nonobese individuals serving as a possible mechanism for increased psoriasis risk. Leptin, an adipocyte secreted hormone that also has a role both in energy management and chronic inflammation through cytokine regulation, has also been shown to be increased in psoriasis patients. Paradoxically, leptin levels may be decreased when using TNF-α blocking agents for treatment of psoriasis, causing decreased satiety and increased weight gain.

Some of the adipokines increased in obesity have also been implicated in helping to promote the development of other disease states in psoriasis. As stated above, obesity results in increases in adipose tissue and resulting increases in adipokines, promoting inflammation, which has been shown to result in insulin resistance. High TNF-α levels have been shown, in mouse models, to decrease efficient glucose utilization, while elevated levels of chemokine CXC ligand 5 have been shown to decrease glucose tolerance of muscle cells. This might help explain the observed higher prevalence of insulin resistance in psoriasis patients, which, in addition to obesity, is an independent risk factor for cardiovascular disease. In addition, both obesity and insulin resistance play key roles in the development of fat accumulation in hepatocytes leading to nonalcoholic fatty liver disease. Nonalcohol fatty liver disease, which is sometimes seen as a hepatocellular consequence of metabolic syndrome, has also shown an increased prevalence in psoriasis patients. This is particularly important, considering the increased alcohol consumption, risk of cirrhosis, and use of possible hepatotoxic mediations (e.g. methotrexate) in psoriasis patients.

Atherogenic dyslipidemia

An additional key metabolic syndrome risk factor that appears to have a direct effect on atherosclerotic disease activity, and thus cardiovascular disease, is atherogenic dyslipidemia. Atherogenic dyslipidemia is a combination of lipoprotein abnormalities including elevations in serum low-density lipoprotein "bad" cholesterol, triglycerides, and apolipoprotein B (apoB), as well as decreased serum HDL-C. Studies of these lipoprotein trends have shown that psoriasis patients tend to have a proatherogenic profile that may be more pronounced in those with more severe/active psoriatic disease.

A Swedish study, however, that attempted to look at the lipid profile of 200 patients at the onset of psoriasis found that HDL-C levels were actually increased when compared with controls. While the study did reveal that very-low-density lipoprotein cholesterol (VLDL) levels were also increased, all other lipoprotein levels were equivalent to controls questioning the correlation of atherogenic dyslipidemia early in the disease process. In addition, recent case–control analyses attempting to evaluate the role of lipid-altering medications, Hmg Co-reductase inhibitors (statins) in particular, found that long-term statin use did not lower a patient's risk of developing psoriasis. The authors did see a decreased risk in those who used short-duration statin, hypothesizing that statins may have an initial protective effect against psoriasis that plateaus over time. Another possibility is that the lifestyle changes (diet and exercise) that often occur during the initiation of pharmacotherapy for dyslipidemia may delay the onset of psoriasis initially more so than the statin itself.

The role of atherogenic dyslipidemia in psoriasis pathogenesis and vice versa is still unclear, though the association between the two entities will be important in understanding future therapeutics and recommendations regarding treatment options that may address both diseases. Clinicians treating psoriasis should also be cognizant of the relationship, as many of the current therapies for psoriasis such as cyclosporine and acitretin are known to affect lipid profiles.

Hypertension

Hypertension affects over 1 billion people worldwide and is expected to increase as the population ages. Blood-pressure classifications and definitions were reported in the seventh report of the Joint National Committee (JNC 7) in 2003

Table 15.2 JNC 7 classifications of blood pressure (BP).

BP class	Systolic BP (mmHg)	Diastolic BP (mmHg)
Normal	<120	and < 80
Prehypertension	120–139	or 80–90
Stage 1 HTN	140–159	or 90–99
Stage 2 HTN	≥160	or ≥100

in order to address the consistent association between blood pressure and cardiovascular disease, and its major role in morbidity and mortality. Table 15.2 shows the classification of hypertension.

The ATP III metabolic syndrome criteria blood-pressure cut-off is 130/85 mmHg. This cut off falls in the JNC 7 defined prehypertension category. Increased risk of hypertension in patients with psoriasis has been reported but, when adjusted for age, gender, person years, and other comorbidities, is small and not affected by psoriasis disease severity. This small but increased risk is usually attributed to the higher rates of obesity and smoking in the patient population, highlighting the psychosocial effects of the disease on lifestyle behaviors. Data from the Nurses' Health Study confirmed the slightly increased risk of hypertension and additionally showed that this risk persisted even after adjustments were made for BMI, physical activity, and smoking.

A recent study that included 12,502 psoriasis patients and matched controls showed a higher prevalence of hypertension in psoriasis patients, which remained significant during multivariate analysis including sex, smoking history, obesity, and nonsteroidal anti-inflammatory drug use. Authors of this study postulated that increased blood-pressure measurements could be related to elevated angiotensin-converting enzyme levels in seen psoriasis patients.

While there are many variables in the development of hypertension, the small increased risk of developing high blood pressure could again point towards the role in chronic inflammation, such as that seen in psoriasis. In addition to this, cyclosporine, a therapy option for those with psoriasis, does carry a risk of hypertension through to the drug's effects on systemic vasoconstriction, though this risk is low, and psoriasis patients are unlikely to be on the medication for long-term treatment.

Inflammatory bowel disease

Inflammatory bowel disease, while comprising several disorders, is notable for two major diseases; Crohn's disease and ulcerative colitis. Crohn's disease is typically thought of as an inflammatory autoimmune disease, with lesions affecting the gastrointestinal tract transmurally anywhere from the mouth to the perianal area (with rectal sparing). Inflammatory changes are seen in a skipwise fashion and, depending on the degree, can lead to extensive fibrosis, intestinal obstruction, and sinus tract formation. Ulcerative colitis inflammation is limited to the colonic mucosal layer, with a majority of patients having rectal involvement. Unlike the skip lesion nature of Crohn's, ulcerative colitis lesions tend to be continuous and extend from the distal bowel proximally. The pathogenesis, and more specifically the role of the immune system in the development of ulcerative colitis, is less understood than it is in Crohn's disease.

There has been shown to be a link between psoriasis and both Crohn's disease and ulcerative colitis, though this association has been most studied with Crohn's disease. The prevalence of psoriasis in patients with Crohn's disease is 9%. When compared and matched with controls, patients with Crohn's disease are more likely to have psoriasis as are their first-degree relatives. Meanwhile, patients with psoriasis have been shown to have an increased prevalence ratio of developing Crohn's disease (and ulcerative colitis for that matter), which is even more pronounced when those patients have psoriatic arthritis. Prevalence rates of Crohn's disease in psoriasis patients might actually be underestimated, as the inflammatory bowel changes may be under-reported in those with asymptomatic disease.

Pathologic similarities in both diseases suggest that both have common immunologic and inflammatory pathways. The intestinal immune system involves a tight balance of defense against pathogenic microbes and tolerance of the "normal" flora that aid in luminal bacterial regulation. Much like psoriasis, the development of inflammatory bowel disease involves upregulation of both the innate and adaptive immune systems leading to an infiltration of the lamina propria with neutrophils, macrophages, dendritic cells, natural killer T-cells, B-cells, and T-cells. The activation and propagation of this cascade are aided by elevations in cytokines such as IL-1β, IFN-γ, and TNF-α, which in turn activate dendritic cells promoting the release of IL-12 and IL-23, the differentiation of Th1 and Th17, and further cytokine and chemokine release (see Chapter 4). TNF-α, a key T1 cytokine, has an important role in the cascade reaction that eventually leads to both psoriasis and Crohn's disease, with demonstrated elevations seen in both psoriatic lesions and the stool and intestinal mucosa of patients with active Crohn's disease.

Infliximab, a monoclonal antibody that works by binding soluble and receptor-bound TNF-α, has been a therapeutic agent for Crohn's patients. After infliximab was shown to provide a significant improvement in a patient who had both psoriasis and Crohn's, a randomized, double-blind, placebo-controlled trial comparing placebo with infliximab was performed in psoriasis patients. Seventy-seven percent of patients in the infliximab group showed at least a 75% improvement in their Psoriasis Area and Severity Index (PASI 75) scores compared with 18% of patient patients in the control group. This helped to further suggest a common inflammatory pathway between the two diseases.

Interestingly, studies with another TNF-α inhibitor have not been as suggestive. Etanercept, an artificially engineered dimeric fusion protein directed against TNF-α, has been shown to be effective for plaque psoriasis. Clinical trials involving etanercept in Crohn's disease, however, have not shown a significant therapeutic benefit. Theories on why pharmaceuticals directed against the same cytokine would have such varied response rates include variability in drug target organ penetration, TNF-α binding, and inflammatory cell modulation. Additionally, this may highlight the different role of TNF-α in these diseases. Comparisons of the utility of other drugs used in both disease states that target the immune system have also shown a spectrum of therapeutic efficacy, with some offering benefit in both diseases (e.g. cyclosporine) and others showing a discordant response (e.g. etanercept).

Familial recurrence of both diseases, as well as the immunologic similarity, has fueled studies attempting to find a shared genetic determinant between the two diseases. Genomic studies have identified several psoriasis susceptibility loci (PSORS1 through PSORS9; see Chapter 5). PSORS1 located on chromosome 6p21 confers an odds ratio of 6.4 for developing disease, and is believed to be the major genetic determinant for developing disease. Also located on chromosome 6p is an HLA antigen region named IBD3, thought to increase the chances of developing Crohn's disease. Neighboring both genes is a region that encodes for TNF-α. Polymorphisms to this region are linked to both psoriasis and Crohn's disease. Gene variants for IL-23 receptor and its p40 (part of IL-12 and IL-23) ligand IL12B, which confer susceptibility to Crohn's disease, also appear to increase psoriasis risk (see Chapter 5). In addition to this, CDKAL1, a gene associated with type 2 diabetes, seemed also to link psoriasis with Crohn's disease.

While not traditionally classified as an inflammatory bowel disease, celiac disease, characterized by intestinal villous atrophy brought on by dietary intolerance of gluten products, has also been linked to psoriasis, though inconsistently. Although the association is not clear, some reports have found that patients with psoriasis with elevated antigliadin antibodies do have an immunohistochemical improvement in psoriatic lesions after being placed on a gluten-free diet, fueling further studies to examine the relationship between the two diseases.

Other inflammatory diseases

Both psoriasis and inflammatory bowel disease can be grouped into a common category of diseases known as immune-mediated inflammatory disease. This classification of diseases includes, but is not limited to, rheumatoid arthritis, insulin-dependent diabetes mellitus, and ankylosing spondylitis. The diseases are noted for dysregulation of the immune system leading to activation of common inflammatory pathways. The inciting event that sets the cascade off is unknown but has been postulated to be dependent on interplay of environmental insults in a genetically susceptible host.

It has been noted that patients with a known diagnosis of one immune-mediated inflammatory disease are more likely than controls to have another immune-mediated inflammatory disease. As discussed above, most of the most compelling evidence has linked psoriasis with inflammatory bowel disease. However, psoriasis patients have also been shown to be more likely to develop rheumatoid arthritis, giant-cell arteritis, and pulmonary fibrosis. In addition to this, immune-mediated inflammatory diseases appear to share common risks of morbidity and mortality. Like psoriasis, studies have shown patients with rheumatoid arthritis to have an increased risk of atherosclerotic cardiovascular-disease-related mortality, postulated due to accelerated atherosclerosis development from chronic systemic inflammation.

Type II diabetes and insulin resistance have also been linked with psoriasis, though it is still mostly unclear if this is a result of increased rates of obesity and associated insulin resistance or an independent risk factor. One study did find that the prevalence of diabetes in psoriasis patients was still elevated, even when correcting for BMI, suggesting that the predisposition could be due to shared immune-mediated inflammation.

Scientists have also used genetic analysis to find a common link between the diseases. HLA alleles appear to be a large factor in developing an immune-mediated inflammatory disease. In addition, genome-wide scans identifying different loci that confer susceptibility to developing psoriasis showed that these loci coincided with loci for other immune-mediated inflammatory diseases such as rheumatoid arthritis, Grave's disease, insulin-dependent diabetes, and inflammatory bowel disease. Researchers are still only beginning to understand the environmental and host factors that determine the phenotypic expression of these susceptibility loci.

Psychosocial aspects

Beyond the physical manifestations, dermatologic disease has long been associated with significant functional, psychological, and social comorbidities. Early studies have suggested that up to 30% of dermatology outpatients and 60% of inpatients had self-reported impairments in mental health, of which 20% had symptoms meeting criteria for having an adjustment disorder. A 1998 survey performed by the National Psoriasis Foundation found that 79% of patients thought that the disease had a negative impact on their life, and over half felt that the disease was significantly disruptive to their daily life.

Psoriasis lesions are most commonly characterized by sharply demarcated plaques with silvery scales, though presentations and body surface involvement are varied. Lesions can be irritable, pruritic, painful, and/or hemorrhagic. In addition to this, patients affected by psoriatic arthritis can experience discomfort and limited mobility from affected joints that can lead to joint deformities and resulting disability. The severity of the symptoms associated with psoriasis has the capacity to disturb a patient's activities of daily living, including, but not limited to, fatigue, sleep disturbances, ambulation restriction, and resulting occupational impairments. The extent to which these physical symptoms affect patients with psoriasis makes the disease comparable with other major chronic medical diseases (e.g. heart disease, depression, cancer, etc.).

The effect of the physical, visible manifestations of psoriasis on the patient psyche is significant and can be debilitating. Self-esteem levels in patients with psoriasis are generally low due to the embarrassment of visible skin lesions. Psoriatic plaque development has a distinct role in patient self image particularly in those afflicted at an early age. As a result, patients spend a considerable amount of time and energy choosing appropriate clothing to cover lesions and preparing for activities where psoriatic skin involvement may be exposed to others (swimming, sports activities, attending social events, etc.). In addition, 75% of psoriasis patients report that they find themselves unattractive and/or sexually unappealing, causing, for some, inhibition of social interactions, detrimental effects on assertiveness, and sexual dysfunction. Psoriasis's effects on patient body image may be based not only on perceived or anticipated stigmatization experiences but also on realized ones. Discrimination by others due to skin lesions is repeatedly shown to be a reality for those with psoriasis. Psoriasis surveys have documented various negative patient experiences, such receiving a poorer service than those without visible skin disease, or even being asked to leave a social establishment because of the visibility of their skin lesions. These experiences only reinforce poor self-esteem patterns and perpetuate psoriasis-related social isolation.

Financially, a diagnosis of psoriasis can also have a negative impact on patients' lives. Taking into account inpatient and outpatient physician encounters and over-the-counter and prescription medication costs, it has been estimated that patients with clinically significant psoriasis spend approximately $648 annually. A multivariate analysis echoed these findings, estimating direct costs of around $600. However, when indirect costs of treatment (i.e. sick days, missed work time, disability payments) were factored in, the total cost per patient per year was roughly $1500. The analysis compared this amount with the approximate combined direct and indirect cost of diverticular disease (estimated to be the costliest of gastrointestinal conditions), which is $1231 per patient per year. These data seem to support the economic burden reported by psoriasis patients on patient surveys, particularly of those patients in lower income brackets.

The burden of disease can manifest itself in different ways, and for some this occurs through behavioral and lifestyle changes. The combination of social isolation, decreased physical activity, and increased economic hardships predisposes patients to the development of obesity as discussed earlier. With the emotional hardships of psoriasis comes increased risk of anxiety and/or depression, as well as a reliance on coping strategies that can also be detrimental to patient health including consumption of a high-fat diet, nicotine use, and/or alcohol abuse. Also, given that the severity of skin involvement does not necessarily correlate with equivalent quality-of-life ratings, there has been increasing awareness that measurements of psoriasis progression/regression should involve addressing the diseases' psychosocial and quality-of-life impact in addition to the physical exam.

Depression

As mentioned before, psoriasis is associated with increased rates of mood disorders such as anxiety and depression. Though the prevalence of depression in patients with psoriasis is approximately 24%, a survey of 2391 Italian patients with psoriasis sent to the Center for Epidemiological Studies-Depression Scale found that 62% of patients had depressive symptomatology. This wide disparity in depression rates could illustrate the underdiagnosis of clinical depression in this patient population. The study found that patients with only a primary or secondary level of education were significantly more likely to have depressive symptomatology than those of a higher education level, as were men younger than 40 when compared with men older than 40. There was also a trend (though not statistically significant) for women to have more symptoms than men.

A British population cohort study confirmed the higher risk of depression and anxiety in psoriasis patients, showing a statistically significant increased risk of depression in patients with severe psoriasis when compared with those with mild psoriasis. The study also built on earlier research showing an alarming increase in suicidality in patients with psoriasis, some of which showed up to 10% of patients expressing a wish for death.

The relationship between psoriasis and depression is often attributed to the psychosocial burden of the disease itself. TNF-α, along with other proinflammatory cytokines involved in the pathogenesis of psoriasis, has also been linked to depression. Elevated concentrations of TNF have been observed in patients with medication-resistant depression as well as acute depression, suggesting that both diseases may have a common physiological link. This relationship might explain the role of immunomodulator therapy in improving psychiatric symptoms in psoriasis patients.

Correlations between psoriasis-associated decreases in quality-of-life indexes and TNF-α inhibitors have been documented in several studies. More specifically, the effectiveness of TNF-α inhibitors in improving psoriasis-associated depression has proven promising. Patients taking etanercept were shown to be more likely than those on placebo to have more than 50% improvement in their Hamilton rating scale for depression or their Beck depression inventory scores. In addition, there was less correlation with improvements in depressive symptoms and PASI scores, which might suggest that depressive symptoms in psoriasis patients may not all be due to objective skin involvement. Adalimumab, the first FDA-approved fully human monoclonal antibody, also works against TNF and has shown benefit in plaque psoriasis. When compared with controls, patients who received adalimumab showed significant reductions in their Zung Self-rating Depression Scale at 12 weeks. It is difficult to determine if the inhibition of TNF improved depression directly or indirectly, as improvements in depressive symptoms did correlate with PASI score improvement, with greater improvements in depressive symptoms occurring in responder groups.

Other proinflammatory cytokines involved in the pathogenesis of psoriasis include IL-12 and IL-23, which induce CD4+ T-cell differentiation into Th1 and Th17 cells, respectively. Biologics inhibiting IL-12 and IL-23 have been proven to improve moderate to severe plaque psoriasis. The ACCEPT trial showed that ustekinumab, an IL-12/23 inhibitor, was better for treatment of psoriasis than etanercept. When compared with placebo, patients on ustekinumab had significantly greater improvements at 12 weeks in both anxiety and depression as measured by the Hospital Anxiety and Depression Scale. In addition to these findings, the analysis also confirmed the prevalence of depression and anxiety in psoriasis patients, with mean reported Hospital Anxiety and Depression Scale scores at baseline being comparable with those of patients with breast cancer and chronic obstructive pulmonary disease.

Although the above studies do not prove the role of inflammatory cytokines in the development of depression, they do highlight the relationship between mood disorders and psoriasis, as well as the need to address patient psychosocial health during psoriasis assessments and follow-ups.

Nicotine use

The World Health Organization reports that tobacco use kills nearly 6 million people yearly and continues to be the leading cause of preventable death worldwide (more than illegal drugs, AIDS, murder/suicide, and road accidents combined). Smoking in particular has been implicated in a wide range of disease states, with the major causes of smoking-related death attributed to atherosclerotic cardiovascular disease, chronic obstructive pulmonary disease, and lung cancer. Smoking is now considered an independent risk factor for the development of atherosclerotic cardiovascular disease.

The Utah Psoriasis Initiative study, which showed increase obesity rates in psoriasis patients as discussed earlier, also showed that the prevalence of smoking was also higher in psoriasis patients than in the general population. While it might be that psoriasis patients are more likely to use cigarette smoking as a coping mechanism for the psychosocial burden of the disease, the Utah study showed that cigarette smoking is not only more prevalent in psoriasis patients but also a possible risk factor for developing disease. Seventy-seven percent of patients in that cross-sectional evaluation started smoking before diagnosis of psoriasis, while only 22% started afterwards. The Nurses' Health Study showed that compared with nonsmokers, the risk of psoriasis was 78% higher among current smokers and 37% higher in past smokers. The risk of developing psoriasis only decreased to near nonsmoker levels after 20 years of cessation. These data built upon earlier observations strongly linking pustulosis palmoplantaris (thought to be a variant of psoriasis) with smoking.

Smoking's effects on the body, and more specifically the skin, are believed to be through its role in delivering oxidative stress. A study aiming to link the role of smoking-induced stress in psoriasis patients found that malondialdehyde levels were significantly elevated and superoxide dismutase levels decreased in both smokers and psoriasis patients when compared with nonsmokers and controls, respectively. The resulting oxidative stress and formation of free radicals through cigarette smoking is thought to stimulate cell-signaling pathways involved in the formation of psoriatic plaques including Janus kinases/signal transducers and activators of transcription (JAK-STAT). In addition to this, the same inflammatory mechanisms that link smoking to atherosclerosis, as well as smoking's effect on gene expression, support the notion that smoking's relationship to psoriasis is multifactoral.

While patients should be aware of the role of cigarette smoke in the development and severity of psoriasis, it is also worthwhile noting the other negative health impacts of cigarette smoking. As has been discussed, cigarette smoking is an independent risk factor for cardiovascular disease. The higher prevalence of smoking in psoriasis patients may help explain the increased risk of cardiovascular disease in this group. Furthermore, cigarette smoking (and even second-hand smoke, for that matter) increases a psoriasis patient's already-higher risk of malignancy.

Alcohol

Alcohol consumption is a common practice worldwide, and some studies have suggested that modest consumption may actually be beneficial to health in some diseases. The difficulty with recommending consumption, even if deemed beneficial, is the potential for abuse and dependence and associated consequence of long-term use (cirrhosis, hepatocellular carcinoma and other malignancies, suicidality, arrhythmias, etc.).

There has been debate on the link of alcohol abuse being a cause or consequence of psoriasis for many years, and demonstrating causality continues to be difficult. Early correlations between heavy drinking and psoriasis even described lesions having a more inflamed and less scaled characteristic similar to psoriasis lesion seen in HIV at the time. Like smoking, alcohol consumption (particularly abuse) appears to be more prevalent in patients with psoriasis and could be associated with worsening of psoriasis severity. In a recent prospective analysis of 1150 cases of incident psoriasis in women, patients who drank 2.3 drinks per week or more had a relative risk of developing psoriasis of 1.72. Authors attempted to determine whether the type of alcoholic beverage made a significant difference and found that only nonlight beer was associated with an increased risk of incident psoriasis (compared with light beer, red wine, white wine, and liquor), suggesting a possible role of a nonalcoholic component of beer, such as gluten, in the associated risk increase. The mechanisms by which alcohol affects disease progression are still mostly unknown, though alcohol's effects on obesity rates, as well as possible direct action on keratinocyte proliferation, have been suggested.

In addition to prevalence information, it also appears that alcohol consumption affects prognosis. Psoriasis patients who consume moderate amounts of alcohol have been shown to have less improvement in psoriasis with treatment, higher rates of deaths from cirrhosis, and higher rates of death from alcohol-related disease. Furthermore, psoriasis patients with cancer have a worse prognosis if previously hospitalized for alcohol-related diseases.

Conclusion

On top of the aesthetic and often debilitating skin manifestations of psoriasis, patients with the disease are at risk for a number of systemic, psychological, and behavioral comorbidities, many of which are life-threatening. Additionally, some of these comorbidities themselves may have a role in the development and progression of psoriasis itself. As research continues to unravel the multidimensional relationships between psoriasis and these diseases, healthcare providers will need to be increasingly aware of the associations in order to improve global health outcomes in this population. Though the growing data associating psoriasis with other chronic diseases may paint a grim prognosis, they also present an opportunity by physicians to address and treat these comorbidities. What is learned from psoriasis and its associated diseases may also offer insight into the development and use of future therapeutics.

Further reading

Alberti, K.G., Zimmet, P. and Shaw, J. (2005) IDF epidemiology Task Force Consensus Group. The metabolic syndrome—a new worldwide definition. *Lancet*, **366**, 1059–1062.

Bremmer, S., Van Voorhees, A.S., Hsu, S. *et al.* (2010) Obesity and psoriasis: from the medical board of the National Psoriasis Foundation. *Journal of the American Academy of Dermatology*, **63**, 1058–1069.

Chobanian, A.V., Bakris, G.L., Black, H.R. *et al.* (2003) The seventh report of the joint national committee on prevention, detection, evaluation and treatment of high blood pressure: the JNC 7 report. *Journal of the American Medical Association*, **289**, 2560–2572.

Gelfand, J.M., Neimann, A.L., Shin, D.B. *et al.* (2006) Risk of myocardial infarction in patients with psoriasis. *Journal of the American Medical Association*, **296**, 1735–1741.

Grundy, S.M., Cleeman, J.I., Daniels, S.R. *et al.* (2005) Diagnosis and management of the metabolic syndrome: an American Heart Association/National Heart, Lung, and Blood Institute Scientific Statement. *Circulation*, **112**, 2736–2737.

Herron M D., Ninckley, M., Hoffman, M.S. *et al.* (2005) Impact of obesity and smoking on psoriasis presentation and management. *Archives of Dermatology*, **141**, 1527–1534.

Kimball, A.B., Gladman, D., Gelfand, J.M. *et al.* (2008) National Psoriasis Foundation clinical consensus on psoriasis comorbidities and recommendations for screening. *Journal of the American Academy of Dermatology*, **58**, 1031–1042.

Krueger, G., Koo, J., Lebwohl, M. *et al.* (2001) The impact of psoriasis on quality of life: results of a 1998 National Psoriasis Foundation patient-membership survey. *Archives of Dermatology*, **137**, 280–284.

Makredes, M., Robinson, D. and Bala, M. (2009) The burden of autoimmune disease: A comparison of prevalence rations in patients with psoriatic arthritis and psoriasis. *Journal of the American Academy of Dermatology*, **61**, 405–410.

Setty, A.R., Curhan, G. and Choi, H.K. (2007) Obesity, waist circumference, weight change, and the risk of psoriasis in women. *Archives of Internal Medicine*, **167**, 1670–1675.

PART VI
Therapeutic management

CHAPTER 16

Therapeutic aim of psoriasis therapy

Sandra Philipp

Psoriasis Research and Treatment Center, Department of Dermatology and Allergy/Institute of Medical Immunology, University Hospital Charité, Berlin, Germany

Psoriasis is a chronic inflammatory disease that affects the skin, nails, and joints, and thus may cause symptoms such as itching, burning, or pain, which can result in impairment of physical functions such as walking or even cause work disability. Psoriasis also negatively impacts psychosocial well-being. The visibility of the lesions often results in feelings of stigmatization, shame, or exclusion, and can have a negative impact on self-confidence and self-image. Trying to hide the affected skin may impede social contacts or even employment opportunities. Overall, the disease can lead to a deterioration of all aspects of life such as personal relationships, leisure activities, social activities, or professional development. Therefore, the primary treatment aim is to enable patients to live a life that is not, or only minimally, impaired by their disease.

Though one may view the ideal treatment aim in rapidly achieving complete remission of the skin or joint complaints, this might not be appropriate in the majority of patients, as this excludes not only patient immanent factors but also safety aspects. First, one has to differentiate between patients with severe flairs that may need a rapid response and patients with a more chronic course of disease that primarily requires effective long-term control. Furthermore, some patients might need high dosages or combinations of treatments to achieve complete clearance, which might in turn lead to adverse effects. Therefore, a careful assessment of the potential benefits and risks should be carried out when choosing an individual therapy.

It is important also to consider the preferences of the patients. Some may be afraid of certain therapies or dislike specific treatments, which may affect the compliance and adherence to the treatment strategy. In conclusion, the optimal treatment aim is not only to obtain rapid improvements in the skin, nails, or joints, and the maintenance of a long-term remission but also to include the tolerability, safety, and practicability of a treatment in order to minimize the impairment of daily life by the disease.

Another interesting aspect with respect to the therapeutic aim is the devising of defined treatment goals in the management of chronic diseases to support and

Psoriasis: Diagnosis and Management, First Edition. Edited by Wolfram Sterry, Robert Sabat, and Sandra Philipp.

promote the standardized use of available therapies and thus optimize the care of the patients. The basis of any goal-oriented strategy is the establishment of the individual treatment goal. To successfully apply the treatment goals, treatment responses have to be monitored regularly, so that prompt adjustment of the therapy may be initiated if these goals are not met. So far, hard outcome measures such as biomarkers, for example, glucose level or HbA1c in diabetes, are not available for psoriasis. Therefore, a European expert consensus group developed treatment goals for patients suffering from moderate to severe psoriasis ("rule of ten") based on changes in Psoriasis Area and Severity Index (PASI) and Dermatology Life Quality Index (DLQI) scores.

The control of the distinct parameters is recommended after an induction period of 16–24 weeks according to the respective treatment and then in regular time intervals. Successful treatment has been determined as an improvement in PASI by at least 75%. Though PASI values often do not correlate well with the DLQI, the proportion of patients achieving PASI 75 corresponds well with the proportion of patients exhibiting a DLQI score of <5, which can be interpreted as an acceptable or good quality of life. In addition, the minimum requirement for therapeutic efficacy has been defined as a reduction in the baseline PASI by at least 50%. If this is not achieved, a modification of therapy appears appropriate, such as dose increase, combination with another treatment, or complete change in therapeutic strategy. If a patient demonstrates an improvement with a PASI reduction of at least 50% but less than 75%, the DLQI should be taken into consideration when deciding whether to maintain or modify the treatment strategy. A DLQI of ≥5 signifies still distinct impaired quality of life and therefore speaks in favor of modifying the therapy, whereas a DLQI of <5 means less deterioration and may allow continuation of the treatment.

The above-defined treatment goals, which also include the patients' perspective by the use of the DLQI, can help physicians to adjust their treatment decision in a comparable manner and thereby supports standardization of care in day-to-day practice. Yet, this tool still has to be validated in subsequent investigations.

Further reading

Kimball, A.B., Gieler, U., Linder, D., Sampogna, F., Warren, R.B. and Augustin, M. (2010) Psoriasis: is the impairment to a patient's life cumulative? *Journal of the European Academy of Dermatology and Venereology*, **24**, 989–1004.

Lebwohl, M. (2005) A clinician's paradigm in the treatment of psoriasis. *Journal of the American Academy of Dermatology*, **53**, S59–S69.

Mrowietz, U., Kragballe, K., Nast, A. and Reich, K. (2011), Strategies for improving the quality of care in psoriasis with the use of treatment goals—a report on an implementation meeting. *Journal of the European Academy of Dermatology and Venereology*, **25** (Supplement 3), 1–13.

Mrowietz, U., Kragballe, K., Reich, K. *et al.* (2011) Definition of treatment goals for moderate to severe psoriasis: a European consensus. *Archives of Dermatological Research*, **303**, 1–10.

CHAPTER 17

Treatment of plaque psoriasis

Topical therapy of psoriasis
Knud Kragballe
Department of Dermatology, Arhus University Hospital, Arhus, Denmark

Phototherapy and photochemotherapy
Erhard Hölzle
Department of Dermatology and Allergology, Klinikum Oldenburg, Oldenburg, Germany

Classical systemic treatments
Peter C.M. van de Kerkhof
Department of Dermatology, Radboud University Nijmegen Medical Centre, Nijmegen, Netherlands

Biologics
Sandra Philipp
Psoriasis Research and Treatment Center, Department of Dermatology and Allergy/Institute of Medical Immunology, University Hospital Charité, Berlin, Germany

TOPICAL THERAPY OF PSORIASIS

Knud Kragballe
Department of Dermatology, Arhus University Hospital, Arhus, Denmark

General principles

Topical treatments may be used for psoriasis of any severity, either as monotherapy for mild disease or in combination with phototherapy and systemic therapy for moderate to severe psoriasis. Because most psoriasis patients suffer from mild disease, the majority of patients with psoriasis receive therapy with a topical agent. Currently, there are no valid scores with cutoff values to define the population of patients eligible for topical versus systemic therapy. In a recent consensus, mild disease was defined as body surface area (BSA) less than 10%, psoriasis area severity index (PASI) less than 10, and dermatology life quality index (DLQI) less than 10. Mild psoriasis defined in this way can usually be controlled by topical therapy. In resistant cases, the addition of phototherapy should be considered. Patients with mild psoriasis, as indicated by the somatic scores BSA and PASI, may present with disease manifestation impairing the quality of life to a degree that systemic therapy is indicated. This includes involvement of visible areas,

Psoriasis: Diagnosis and Management, First Edition. Edited by Wolfram Sterry, Robert Sabat, and Sandra Philipp.

major parts of the scalp, genitals, palms, and/or soles, significant nail involvement, severe pruritus, and presence of recalcitrant plaques.

To improve treatment outcomes from topical therapy, it is important not only to choose among the available treatments but also to select patients suitable for topicals. Factors involved in patient and drug selection include the following:

- patient selection:
  - location of psoriasis;
  - severity of skin lesions;
  - response to previous therapy;
  - patients acceptance of benefit–risk profile of therapy;
  - patient preferences;
  - treatment cost;
- drug selection:
  - drug class;
  - strength;
  - vehicle;
  - frequency of application;
  - monotherapy or combination therapy;
  - treatment duration.

Patient selection depends on body location, characteristics of skin lesions, response to previous therapies, patient acceptance of the benefit–risk profile, patient preferences and expectations, and treatment costs. Psoriasis on the palms and soles requires a treatment strategy different from that of facial psoriasis. Patient fear of side-effects from topical corticosteroids has a negative impact on adherence. Topical treatment regimens for psoriasis can be complex and difficult to follow over longer periods of time. Patient preferences for different vehicles affect their use, and careful instructions may be required, including guidance by trained nurses in a day-care setting.

To select a proper topical agent, it is important to know which factors determine the safety and efficacy of the respective topical agent. The bioavailability of a topical agent is dependent on the type of psoriasis, the drug metabolism in the skin, the vehicle, the barrier function, the specific location of psoriasis, the drug concentration, and the frequency of application. Although there is some disturbance of barrier function in lesional psoriatic skin as evidenced by increased transepidermal water loss, barrier recovery following tape stripping is still fully functional. In normal skin, molecules with a molecular weight above 500 Da are not capable of crossing the stratum corneum (the 500 Da rule). The fact that topical tacrolimus (molecular weight 802 Da) is not effective for treating psoriasis lesions on trunk and extremities but is effective for atopic dermatitis illustrates that the epidermal barrier is to some extent conserved in psoriasis. The lipophilicity of a molecule may also result in increased skin penetration. The barrier function of the skin is based not only on the physicochemical properties of the stratum corneum but also on the presence of drug-metabolizing enzymes. Most drugs are inactivated by cytochrome P450 enzymes. Moreover, expression of drug-metabolizing enzymes is increased in psoriasis.

Topicals are available in various vehicles, including creams, ointments, lotions, gels, solutions, drugs, shampoos, and tape. In this context, it is important to realize that the vehicle can have a therapeutic effect by itself. In some clinical studies, response rates of over 30% have been reported with the vehicle alone. It is generally assumed that ointments are more effective than creams and other water-containing formulations. Lipid-rich occluding vehicles may enhance bioavailability by facilitating penetration of the drug. Accordingly, betamethasone and mometasone ointments are classified as being more potent than the respective creams. This superiority of ointment as a vehicle has recently been questioned. The bioavailability of betamethasone valerate from topical formulations was assessed in relation to the lipid content of the formulation. It was found that the efficacy of betamethasone valerate with a low-lipid-content formulation was greater than that of high-lipid content formulations, and low-lipid-content formulations were associated with a higher degree of blanching. These results suggest that earlier claims of superior efficacy of cream formulations are not only due to increased adherence with cosmetically more acceptable formulations.

Individual vehicle ingredients can be added to enhance bioavailability of a topical agent. A classical example is propylene glycol, which has been shown to increase percutaneous absorption of hydrocortisone through the skin by 12-fold. By addition of prophylene glycol to betamethasone dipropionate, the potency ranking is changed from potent to superpotent.

The role of the location of psoriasis in determining bioavailability is underscored by the therapeutic response to topical tacrolimus of facial and intertriginous lesions, but not of trunk/limb lesions. The scalp skin has distinct properties that affect drug penetration. It is covered by hair and contains pilosebaceous glands, and these two factors may explain the higher resistance of scalp psoriasis to steroid efficacy as well as side-effects such as atrophy. Psoriasis of the nails is extremely recalcitrant to topical treatment because the nail bed and matrix are poorly accessible for traditional topical drug formulations.

There is a paucity of pharmacokinectic data dealing with the optimal dose–response characteristics of topical agents. In a study of topical bioavailability of triamcinolone acetonide, the dosing frequency of application on the forearms of volunteers was studied. The application of higher triamcinolone doses multiple times resulted in a higher drug levels in the first few hours after application. However, after 24 h, the drug levels were independent of the dosing frequency.

A critical aspect of response to topical therapy is adherence. Studies addressing this topic show that up to 40% of psoriasis patients are self-admittedly nonadherent. Adherence is better early in the course of treatment and more likely when topical agents are used only once daily. Poor adherence to treatment is considered to explain insufficient treatment outcomes. The reasons why patients do not use their medication as directed include intolerance to medication, lack of therapeutic response, inconvenient vehicle, time constraints, use of topicals in the setting of extensive disease, and fear of side-effects. Also, cost and unclear instructions are important factors. It is, therefore, important to prescribe topical treatment regimens as simply as possible, to allow for patients' preferences regarding vehicle, and to provide instructions and guidance; where available, this may involve instruction by a nurse. The best results are obtained when the dermatologist shows an interest in their patient's disease. This involves a thorough skin examination and a commitment to follow up on the prescribed treatment.

For the topical management of psoriasis, a number of drugs are available:

- corticosteroids;
- vitamin D analogs;
- retinoids;
- tar products;
- dithranol/anthralin;
- calcineurin inhibitors.

Corticosteroids are also available in combination with the vitamin D analog calcipotriol and salicylic acid. Corticosteroids and calcipotriol are considered to be the most useful topical agents. Clinically rigorous assessments according to the current standards of evidence-based medicine, including placebo-controlled studies and head-to-head comparisons, are restricted to vitamin D analogs and some of the corticosteroids. In particular, the evidence behind the usage of topicals for the long-term management of psoriasis is lacking except for vitamin D analogs and superpotent corticosteroids. Therefore, it is not possible to define and recommend a therapeutic ranking list from currently available evidence-based data. Also, the availability of the various topicals varies between and within different countries. Topicals are used for chronic plaques and acute guttate lesions as well as pustular lesions. It should, however, be emphasized that the clinical studies have almost exclusively been conducted in chronic plaque psoriasis.

Corticosteroid

Corticosteroids are believed to act by binding to the cytosolic glucocorticosteroid receptor. Activated glucocorticosteroid receptors then modulate a number of nuclear transcription factors including the nuclear factor kappa-B transcription elements. A wide range of favorable and potentially unfavorable biological responses from corticosteroids have been identified, including direct effects on dendritic cell differentiation and function, lymphocyte apoptosis, toll-like receptor regulation, cytokine inhibition, collagenase, and elastase expression. These actions result in anti-inflammatory, antiprofilerative, immunosuppressive, and vasoconstrictive effects. Corticosteroids are available in many strengths and formulations which allows for diversity of use.

A number of factors determine the safety and efficacy of different corticosteroids, including also the corticosteroid molecule itself. Halogenation of corticosteroids markedly increased the efficacy. Halogene substitution of the C6, C9, or C21 side chain of the corticosteroid molecule can increase both the efficacy and the side-effects. The lipophilicity of the molecule also results in an increased permeation. Potency is classified according to the Stoughton–Cornell system on the basis of a vasoconstriction assay and clinical activity. Classification systems differ by country as shown in Table 17.1. In this context, it is important to notice that corticosteroids in the US and UK are classified in order of decreasing potency, while the opposite is the case for the German/Nordic classification. For practical purposes, corticosteroids are in the following categorized as having low, moderate, high, or superhigh potency. Corticosteroids of low to moderate potency are mainly used on face and intertriginous areas and in children, whereas high-potency corticosteroids are typically used as initial therapy on other areas in adults. Superpotent corticosteroids are mainly used for persistent plaques and for palms and soles. Daily use in the initial treatment phase may result in rapid improvement within 4 weeks in up to 46–56% for potent corticosteroids (betamethasone dipropionate) and in up to 68–89% for superpotent corticosteroids (clobetasol).

Topical corticosteroids can be associated with many potentially untoward effects including cutaneous atrophy, formation of teleangiectasia, development of striae, steroid rosacea and perioral dermatitis, hypothalamic–pituitary–adrenal (HPA) axis suppression, and skin infections. Striae are permanent and difficult to treat, while teleangiectasia and atrophy may be long-lasting or permanent. The potential for side-effects is often associated with prolonged and/or widespread use and usually correlates with increased clinical potency. The face and the intertriginous areas are particularly sensitive to these effects. Systemic absorption of corticosteroids may lead to laboratory evidence of adrenal suppression, and risk factors include high-potency corticosteroids, occlusive or prolonged treatment duration, and use in thin-skinned areas. Children are more susceptible to these systemic side-effects, because of their smaller body mass in relation to their surface area involved. However, nonreversible secondary adrenal insufficiency has not been documented.

Table 17.1 Comparison of corticosteroid potency classifications in the US, UK, and Germany/Nordic countries.

Potency	US Classification	UK Classification	German/Nordic Classification
Superpotent	I	I	IV
High potency	II/III	II	III
Moderate potency	IV/V	III	II
Low potency	VI/VII	IV	I

To choose the appropriate corticosteroid, the first consideration is the corticosteroid strength. This depends on the location of psoriasis and the lesion severity. Then, one has to take into account the individual patients' characteristics; e.g. potent corticosteroids may be avoided in children and elderly patients because of a higher risk for skin atrophy. Finally, the vehicle is chosen; this depends on the location of psoriasis as well as the patient's preference. As initial therapy, corticosteroids of lower potency are mainly used on the face and intertriginous areas, and in children, whereas moderate to potent corticosteroids are used on all other areas in adults. Superpotent corticosteroids are mainly used on the palms and/or soles and other refractory plaques. Initially, corticosteroids may be applied twice daily, but there are no data supporting the notion that more frequent applications lead to better or faster improvement. To optimize adherence, application once daily is often recommended. For potent corticosteroid treatment, 4–8 weeks of everyday use is acceptable. Longer continuous use requires supervision. In general, the amount of corticosteroids should not ecceed 50–60 g per week. To help patients dose their topical corticosteroids, the fingertip unit concept or dosing devices may be used. Whenever topical corticosteroids must be discontinued, they should be tapered off because abrupt discontinuation may lead to a rebound (see below).

Generally, it is assumed that ointments are more effective than creams and other water-containing formulations of corticosteroids. This is reflected in the US classifications where ointments are classified as more potent than creams. This concept has recently been challenged by the finding that betamethasone valerate in a low-lipid vehicle resulted in a higher degree of blanching than a high-lipid vehicle. It is recommended that the vehicle for corticosteroids be chosen according to the patient's preferences. To increase adherence, the optimal choice is generally the vehicle the individual patient most likely will use.

Rebound and tachyphylaxis are concerns when dealing with corticosteroid therapy. Rebound represents a rapid and atypical recurrence of disease upon discontinuation of treatment. After superpotent corticosteroids, even pustular transformation of psoriasis can occur. Although reported, the frequency and severity of such events have not been adequately studied. Tachyphylaxis is a progressive loss of efficacy on continued use of treatment. Tachyphylaxis was identified by du Vivier and Staughton and recently reviewed by Feldman. It is believed that nonadherence to treatment to some extent may explain tachyphylaxis.

While corticosteroid treatment usually is simple and effective in the initial phase of therapy, it is a challenge to use the potent corticosteroids for long-term management of psoriasis without causing cutaneous side-effects. Strategies to improve safety for long-term use of corticosteroids include treatment regimens that minimize side-effects, combination with other topical agents, following package-insert recommendations, careful consideration of use in vulnerable areas, and conservative use in children. A modification in daily dosing is necessary when patients require long-term therapy. One regimen is weekend or pulse therapy where three or four consecutive superpotent corticosteroid doses of 12 h intervals are applied on weekends, following a successful initial cleared or almost cleared therapeutic response to daily superpotent corticosteroid use. Using this treatment regimen, many patients can maintain remission without evidence of skin atrophy.

Combining topical corticosteroids with other topical agents is another strategy to increase efficacy with fewer side-effects. Sequential polytherapy with a superpotent corticosteroid in combination with a vitamin D analog can maximize short-term efficacy and minimize side-effects in long-term treatment. A simpler combination is the fixed combination of calcipotriol and betamethasone dipropionate. In a prospective, double-blind, parallel group study, there was no increase in corticosteroid-related side-effects after treatment for 1 year with this combination product. Because treatment was used as needed, these results likely reflect intermittent long-term use. The fixed combination of calcipotriol and betamethasone dipropionate is also available as a gel, making it possible for patients to switch to a cosmetically more acceptable formulation for long-term treatment.

Because of its keratolytic effect, salicylic acid can be used for the descaling of psoriatic lesions. Also, salicylic acid has been shown to enhance the efficacy of corticosteroids by increasing their penetration. These observations have led to the development of products combining corticosteroids with salicylic acid. Betamethasone dipropionate combined with 3% salicylic acid has a similar efficacy to that of clobetasol in comparative trials. Fixed dose combinations of salicylic acid 3% and betamethasone dipropionate are available as ointment and lotion in some markets. These formulations are particularly recommended for applications to limited skin areas for thick scaly plaques. Salicylic acid is generally safe. However, systemic salicylic acid toxicity can occur after long-term use on large skin areas.

Some topical corticosteroids are alleged to have an improved benefit–risk profile. Thus, mometasone fourate has limited penetration, and fluticasone propionate is rapidly metabolized to inactive products so that the duration of the effect on the skin is minimized. In both instances, the safety profile should be improved; however, the efficacy may also be decreased due to limited penetration and rapid breakdown, respectively.

Vitamin D analogs

Vitamin D analogs bind to the nuclear vitamin D receptor, and following dimer formation with members of the nuclear receptor superfamily, the receptor activation results in modulation of genes involved in epidermal proliferation, inflammation and keratinization. At present, there are three vitamin D analogs available for the treatment of psoriasis, calcitriol, tacalcitol, and calcipotriol, although not all are universally available.

Calcitriol is the hormonally active form of vitamin D. A dose of 3 μg/g calcitriol ointment applied twice daily is effective and safe for the short-term treatment of psoriasis. Calcitriol may be particularly useful for facial and intertriginous psoriasis because of its less irritative potential. Treatment with calcitriol may be continued according to clinical need, although the long-term efficacy and safety are only established in open-label treatment applied intermittently for 1 year.

Tacalcitol is a synthetic vitamin D analog. Tacalcitol ointment 4 μg/g applied once daily is effective and safe for short-term treatment. Formulated in an emulsion, tacalcitol has been found to be efficacious as well as well tolerated for the treatment of scalp psoriasis. Long-term efficacy and safety have been reported in an open-label study.

Calcipotriol (or calcipotriene in the USA) is a synthetic vitamin D analog with a low calcemic effect. It is the most extensively studied vitamin D analog for psoriasis. Calcipotriol ointment and cream 50 μg/g applied twice daily is effective and tolerated in adults and children for short-term as well as long-term treatment. Treatment with calcipotriol is safe in amounts up to 100 g per week. Because of its irritating potential, calcipotriol cream should be used with caution on the face and intertriginous areas. Treatment is frequently continued on a maintenance basis. Long-term efficacy and safety are established in a controlled study allowing therapy as needed for 1 year.

To improve the benefit–risk profile, the vitamin D analogs are sometimes used in combination with a topical corticosteroid. The rationale behind this combination is that the corticosteroid component inhibits vitamin D-induced skin irritation and that the combination improves efficacy, thereby decreasing the total amount of corticosteroids used. Calcitriol ointment 0.03% in combination with betamethasone valerate (each applied separately once daily) is as efficacious as twice-daily betamethasone valerate, thereby achieving a corticosteroid-sparing effect. Several studies have shown that a combination of calcipotriol in the morning and a corticosteroid in the evening is more effective than either agent administered as monotherapy and that reduced skin irritation may be achieved. Unfortunately, a number of corticosteroids cannot be mixed with calcipotriol because the drugs are incompatible and will degrade when mixed. The development of a new ointment vehicle has made it possible to combine calcipotriol and betamethasone dipropionate in a single vehicle. The combination of calcipotriol and betamethasone dipropionate has proven to be superior to either individual component for short-term therapy. Also, the tolerability (skin irritation) is similar to that of corticosteroid alone. While calcipotriol alone is approved for long-term treatment, concern prevails over the long-term use of topical corticosteroids because of the potential for steroid-related side-effects. It is, therefore, reassuring that a long-term study for 52 weeks' duration showed no increase in steroid-related side-effects. Furthermore, efficacy was maintained in patients that were allowed to use the combination product on average for up to 1 year.

The combination of calcipotriol and betamethasone dipropionate has also become available as a lipophilic gel formulation for scalp psoriasis as well as psoriasis on the trunk and limbs. Being cosmetically more acceptable, the two-compound gel may be preferable for the long-term topical treatment of psoriasis.

Tazarotene

Tazarotene is a synthetic retinoid with a selective affinity for the retinoic acid receptor. It has been shown to have antiproliferative and anti-inflammatory activities. Teratogenic aspects of topical tazarotene are only of concern if more than 20% of the BSA is treated. Tazarotene (0.05% or 0.01%) is available as gel and cream formulations. Although effective for short-term therapy, tazarotene often results in significant skin irritation such as pruritus, erythema, burning, and desquamation within, and especially in the periphery of, the treated lesions. This skin irritation may be decreased by applying tazarotene in conjunction with a topical corticosteroid. Tazarotene can protect against corticosteroid-induced skin atrophy. This clinically relevant observation remains, however, to be fully explored.

Dithranol (anthralin)

Dithranol (anthralin) is 1,8-dihydroxy-9-anthrone. It induces a cascade of free radicals in the skin resulting in antiproliferative effects and modulation of inflammation in psoriasis. The inhibition of adenosine triphosphate leads to damage of mitochondria and thereby may account for additional antiproliferative effects of dithranol. Depending on the market, dithranol is available as a cream, ointment, and paste. The dithranol molecule is unstable, and standardization of dithranol formulations is poor. Although a time-honoured treatment, there is a shortage of evidence to substantiate the efficacy and safety of this treatment. Because of its irritating and staining effects, dithranol is primarily used as treatment for patients in a day-care setting.

There exist two treatment regimens for dithranol: classical 24 h therapy and short contact therapy. With classical therapy, a low concentration (0.1%) is applied initially twice daily without being washed off. According to the degree of skin irritation, the concentration of dithranol is doubled every 3 days; thereby, a concentration of 1–3% may be reached. With the short contact therapy, dithranol 1% cream is applied to lesions for 5–10 min and then removed by rinsing with warm water. The exposure time is gradually extended to 10–30 min depending on the skin irritation. The use of dithranol in hospital base or day-care clinics with trained personal can be highly effective. There is no evidence for long-term cutaneous or systemic toxicity with dithranol therapy.

Tar

Tars are distillation products of organic material, including wood, shale, and coal. Tars, in particular, coal tar, have been used for psoriasis for more than 100 years. Coal tar has several hundred chemical constituents. Its exact mode of action is unknown, although it has antiproliferative effects and modulates inflammatory processes in psoriasis. Being a natural mixture of many chemicals, the standardization of tar products is poor. Side-effects of tar include immediate and long-term effects. Messiness, staining, odour, irritation, allergic and phototoxic skin responses, folliculitis, and bronchoconstriction in asthmatic patients are the most important immediate side-effects. Although occupational exposure to coal tar is associated with an increased risk of lung, scrotal, and skin cancer, carcinogenicity following coal tar applications in psoriasis and atopic dermatitis remains unsubstantiated. However, used in combination with phototherapy, coal tar is implicated as a risk factor for carcinogenicity.

In addition to crude coal tar, tar can be applied in solution, cream, and shampoo. Despite a shortage of controlled studies supporting the efficacy of coal tar, coal tar has traditionally been considered to have a longer-lasting effect than topical corticosteroids. To overcome the limitations of traditional coal tar preparations, new formulations have been developed. One of these contains liquor carbonis distillate 15%, equivalent to 2.3% coal tar, in a liquid wax vehicle designed to be easy to apply and to have reduced odour and staining properties. After application twice daily for 12 weeks, this formulation was found to be effective as well as well tolerated and cosmetically acceptable compared with calcipotriol cream. Despite this apparent progress, it is difficult to imagine that tar will regain its position as a first-line topical therapy for psoriasis.

Calcineurin inhibitors

Calcineurin inhibitors developed for topical treatments of atopic dermatitis include tacrolimus and pimecrolimus. Calcineurin inhibitors inhibit T-cell activation by inhibition of dephosphorylation of cellular nuclear factor of activated T-cell.

While tacrolimus and pimecrolimus are not effective for treatment of psoriasis on trunk and limbs in adults, they are effective in flexural and facial psoriasis. Compared with topical corticosteroids, calcineurin inhibitors may be attractive for treatment of psoriasis in face and skin folds, in particular, when treatment for longer periods of time is required. It should be stressed, however, that neither tacrolimus nor pimecrolimus is currently licensed for the treatment of psoriasis.

Comparative efficacy and safety of topical treatments

It is difficult to compare the various topical treatments of psoriasis because clinically rigorous assessments according to the current standards of evidence-based medicine, including placebo-controlled studies and head-to-head comparative studies, are largely restricted to vitamin D analogs and superpotent corticosteroids. In 2009, a Cochrane review of topical psoriasis therapy included 131 randomized trials with 21,448 participants. The evidence from these trials indicates that most of the topical treatments improve psoriasis. However, it was not possible to assess the performance of treatments at different levels of disease severity. The evidence suggests that vitamin D products are more effective than vehicle alone. Potent and superpotent corticosteroids are also effective, and superpotent corticosteroids are more effective than either potent corticosteroid or vitamin D products. The effectiveness of dithranol and tazarotene appears to be similar to that of vitamin D products. Although vitamin D and potent corticosteroids are equally effective for treating psoriasis of the body, potent corticosteroids appear to be more effective than vitamin D for treating psoriasis of the scalp. Combined treatment of vitamin D and corticosteroids is more effective than either vitamin D alone or corticosteroids alone. Vitamin D is more effective than coal tar, while findings on the relative effectiveness of vitamin D and dithranol were mixed. Occlusion enhanced the effectiveness of vitamin D as a twice-daily dose compared with once-daily application.

Management of psoriasis on scalp, face, flexures, palms, soles, and nails

Psoriasis on the scalp, face, skin folds, palms, soles, and nails may require special consideration because the efficacy and safety of topicals may be different.

Scalp psoriasis is difficult to treat because the surface skin of the scalp skin is relatively inaccessible, thus reducing the effectiveness of topical therapies. Also, patients' satisfaction with currently available treatments is low, primarily due to the lack of efficacy and difficulty in applying treatment. Convenience and a non-greasy formulation rank high on patients' wishes for an ideal treatment. For the treatment of scalp psoriasis, the vehicle used can be either rinsed as a shampoo or left on the scalp, typically overnight. Topical corticosteroids are the mainstay of treatment for scalp psoriasis. Corticosteroids delivered as ointments are considered to be more potent than those delivered with other vehicles. Recent studies, however, have found that vehicles such as lotions increase the ability of the active ingredients to penetrate the skin. Also, clobetasol propionate and betamethasone valerate have become available as shampoo and low-residue foam vehicle. Delivered in such vehicles, the treatment becomes more convenient, which might improve patients' adherence. Clobetasol shampoo, used initially once daily and for maintenance twice weekly, has been demonstrated to be safe and effective for scalp psoriasis. A lipophilic gel combining betamethasone dipropionate and calcipotriol is available for use on the scalp. This two-compound gel is more effective than either monotherapy and does not require pretreatment with descaling formulations. Furthermore, it has been shown to be effective and safe for long-term treatment for up to 1 year. In patients with thick scaling psoriasis, keratolytic agents, in particular salicylic acid, may be beneficial. Keratolytics may be used at the start of the treatment to remove scales and thereby improve penetration of other topical therapies. Also, salicylic acid is used in fixed combination with betamethasone dipropionate. Salicylic acid should not be mixed with vitamin D analogs due to chemical incompatibility. In very thick scaly scalp psoriasis, petrolatum or plant oil may be applied at bed time, sometimes occluded overnight with a shower cap, and washed off in the morning. After removal of scales, a topical agent in a more convenient vehicle may be used.

Psoriasis of face and flexures may be difficult to treat because of the increased risk of corticosteroid-related side-effects including skin atrophy. Therefore, only low- to moderate-potency corticosteroids are recommended. In patients requiring treatment for longer time periods, vitamin D analogs and calcineurin inhibitors should be considered. Among the vitamin D analogs, calcitriol causes less skin irritation than calcipotriol. Because of their minimal irritative potential, the calcineurin inhibitors tacrolimus and pimecrolimus may be first-line treatment for facial and flexural psoriasis, particularly when long-term treatment is required. Bacterial overgrowth and candida infection can occur in intertriginious psoriasis. However, antimicrobial therapy should only be added to the antipsoriatic treatment if clinical signs of infection are present.

Palmoplantar psoriasis appears in plaque-type- and pustular-type psoriasis, both being relatively resistant to topical therapy. A superpotent corticosteroid alone or a potent corticosteroid in combination with calcipotriol can be tried. Occlusion of the corticosteroid under plastic or a hydrocolloid dressing increases the speed and degree of improvement of palmo-plantar psoriasis. However, fast recurrence is usually the case. In recalcitrant patients, the impaired quality of life can justify systemic therapy.

The effects of topical agents are usually disappointing in nail psoriasis. Topical corticosteroids and calcipotriol alone or in combination may be tried. Alternatively, corticosteroids may be injected into the nail fold or nail bed. Innovations in corticosteroid formulation are provided in nail lacquers. In a small study, 8% clobetasol nail lacquer improved nail psoriasis after only 4 weeks of treatment. In severe nail psoriasis, systemic therapy should be considered.

Further reading

Brown, K.K., Rehmus, W.E. and Kimball, A.B. (2006) Determining the relative importance of patient motivations for nonadherence to topical corticosteroid therapy in psoriasis. *Journal of the American Academy of Dermatology*, **55**, 607–613.

Cornell, R.C. and Stoughton, R.B. (1985) Correlation of the vasoconstriction assay and clinical activity in psoriasis. *Archives of Dermatology*, **121**, 63–67.

Horn, E.J., Domm, S., Katz, H.I., Lebwohl, M., Mrowietz, U. and Kragballe, K. (2010) Topical corticosteroids in psoriasis: strategies for improving safety. *Journal of the European Academy of Dermatology and Venereology*, **24**, 119–124.

Jemec, G.B., Ganslandt, C., Ortonne, J.P., *et al.* (2008) A new scalp formulation of calcipotriene plus betamethasone compared with its active ingredients and the vehicle in the treatment of scalp psoriasis: a randomized, double-blind, controlled trial. *Journal of the American Academy of Dermatology*, **59**, 455–463.

Katz, H.I., Prawer, S.E., Medansky, R.S. *et al.* (1991) Intermittent corticosteroid maintenance treatment of psoriasis: a double-blind multicentre trial of augmented betamethasone dipropionate ointment in a pulse dose treatment regimen. *Dermatologica*, **183**, 269–274.

Kragballe, K., Austad, J., Barnes, L. *et al.* (2006) A 52-week randomized safety study of a calcipotriol/betamethasone dipropionate two-compound product (Daivobet/Dovobet/Taclonex) in the treatment of psoriasis vulgaris. *British Journal of Dermatology*, **154**, 1155–1160.

Kragballe, K. (2009) Management of difficult to treat locations of psoriasis. In: N. Yawalkar (ed.), Vol. **38**, pp. 159–170. *Management of Psoriasis. Current Problems in Dermatology*. Karger, Basel.

Kragballe, K. (2009) Management of difficult to treat locations of psoriasis: scalp, face, flexures, palm/soles and nails. *Current Problems in Dermatology*, **38**, 159–170.

Mason, A.R., Mason, J., Cork, M., Dooley, G. and Edwards, G. (2009) Topical treatments for chronic plaque psoriasis. *Cochrane Database of Systemic Reviews*, **3**, CD005028.

Nast, A., Kopp, I.B., Augustin, M. *et al.* (2007) Evidence-based (S3) guidelines for the treatment of psoriasis vulgaris. *Journal der Deutschen Dermatologischen Gesellschaft*, **5** (Supplement), 1–119.

van de Kerkhof, P.C. (1992) Dithranol treatment for psoriasis: after 75 years still going strong. *European Journal of Dermatology*, **1**, 79–88.

PHOTOTHERAPY AND PHOTOCHEMOTHERAPY

Erhard Hölzle

Department of Dermatology and Allergology, Klinikum Oldenburg, Oldenburg, Germany

History

Phototherapy

Therapy of skin diseases with sunlight (heliotherapy) dates back to ancient times and was known in ancient Greece and Egypt. In recent times, Goeckerman was the first to treat psoriasis with sunlight exposures in combination with topical tar application. A combination of topical anthralen with a tar bath and successive ultraviolet B (UVB) irradiation was introduced by Ingram and became known as the "Ingram Scheme," which remained a standard therapeutic regimen for decades.

In 1981, Parish and Jaenicke demonstrated that wavelengths shorter than 296 nm were almost ineffective, but the 304–313 nm bands exerted an optimal efficacy even when suberythemogenic doses were used. New fluorescent lamps were developed (Philips TL 01) to match this therapeutic action spectrum. These fluorescent tubes, today known as 311 nm narrow-band UV (NB-UVB) sources, led to a breakthrough in phototherapy, and these lamps are now regarded as the standard in UV treatment of psoriasis and other UV-responsive skin disorders.

Balneophototherapy

In balneophototherapy, saline baths are combined with UVB irradiation. The approach follows the climatotherapy that is practiced in the resorts of the North Sea, Baltic Sea, and Dead Sea. Mostly industrial NaCl is used but various combinations are designed in an attempt to imitate Dead Sea water.

Photochemotherapy

The principal of photochemotherapy was already known in ancient Egypt. El Mofty in 1948 described the mechanism of this popular Egyptian folk medicine mainly used to treat vitiligo. He indentified furocoumarins as the active ingredients in the used plants. Parish *et al.*, at Harvard University in Boston, developed systemic photochemotherapy combining 8-methoxypsoralen with whole-body ultraviolet A irradiation (PUVA). This was made possible by the development of new high-intensity UVA fluorescent tubes suitable for whole-body exposure. This classical type of photochemotherapy became the standard in the United States and spread across Central Europe. In Scandinavia, bath PUVA therapy with trimethylpsoralen was used from the beginning. In the 1980s, the use of PUVA baths with 8-methoxypsoralen has enjoyed a renaissance in Central Europe and in the United States because it is much better tolerated than oral 8-methoxypsoralen.

Requirements for phototherapy and photochemotherapy

There are several technical and procedural requirements, and the key points of these are listed below.

Technical requirements:

- Light sources should be maintained properly and calibrated monthly to ensure accurate dosimetry.
- Room temperature should be relatively uniform, and air conditioning might be required in warmer climates. Irradiation apparatuses should be arranged in a way that ensures patients' privacy.
- On the other hand, nursing personnel always must be able to communicate with the patients.
- The bath facilities used for balneophototherapy should be in the proximity of the light sources.
- The medical personnel must be familiar with the technical aspects of the light sources, phototherapy protocols, and physiological and pathological cutaneous

reactions to UV irradiation. If a consultation is required, a physician must always be immediately available.

Procedural requirements:

- Indications and contraindications have to be carefully considered. Absolute contraindications include genetic disorders with increased photosensitivity and increased carcinogenic risk such as xeroderma pigmentosum, Cockayne's syndrome, and Bloom's syndrome.
- Relative contraindications represent seizures, necessary but potentially photo-sensitizing medications, atypical nevi, and a history of skin cancer or genuine photosensitivity. In these cases, special care must be taken, including close supervision and modified therapeutic schemes.
- The patient must be informed about the details of the planned therapy, the side-effects to be expected, and the long-term risks. He should give informed written consent, at least, if photochemotherapy is conducted.
- UV doses administered should be measured in J/cm^2 and documented in a permanent record. After each course of therapy, the number of treatments and total UV dose should once again be recorded.
- During a treatment course, patients should be regularly examined by a physician, preferably weekly. Response to therapy, side-effects, and accompanying therapy should be noted.
- Eye protection during UV exposure is an absolute prerequisite of UV therapy. If areas with chronic sun exposure, such as head, neck, back of the hands, are not affected by psoriatic lesions, they should be shielded during irradiation.
- In children, phototherapy is generally possible. However, the child must wear eye protection and be capable of cooperating with the treating protocol. Indications have to be considered carefully. Photochemotherapy should be an exemption. Oral photochemotherapy should not be used below the age of 16, and PUVA-bath therapy not below the age of 10 years. It is advisable to apply doses in the suberythema range, and cumulative doses should be kept as low as possible.

Phototherapy

Action spectra

In general, NB-UVB is used for treating psoriasis, and its efficacy is almost equal to that of PUVA therapy. As an alternative, broadband UVB (BB-UVB) may be employed, but several studies have documented the superiority of NB-UVB over BB-UVB in terms of efficacy and tolerability. As far as the presumed carcinogenic risk is concerned, both spectra are fairly similar in their potential risks. One advantage of NB-UVB, however, is its efficacy even in the suberythemogenic dose range. As a consequence, cumulative erythema doses for induction of skin clearance are lower, and so the carcinogenic risk is decreased.

Practical approach

Before starting phototherapy, it is recommended that the individual minimal erythema dose (MED) be determined using the type of UV source with the same emission spectrum as that of the source used for treating the patient. Alternatively the starting doses can be selected using a standard scheme based on the photo-skin type of the patient (Table 17.2).

The usual starting dose should be 70% of the individual MED. Since erythema after UVB irradiation peeks between 18 and 24 h, doses can be adjusted at each session. The increase varies between 10 and 30%, depending on the erythema response of the patient. The goal is to induce slight erythema, showing that the UV dose applied is as close as possible to the MED of the patient. If erythema persists, increments have to be lowered; if it is associated with burning, treatment must be interrupted, or at least any afflicted areas must be kept covered during successive irradiation until discomfort has subsided. Edema or blisters require complete cessation of UV treatment (Table 17.3) and should involve appropriate therapy to relieve symtoms.

After the skin has completely cleared, a long-lasting maintenance therapy is not indicated. This would only increase cumulative UV doses and has no or little effect in preventing recurrences. The idea is to achieve skin clearance as rapidly as possible with the lowest cumulative UV doses by combining phototherapy with

Table 17.2 Starting doses for UVB phototherapy.

Skin type	Broadband UVB (mJ/cm^2)	Narrowband UVB (311 nm) (mJ/cm^2)
I	20	200
II	30	300
III	50	500
IV	60	600

Table 17.3 Routine therapy plan for UVB phototherapy (broad spectrum and 311 nm).

Step 1	Determine MED	Reading after 24 Std.	
Step 2	Start therapy	First dose	70% of MED or follow standard plan
Step 3	Continue therapy 3–5 times weekly	No erythema	Increase by 30%
		Minimal erythema	Increase by 15–20%
		Persistent erythema	No change, consider reduction
		Painful erythema edema, blisters	No UVB until symptoms have resolved
Step 4	Restart therapy	Wait until symptoms have resolved	Reduce last dose by 50%, further increases by only 10%

topical and/or systemic agents. If phototherapy does not appear to be sufficiently effective, it might be wise to use other forms of therapy.

Balneophototherapy combines UVB irradiation with saline baths. For psoriasis treatment, 20% solutions of sodium chloride are mainly used, and the patient's skin is soaked for 15–20 min at a temperature of 37 °C. Oil can be added to the bath, and irradiation is performed immediately after the bath. By using a plastic sheet in the tub, the amount of saline solution needed can be reduced. A large sheet is placed over the tub, which is partially filled with water. Then, the patient lies on top of the sheet on which the saltwater is added.

Combination treatments

In treating psoriasis, a combination of UVB with topical and/or systemic agents is desirable. This accelerates the clearance of skin lesions and keeps cumulative UVB doses lower. As topical agents, corticosteroids, vitamin D_3 analogs, or anthralen may be used.

The most common systemic drug combined with UVB irradiation is the retinoid acitretin. This enhances the efficacy, particularly in hyperkeratotic lesions and palmoplantar psoriasis, and, as it does so in PUVA therapy, it may reduce the carcinogenic potential of UVB phototherapy. UVB also can be combined with methotrexate (MTX), but there is limited experience in using it with fumaric acid. Combination with cyclosporine should be avoided because this may enhance the carcinogenicity of UV irradiation.

Photochemotherapy

Treatment regimens

Photochemotherapy uses the combination of 8-methoxypsoralen and UVA (PUVA). The photosensitizer can be applied orally via tablets or topically using solutions of 8-methoxypsoralen (0.5–1.0 mg/L). In special cases, if only circumscribed lesions are to be treated, cream PUVA might be used (0.0006–0.005% 8-MOP in a standardized cream base). In Scandinavia, trimethylpsoralen (0.33 mg/L) is used for PUVA baths.

Bath PUVA has been shown to be as effective as oral PUVA but is much better tolerated. Topical toxicity is related to dose-dependent phototoxic skin reactions and can be avoided by lower starting doses and careful dose increments. Systemic adverse effects are virtually absent.

Indications and contraindications

PUVA is indicated in moderate to severe plaques psoriasis and in pustular, palmoplantar, as well as generalized psoriasis. Oral PUVA should not be used before the age of 16 years, and topical PUVA might be used in children above 10 years. In childhood, photochemotherapy should be restricted to selected cases and should be performed with special caution. Because of potential acute and chronic side-effects, in any case, photochemotherapy must be used carefully. As is the case with phototherapy, PUVA can be combined with topical and systemic treatments to minimize side-effects and enhance efficacy. Patients should be informed about the principle of the procedure and should be particularly advised with regard to eye protection and additional UV exposure by sun or solaria. Full compliance of the patient is a prerequisite for photochemotherapy.

Absolute and relative contraindications of UV therapy were mentioned earlier in the list of procedural requirements. Further potential contraindications for PUVA include previous treatment with arsenic or ionizing radiation, use of photosensitizing medications that cannot be withdrawn, and chronic liver disease interfering with metabolism of 8-methoxypsoralen, thus making the sensitization phase irregular. PUVA is contraindicated in combination with cyclosporine. High total UV doses should be avoided, and it is recommended that PUVA be restricted to 150–200 treatment sessions.

Practical approach

In systemic PUVA, 8-methoxypsoralen is orally administered in tablets 2 h before irradiation. The dose is 0.6 mg/kg body weight. Using a PUVA bath, concentrations vary between 0.5 and 1.0 mg/L. The patient is soaked for 15–20 min, and the temperature of the solution should be 37 °C. Irradiation is performed immediately after bathing. If cream PUVA is performed, the application time of the cream should be 1 h, and irradiation should follow immediately after removal of the cream.

Patients must be advised to protect their skin from sun exposure and avoid artificial UV sources while their skin is photosensitized. After systemic administration of 8-methoxypsoralen, photosensitivity lasts for about 8–10 h. After PUVA bath, the skin is photosensitized for about 1–2 h, and after application of an 8-methoxypsoralen-containing cream, photosensitization may last up to 3 h.

In oral photochemotherapy, patients must wear UV-protective eye glasses during the entire period of photosensitization. The glasses must filter out UVA and UVB completely and should not be darkened, since glasses must also be worn on cloudy days as well as indoors.

Initially, the minimal phototoxic dose (MPD) should be determined. The starting dose of UVA should be 50–70% of the MPD or should follow a standard plan depending on the photo-skin type of the patient (Table 17.4). Determination of the MPD is fairly comparable with MED testing. Besides the use of a UVA spectrum identical to that of the therapeutic unit, it is also important to administer or apply the photosensitizer at the same dose and/or concentration, as it will be used for therapy. The test is read 72–96 h after exposure. The MPD determination is exactly reproducible for bath PUVA but varies for cream and oral PUVA, as the skin absorption and metabolism of 8-methoxypsoralen might differ among patients.

Table 17.4 Starting dosages for photochemotherapy.

Skin type	Oral PUVA (J/cm^2)	Bath PUVA (1.0 mg/L 8-MOP) (J/cm^2)
I	0.3	0.2
II	0.5	0.3
III	0.8	0.4
IV	1.0	0.6

Table 17.5 Routine approach to photochemotherapy.

			Oral PUVA	Bath PUVA
Step 1	Determine MPD		Read after 72–96 h	Read after 96 h
Step 2	Start therapy	Initial dose	50–70% of MPD or follow standard plan (Table 17.4)	30% of MPD or follow standard plan (Table 17.4)
Step 3	Continue 2–4 times weekly	No erythema	Increase by maximum 30% 2 times weekly	
		Minimal erythema	No increase	
		Persistent asymptomatic erythema	No increase, consider reduction	
		Painful erythema, edema, blisters	No PUVA until resolution	
Step 4	Restart therapy	Wait until symptoms have resolved	Reduce last dose by 50%, further increases by only 10%	

During the initial treatment phase, which lasts until complete remission, ideally four treatment sessions per week are scheduled. At a minimum, two may be performed. Dose increments should not be made more than twice weekly and never sooner than 72 h after a previous increase because of the delayed onset of PUVA erythema. There are no fixed rules, but the improvement in skin involvement and the individual tolerance of photochemotherapy are weighed up against each other. As in UVB treatment, a faintly visible erythema is considered to be ideal. Because of the risks of cumulative phototoxic overdoses, a patient should not be treated on more than two successive days. A typical schedule is to treat on Monday and Tuesday, and on Thursday and Friday. Recommendations for dose adjustments are given in Table 17.5.

Since bath PUVA causes more photosensitivity, lower UVA doses can be used. In addition, photosensitivity might increase during the first week so that MPD can decrease by as much as 50%. After that, the MPD normalizes again. After skin lesions have cleared, it might be useful to continue therapy on a reduced schedule. The value of a prolonged interval therapy or maintenance therapy is, however, poorly documented and not universally accepted.

Combination treatments

Photochemotherapy can be combined with topical therapy, preferably corticosteroids. Anthralen should be used with care, because it is potentially irritating, as are vitamin D analogs.

A combination with systemic agents is also possible, and the classical drug to be combined with PUVA is acitretin. This enhances the therapeutic effect of PUVA but also might decrease the carcinogenicity of photochemotherapy. PUVA can be combined with MTX, and it reduces the number of treatments and cumulative UVA doses needed for clearing skin lesions. Concerning fumaric acid, there is insufficient experience.

PUVA must not be combined with cyclosporine. It has been observed that PUVA, in combination with cyclosporine, enhances carcinogenicity, even if the treatments are applied successively.

Mechanisms of phototherapy and photochemotherapy

Immune suppression, altered cytokine expression, and cell-cycle arrest may contribute to the therapeutic effect of UV radiation in psoriasis.

As a consequence of formation of DNA photoproducts, mainly pyrimidine dimers, UVB reduces DNA synthesis and modulates cell cycle via induction of p53. This leads to a decrease in the accelerated epidermopoiesis and thus an improvement of psoriasis plaques.

An additional mechanism of action is modulation of the immune response with the net effect of immunosuppression, which has also been linked to the formation of pyrimidine dimers. The UV-induced release of interleukins 6 and 10 from keratinocytes is responsible for systemic symptoms of sunburn. This mechanism may also be involved in the therapeutic action of UVB. There is evidence that not only nuclear DNA damage but also UV effects on cell membranes and cytoplasmic targets contribute to biological effects of UV radiation.

In balneophototherapy, it is assumed that the saline solution changes the optical properties of the stratum corneum resulting in a lowered MED and, in addition, probably elutes proinflammatory mediators from the stratum corneum. Mg ions, which are abundant in Dead Sea water, are found to cause depletion and functional perturbation of human epidermal Langerhans cells.

PUVA induces crosslinks via photoaddition of psoralen to DNA, which leads to cell-cycle arrest and apoptosis of keratinocytes. PUVA-induced apoptosis is even more pronounced in lymphocytes than in keratinocytes, which may explain the high potency of PUVA in treating T-cell lymphoma, but also may be responsible for its effect in inflammatory skin diseases.

Besides psoralen-DNA photoproducts, other photochemical reactions may contribute to the phototoxicity. Photo-activated psoralens can react with oxygen to form reactive oxygen species such as singlet oxygen. This causes membrane damage and may activate the arachidonic acid metabolic pathway. Both may be responsible for the therapeutic effect as well as phototoxic side-effects.

Risks and side-effects of phototherapy and photochemotherapy

The most common side-effects are UV-induced sunburn-like reactions or excessive phototoxic reactions after PUVA. If eye protection is inadequate, acute conjunctivitis and keratitis may result. Chronic exposure from PUVA theoretically leads to cataracts. But despite the experimental data on animals indicating a risk of premature cataract formation, clinical evaluation has shown no increase in lens opacities, even in patients who have not worn eye protection.

A special problem of photochemotherapy might be the induction of PUVA pruritus, which is very difficult to treat and sometimes necessitates a cessation of PUVA. Rarely, acral blisters occur, probably caused by loosening of the dermoepidermal junction as in pseudoporphyria. Systemic toxicity caused by 8-methoxypsoralen includes nausea, dizziness, and headache.

One feature of chronic skin damage from UVB phototherapy and photochemotherapy is accelerated cutaneous aging (photoaging), and actinic lentigines, actinic keratoses, and cutaneous malignancies may also be induced. After UVB phototherapy, so far no enhanced risks for squamous or basal cell carcinomas have been observed, and this was also confirmed for NB-UVB. Enhancement of UV carcinogenesis by additional topical tar applications is, however, possible.

The prospective American PUVA follow-up study and clinical studies in Europe have shown a significant risk of squamous-cell carcinoma after PUVA with high cumulative doses or high numbers of treatment sessions, respectively. PUVA nowadays is performed more carefully in several ways. Patients are selected more carefully, treatment schedules are improved, and by using combination therapy and avoiding maintenance therapy, cumulative doses can be substantially reduced. Bath PUVA does not seem to enhance carcinogenicity. No substantial risk of inducing malignant melanoma by PUVA therapy has been observed.

Further reading

Goeckerman, W.H. (1925) The treatment of psoriasis. *Northwest Medicine*, **24**, 229–231.

Hannuksela-Svahn, A., Sigurgeirsson, B., Pukkala, E. *et al.* (1999) Trioxsalen bath PUVA did not increase the risk of squamous cell skin carcinoma and cutaneous malignant melanoma in a joint analysis of 944 Swedish and Finnish patients with psoriasis. *British Journal of Dermatology*, **141**, 497–501.

Ingram, J.T. (1953) The approach to psoriasis. *British Medical Journal*, **II**, 591–594.

Lowe, N.J., Weingarten, D. and Moly, L.S. (1986) PUVA therapy for psoriasis: comparison of oral and bathwater delivery of 8-methoxypsoralen. *Journal of the American Academy of Dermatology*, **14**, 754–760.

Parrish, J.A., Fitzpatrick, T.B., Tanenbaum, L. and Pathak, M.A. (1974) Photochemotherapy of psoriasis with oral methoxsalen and longwave ultraviolet light. *New England Journal of Medicine*, **291**, 1207–1211.

Parrish, J.A. and Jaenicke, K.F. (1981) Action spectrum for phototherapy of psoriasis. *Journal of Investigative Dermatology*, **76**, 359–362.

Stern, R.S., Liebman, E.J. and Vakeva, L. (1998) Oral psoralen and ultraviolet-A light (PUVA) treatment of psoriasis and persistent risk of nonmelanoma skin cancer. PUVA follow-up study. *Journal of the National Cancer Institute*, **90**, 1278–1284.

Van Weelden, H., De La Faille, H.B., Young, D. and Van der Leun, I.C. (1988) A new development in UVB phototherapy of psoriasis. *British Journal of Dermatology*, **119**, 11–19.

CLASSICAL SYSTEMIC TREATMENTS

Peter C.M. van de Kerkhof

Department of Dermatology, Radboud University Nijmegen Medical Centre, Nijmegen, Netherlands

Psoriasis is an immune-mediated polygenic skin disease. Various environmental trigger factors, such as trauma, infections, or medications, may elicit a psoriatic phenotype in predisposed individuals. Psoriasis not only affects the skin; in up to 30% of patients, psoriatic arthritis (PsA) occurs. In patients with moderate to severe psoriasis, comorbidities may complicate psoriasis. In particular, the relative risk for metabolic syndrome and cardiovascular disease is increased in these patients. Therefore, psoriasis should be regarded as a systemic disease.

The impact of psoriasis on quality of life is significant, given its chronicity and prevalence (up to 2% of the population). Pruritus, scaliness, and visible plaques are the signs and symptoms of most concern. In surveys, the majority of psoriatic patients indicate a serious impairment in their quality of life.

Therefore, it remains important to use the entire armamentarium of treatments in patients with psoriasis and to provide an adequate solution for the problems the patient experiences and beyond to provide adequate management of psoriasis as a systemic disease.

In this chapter, the classical systemic treatments are presented. First, we will address the general indication for systemic treatments. Then, we will provide relevant data on the available systemic treatments. Finally, we will present some guidance to position the available treatments in everyday practice.

When to consider a systemic treatment for your patient

Before considering a specific treatment in an individual psoriatic patient, it is important to exclude triggering factors of psoriasis: focal infections, medications and psychological stress. In case immunosuppressive treatments are prescribed in patients with an infection, not only is the chance of eliminating the trigger missed but also the patients may run the risk of an exacerbation of the infection. The choice of starting a systemic treatment should be based on the severity of psoriasis as a skin disease and the comorbidities. With respect to the assessment of severity of psoriasis, the objective severity, quality of life, and historical severity have to be reconciled:

- Objective severity: The area of involvement and the degree of erythema, induration, and desquamation of the cutaneous lesions have to be assessed. PASI is the scoring system that is used in clinical research and in many centers to assess disease severity in real clinical practice (see chapter 14). In a third of patients with psoriasis, the disease is moderate to severe, and a systemic treatment may be indicated.
- Quality of life: The impact of psoriasis on quality of life can be measured by various questionnaires (e.g. DLQI, Skindex29, see chapter 14).
- Responsiveness to previous treatments: Individual patients report a wide variation with respect to their clinical response to various treatments. For example, some patients with widespread disease may experience excellent improvement with a topical therapy, whereas patients with localized disease may prove recalcitrant to high-dose systemic treatments.

Concerning an individual patient, all different aspects have to be considered, and the decision to prescribe a systemic treatment and not a topical or UV therapy thus represents an individualized approach.

With respect to comorbidities, it remains of practical importance to be aware of early signs of arthritis. Arthritis in a patient is a very important indication for a systemic treatment, in order to prevent bone destruction. Metabolic syndrome is more frequent in patients with moderate to severe psoriasis, and patients with psoriasis have an increased risk of cardiovascular events.

In patients with signs and symptoms of the metabolic syndrome, it is important to treat psoriasis: It is highly likely that a reduction in the extensive inflammation of the lesional psoriatic skin will be beneficial for the further development of the metabolic syndrome, and certainly the cleared skin will help to motivate the patient to improve their lifestyles. Another consideration is the definition of treatment goals (see chapter 16) in plaque psoriasis. An international working group defined an important consensus: The change in PASI from baseline until the time of evaluation (ΔPASI) and the absolute DLQI were used. After induction and during maintenance therapy, treatment can be continued if the reduction in PASI is ≥75%. The treatment regimen should be modified if the improvement in PASI is <50%. In a situation where the therapeutic response improved ≥50% but <75%, as assessed by PASI, therapy should be modified if the DLQI is >5 but can be continued if the DLQI is ≤5.

In summary, treatment selection is a multivariable decision process and not a simple stepwise therapeutic ladder. If topical therapies and photo(chemo) therapy do not provide adequate improvement, or if comorbidities require treatment, a systemic agent is indicated.

Available systemic treatments

S-3 guidelines on the use of systemic treatments have been realized by a working group of the European Dermatology Forum.

MTX

In 1971, amethopterin (methotrexate, MTX) was approved by the FDA as a treatment for psoriasis. Although MTX causes a temporary inhibition of keratinocyte proliferation during the first 24h after a therapeutic dose, the effect of MTX on lymphocytes, circulating and cutaneous, is likely to be more relevant. Folate-pathway enzyme-gene polymorphisms may be associated with MTX efficacy and MTX induced livertoxicity in patients with psoriasis. However, in patients with psoriasis, the relevance of these polymorphisms is not yet clear.

For more than four decades, MTX has been a first-line systemic therapy for psoriasis, as it is highly efficacious for severe disease and all clinical variants of psoriasis. In chronic plaque psoriasis, initial improvement is observed between 1 and 7 weeks, and maximal improvement can be expected after 8–12 weeks of treatment. Initial clinical efficacy is highly dependent on the choice of a low-dose initiation with gradual dose increments or a high-dose initiation. The dosages of MTX range between 5 and 25 mg per week and are administered as a single weekly dosage or divided dose with three doses in 12 h intervals. Associated potential side-effects restrict its use to severe involvement resistant to topical treatments and photo(chemo)therapy and/or situations in which these are contraindicated. Folic acid supplementation during MTX is advised. It is mandatory that the guidelines for MTX be strictly followed.

In the European guidelines, the mechanism of action, pharmacology, and safety issues of MTX have been presented, and important side-effects, contraindications, instructions for use, and laboratory controls have been clearly outlined (Tables 17.6–17.8).

The instructions for the use of MTX and necessary measures are as follows:

- pretreatment:
  - history and clinical examination;
  - objective assessment of the disease (such as PASI/BSA/PGA; arthritis);
  - HRQoL (such as DLQI/Skindex-29 or -17);
  - laboratory parameters (see table 17.8);

Table 17.6 Overview of important side effects of MTX.

Very frequent	Nausea, malaise, hair loss
Frequent	Elevated transaminases, bone marrow suppression, gastrointestinal ulcers
Occasional	Fever, chills, depression, infections
Rare	Nephrotoxicity, liver fibrosis, cirrhosis
Very rare	Interstitial pneumonia, alveolitis

Table 17.7 Important contraindications/restrictions on use of MTX.

Absolute contraindications	Relative contraindications
Severe infections	Kidney or liver disorders
Severe liver disease	Old age
Renal failure	Ulcerative colitis
Conception (men and women/breastfeeding)	History of hepatitis
Alcohol abuse	Lack of compliance
Bone marrow dysfunctions/haematologic changes	Active desire to have a child for women of childbearing age and men
Immunodeficiency	Gastritis
Acute peptic ulcer	Diabetes mellitus
Significantly reduced lung function	Previous malignancies
	Congestive heart failure

Table 17.8 Lab controls during treatment with MTX.

	Period in weeks/months			
Parameter	**Pretreatment**	**After first week**	**During first 2 months, once every 2 weeks**	**Thereafter, every 2–3 months**
Blood count	x	x	x	x
Liver enzymes	x		x	x
Serum creatinine	x		x	x
Urine sediment	x		x	x
Pregnancy test (urine)	x			
HBV/HCV	x			
Serum albumin	x		x	x
PIIINP where available	x		Every 3 months	

Further specific testing may be required according to clinical signs, risks, and exposure.

  - chest X-ray;
  - contraception in women of child-bearing age (starting after menstruation), and also in men;
  - if abnormalities in liver screening are found, refer patient to specialist for further evaluation;
- during treatment:
  - objective assessment of the disease (such as PASI/BSA/PGA; arthritis);
  - HRQoL (such as DLQI/Skindex-29 or -17);
  - check concomitant medication;
  - clinical examination;
  - laboratory controls (see table 17.8);
  - contraception in women of child-bearing age, and also in men;

  - 5 mg of folic acid once weekly 24 h after MTX [evidence for the recommendation is scarce; thus, some of the voting experts felt that flexibility in the dosing of folic acid is warranted, suggesting dosing of 1–5 mg of folic acid per day (7 days a week) or 2.5 mg of folic acid once weekly 24 h after MTX];
- post-treatment:
  - women must not become pregnant and men must not conceive when they are taking the drug and for at least 3 months thereafter.

Hepatotoxicity is a side effect of MTX that requires adequate controls. A liver biopsy before treatment in patients at risk for liver impairment and subsequently after cumulative doses of 2 gr has been the approach for many years. Evidence is available showing that repeated measurements of blood procollagen III N-terminal peptide (PIIINP) levels can indicate the development of liver fibrosis, which permits a restriction of liver biopsies to those patients with increases of PIIINP. Additionally, imaging techniques like high-resolution sonography have been improved and can help to detect fibrosis. The question arises whether the occurrence of liver fibrosis/cirrhosis may be more frequent in psoriatic patients as compared with patients with rheumatoid disease. An increased frequency of nonalcoholic fatty liver disease (NAFLD) has been shown in psoriatic patients as compared with a control population, and an association with parameters for the metabolic syndrome was shown. Such patients with NAFLD are at increased risk for development of liver cirrhosis.

As MTX has an immunomodulatory effect, the question of the extent to which MTX may increase the frequency of malignancies has been addressed. MTX has been available for the treatment of psoriasis for four decades, and two studies have shown that there is no indication for an increased risk for malignancies in MTX-treated psoriatic patients.

Cyclosporine

Cyclosporine is a cyclic undecapeptide that was isolated from the fungus *Tolypocladium inflatium* by Gams in 1970. Cyclosporine is a highly effective treatment for severe psoriasis. As a calcineurin inhibitor, it prevents T-lymphocyte activation from being translated into the release of effector cytokines such as IL-2. Cyclosporine can be used safely, provided that the guidelines are strictly followed. Cyclosporine should be given for a maximum of 1–2 years in view of its nephrotoxic effects. An alternative is an intermittent schedule using multiple short courses of a few weeks' duration.

The pronounced efficacy of cyclosporine has been clearly shown in several studies. The European multicenter dose-finding studies have shown that dosages of 1.25, 2.5–3, and 5 mg/kg/day of cyclosporine resulted in PASI reductions of 35%, 57%, and 86%, respectively. An improvement in the PASI of 75% was achieved in 24%, 52%, and 88% of patients. Efficacy of cyclosporine has been demonstrated in all variants of psoriasis, including nail psoriasis and less so psoriatic arthropathy. The improvement is observed within a few weeks. In general, a PASI reduction of 60–70% can be reached within 4 weeks of treatment. During long-term treatment, there are no signs of tachyphylaxis. Cyclosporine can produce a dramatic rapid improvement of psoriasis, but this must be balanced by the need to have an appropriate replacement therapy, given the need to ultimately stop cyclosporine therapy.

Important side-effects, contraindications, instructions for use, and laboratory controls have been listed in the European guideline (Tables 17.9–17.11). The following measures are necessary in the use of cyclosporine.

Table 17.9 Overview of important side effects of cyclosporine.

Very frequent	None
Frequent	Renal failure (dose-dependent); danger of irreversible renal damage (long-term therapy); hypertension; gingival hyperplasia; reversible hepatogastric complaints (dose-dependent); tremor; weariness; headache; burning sensation in hands and feet; reversible elevated blood lipids (especially in combination with corticosteroids); hypertrichosis
Occasional	Seizures, gastrointestinal ulcerations, weight gain, hyperglycemia, hyperuricemia, hyperkalemia, hypomagnesemia, acne, anemia
Rare	Ischemic heart disease, pancreatitis, motor polyneuropathy, impaired vision, defective hearing, central ataxia, myopathy, erythema, itching, leukopenia, thrombocytopenia
Very rare	Microangiopathic haemolytic anemia, haemolytic uremic syndrome, colitis (isolated cases), papillary edema (isolated cases), idiopathic intracranial hypertension (isolated cases)

Table 17.10 Important contraindications/restrictions on the use of cyclosporine.

Absolute contraindications	Relative contraindications
Impaired renal function	Previous potential carcinogenic therapies (e.g. arsenic, PUVA >1000 J/cm^2)
Insufficiently controlled arterial hypertension	Psoriasis triggered by severe infection or drugs (beta-blockers, lithium, antimalarial drugs)
Severe infectious disease	Significant hepatic diseases
History of malignancy (possible exceptions: treated basal-cell carcinoma, history of squamous carcinoma in situ)	Hyperuricemia
Current malignancy	Hyperkalemia
Simultaneous PUVA therapy	Simultaneous therapy with nephrotoxic drugs
	Simultaneous phototherapy (SUP, except PUVA, see above)
	Simultaneous use of other systemic immunosuppressive agents
	Simultaneous use of systemic retinoids or therapy with retinoids in the last four weeks prior to planned onset of therapy with cyclosporine
	Drug of alcohol-related diseases
	Long-term previous treatment with methotrexate
	Pregnancy/breastfeeding
	Vaccination with live vaccines
	Epilepsy
	Current treatment with castor oil preparations

Table 17.11 Lab controls during treatment with cyclosporine.

Diagnostics	Period in weeks					
	Pretreatment	2	4	8	12	16
Full blood count[a]	x	x	x	x	x	x
Liver values[b]	x	x	x	x	x	x
Electrolytes[c]	x	x	x	x	x	x
Serum creatine	x	x	x	x	x	x
Urine status and sediment	x		x			x
Uric acid	x		x	x	x	x
Pregnancy test (urine)	x					
Cholesterol, triglycerides	x[d]			x		x
Magenesium[e]	x			x		x

[a]Erythrocytes, leukocytes, platelets.
[b]Transaminases, AP, gGT, bilirubin.
[c]Sodium, potassium.
[d]Recommended 2 weeks before and on the day of treatment initiation (fasting).
[e]Only with indication (muscle cramps).
Further specific testing may be required according to clinical signs, risks, and exposure.

For pretreatment:

- objective assessment of the disease (such as PASI/BSA/PGA; arthritis);
- HRQoL (such as DLQI/Skindex-29 or -17);
- history and clinical examination should focus on previous and concomitant diseases (e.g. severe infections; malignancies, including cutaneous malignancies; renal and liver diseases) and concomitant medications;
- measurement of blood pressure on two separate occasions;
- laboratory controls (see table 17.11);
- reliable contraception (cave: reduces efficacy of progesterone-containing contraceptives);
- regular gynecologic screening according to national guidelines;
- consultation on vaccination; susceptibility to infections (take infections seriously, seek medical attention promptly); drug interactions (inform other treating physicians about therapy); avoidance of excessive sun exposure; use of sunscreens.
- during treatment

In uncomplicated long-term therapy with low-dose cyclosporine (2.5–3 mg/kg daily), follow-up intervals may be extended to 2 months or longer. Shorter intervals may be needed in patients with risk factors or dose increases, or those who must take concomitant medications that are likely to contribute to adverse drug reactions. In selected patients with intermittent and short-term treatment, less strict monitoring (regular checking of blood pressure and creatinine level) may be sufficient:

- objective assessment of the disease (such as PASI/BSA/PGA; arthritis);
- HRQoL (such as DLQI/Skindex-29 or -17);

- clinical examination should focus on status of skin and mucous membranes (increase in body hair, gingival changes), signs of infections, and gastrointestinal or neurological symptoms;
- repeat recommendation for sun avoidance and sun protection;
- check concomitant medication;
- measurement of blood pressure;
- laboratory controls (see table 17.11);
- reliable contraception;
- regular gynecologic screening according to national guidelines (a consensus, defined as agreement by at least 75% of the voting experts, could not be reached for this point; the percentage of positive votes in this case was 58%);
- if creatinine is significantly elevated and/or patient on therapy for >1 year, perform creatinine clearance (or creatinine-EDTA clearance where available);
- determination of the cyclosporine level is recommended in individual cases.

For post-treatment:

- after discontinuation of cyclosporin, patients should be followed up for skin cancer, especially in case of extensive prior therapeutic or natural UV exposure.

The occurrence of kidney impairment is of major concern during long-term treatment. Therefore, it is important to pay attention to kidney function. Creatinine clearance should be estimated using the Cockroft–Gault formula:

$$\frac{(140 - \text{age in years}) \times (\text{weight in kilograms})}{\text{serum creatinine}\,(\text{mg}/100\ \text{mL}) \times 72}$$

In elderly patients and patients with a history of hypertension, the risk of renal impairment and hypertension is increased.

An interesting observation is the fact that weight loss improves the response of obese psoriatic patients to low-dose cyclosporine. Cyclosporine treatment in psoriatic patients has been reported to increase the frequency of squamous-cell carcinomas. The underlying mechanism is not mutagenesis but a decrease in the immunosurveillance of the skin. In particular, psoriatic patients who have been exposed to high cumulative doses of UV radiation are at risk for development of cutaneous malignancies.

Systemic retinoids

By the 1930s, vitamin A deficiency was known to cause hyperkeratosis of the skin (phrynoderma). Thirty years later, modifications of the vitamin A molecule resulted in the discovery of the so-called first generation of retinoids: all-*trans*-retinoic acid and 13-*cis*-retinoic acid. Further research resulted in the development of the second generation of retinoids, the monoaromatic retinoids, etretinate, and its free metabolite acitretin. Etretinate (which is no longer available) and acitretin are effective treatments for psoriasis as well as disorders of keratinization and cutaneous lupus.

The efficacy of acitretin monotherapy in chronic plaque psoriasis is limited, with approximately 70% of patients achieving a moderate or better response. In 23.1%

of patients treated with 50 mg of acitretin per day, ≥75% improvement in the PASI was observed over 8 weeks of treatment. Combination treatment with photo(chemo) therapy and/or vitamin D_3 analogs results in a substantial improvement in clinical response. Maximal therapeutic efficacy is reached after 2–3 months. Acitretin has been shown to be an effective maintenance therapy. As monotherapy, acitretin has been shown to be highly effective in erythrodermic and pustular psoriasis. Its efficacy in nail psoriasis and PsA has been shown to be only modest.

Important side-effects, contraindications, instruction for use, and laboratory controls have been summarized in the European guidelines (Tables 17.12–17.14). The instructions for the use of retinoids and necessary measures are as follows:

- Pretreatment
  - objective assessment of the disease (such as PASI/BSA/PGA; arthritis);
  - HRQoL (such as DLQI/Skindex-29 or -17);
  - history and clinical examination should focus on musculoskeletal problems; if patient reports complaints, a further imaging investigation may be performed;
  - exclude pregnancy/breastfeeding; patients must be informed explicitly and extensively about the teratogenic risk of the medication, the necessity of

Table 17.12 Overview of important side effects of retinoids.

Very frequent	Vitamin A toxicity (xerosis, cheilitis)
Frequent	Conjunctival inflammation (attention: contact lenses), hair loss, photosensitivity, hyperlipidemia
Occasional	Muscle, joint, and bone pain, retinoid dermatitis
Rare	Gastrointestinal complaints, hepatitis, jaundice; bone changes with long-term therapy
Very rare	Idiopathic intracranial hypertension, decreased color vision, and impaired night vision

Table 17.13 Important contraindications/restrictions on use of retinoids.

Absolute contraindications	Relative contraindications
Severe renal or hepatic dysfunction Hepatitis Woman of child-bearing age: pregnancy, breastfeeding, desire to have children, or insufficient guarantee of effective contraceptive measures up to 2 years after discontinuation of therapy	Alcohol abuse Diabetes mellitus Wearing contact lenses
Excessive alcohol abuse Comedication that is contraindicated Blood donation	Childhood History of pancreatitis Hyperlipidemia (particularly hypertriglyceridemia) and drug-controlled hyperlipidemia Arteriosclerosis

Table 17.14 Lab controls during treatment with retinoids.

Parameter	Period in weeks						
	Pretreatment	1	2	4	8	12	16
Blood count[a]	x				x		x
Liver enzymes[b]	x			x	x		
Serum creatine	x						
Pregnancy test (urine)	x			Monthly up to 2 years after therapy			
Fasting blood sugar	x						
Triglycerides, cholesterol, HDL	x			x			x

Further specific testing may be required according to clinical signs, risks, and exposure.
[a] Hb, Hct, leukocytes, platelets.
[b] AST, ALT, AP, γGT.

effective long-term contraception, and the possible consequences of a pregnancy while taking retinoids; written documentation of this informational interview;
- inform patients about the specific risk of alcohol;
- note that during and up to 1 year after treatment, blood donation is not permitted;
- laboratory controls (see table 17.14).

- During treatment:
  - objective assessment of the disease (such as PASI/BSA/PGA; arthritis)
  - HRQoL (such as DLQI/Skindex-29 of -17)
  - take capsules with a fatty meal or with whole milk;
  - avoidance of pregnancy is mandatory; start treatment on second or third day of the menstrual cycle, after satisfactory contraception for at least 1 month prior to treatment; double contraception is recommended (e.g. condom + pill; IUD/Nuva Ring + pill; cave: no low-dosed progesterone preparations/minipills) during and up to 2 years after the end of therapy; effectiveness of oral contraceptives is reduced by acitretin;
  - avoidance of alcohol;
  - ask patient about spine and joint complaints at follow-up visits; if a patient reports complaints, further imaging investigation may be performed;
  - laboratory controls (see table 17.14);
  - double contraception, as described above, is recommended;
  - patients must not donate blood for up to 1 year after the discontinuation of therapy.

In patients with chronic plaque psoriasis, 0.5 mg/kg/day is the initial dosage, which can be increased depending upon the clinical response and side-effects. For erythrodermic psoriasis, the initial dosage is 0.25 mg/kg/day, and in pustular psoriasis, the dose should be maximized, that is, doses up to 1 mg/kg/day. In patients with chronic plaque psoriasis, a mild cheilitis (just perceived by the patient) is the goal, whereas in patients with pustular psoriasis, the target dosage is reached when patients experience a cheilitis that is still tolerable.

A major problem with systemic retinoids is their teratogenicity, and separation of this from their therapeutic effects has never been achieved.

Fumarates

Since 1959, fumarates have been known in the treatment of psoriasis, and in 1994, approval was obtained in Germany. Dimethyl fumarate is considered to be the active ingredient. As a mode of action, a shift in the balance of oxidized to reduced glutathione has been suggested, interfering with NF-kappa B mediated transcription of tumor necrosis factor alpha (TNF-α) and interleukin 8 and adhesion molecules (ICAM-1). Other hypotheses include interference with dendritic cells and a shift of Th1 to Th2-type cytokines.

Dimethyl fumarate requires a low-dose initiation with stepwise dose increments with a maximum dose of 720mg/day. The efficacy of dimethyl fumarate has been shown in controlled studies. A 50–80% reduction in PASI has been reported in various studies after 16 weeks of treatment. The efficacy is comparable with MTX in daily practice. Long-term treatment resulted in sustained efficacy. During 44 months of treatment, 83% of 984 psoriatic patients remained markedly improved or clear.

Important side-effects, contraindications, instructions for use, and laboratory controls have been listed in the European guidelines (Tables 17.15,17. 16). It is important to realize that absolute lymphocyte counts have to be monitored in order to avoid prolonged periods of lymphopenia, which may be associated with the development of progressive multifocal leukencephalopathia. The instructions for the use of fumaric acid esters and necessary measures are as follows:

- pretreatment:
  - objective assessment of the disease (such as PASI/BSA/PGA; arthritis);
  - HRQoL (such as DLQI/Skindex-29 or -17);
  - history and clinical examination;
  - laboratory controls (see table 17.16);
- during treatment:
  - objective assessment of the disease (such as PASI/BSA/PGA; arthritis);
  - HRQoL (such as DLQI/Skindex-29 of -17);
  - clinical examination;
  - laboratory controls (see table 17.16).

Table 17.15 Overview of important side effects of fumaric acid esters.

Very frequent	Diarrhea, flush
Frequent	Abdominal cramps, flatulence, lymphocytopenia, eosinophilia
Occasional	Nausea, dizziness, headache, fatigue, proteinuria, increase in serum creatinine, increase in liver enzymes
Rare	Isolated increases in ALT or bilirubin

Table 17.16 Lab controls during treatment with fumaric acid esters.

Parameter	Period in weeks/months		
	Pretreatment	Months 1–6 every 4 weeks	As of month 6; thereafter, every 4 weeks
Blood count (+differential blood count)	x	x	x
Liver enzymes	x	x	x
Serum creatinine	x	x	x
Urine sediment	x	x	x
Pregnancy test	x		

Further specific testing may be required according to clinical signs, risks, and exposure.

Fumarates are prescribed in some European countries. Treatment may be limited by gastrointestinal adverse effects and flush symptoms. Long-term treatment is possible in view of the excellent safety.

Positioning the systemic treatments

Table 17.17 lists several major characteristics of classical systemic treatments that may help to make the right selection of a treatment in the individual patient. In the selection of a systemic treatment for an individual patient, the existence of relative and absolute contraindications has to be considered. For example, photo(chemo)therapy will not be chosen for patients with a history of excessive exposure to UV radiation, but these same patients could be excellent candidates for retinoid therapy (considering its anticancer effects). MTX is contraindicated in patients with excessive alcohol intake or active hepatitis, while cyclosporine is contraindicated in patients with renal insufficiency or hypertension.

An important issue is whether a maintenance treatment is needed or desired. Photo(chemo)therapy and cyclosporine are not adequate as maintenance treatments, whereas MTX, acitretin, and fumarates are adequate for long-term control of psoriasis. However, long-term use of these systemic treatments is restricted by their cumulative toxicity potential. If neither photo(chemo)therapy nor classical systemic treatments provide adequate improvement, treatment with a biologic agent is indicated.

As the risk for malignancies is increased in the population of patients with severe psoriasis, it is important that not only immunosupressive and immunomodulatory treatments be available, but also treatments without immunosuppressive effects should be available for patients with psoriasis.

Table 17.17 Preferential use of classical systemic therapies.

Acitretin	Cyclosporine	Methotrexate	Fumarates
Woman of childbearing age willing to use contraception for at least 2 years	Potent immunosuppressive	Immunomodulatory drug	Immunomodulatory drug
Combination treatment often required in chronic plaque psoriasis	Highly effective in severe disease	Liver toxicity and haematosuppression	Rare liver toxicity and haematosuppression
Not immunosuppressive	Not to be used as continuous long-term treatment	Long-term continuous treatment possible	Long-term continuous treatment possible
Long-term continuous treatment possible	Can exacerbate hypertension and hypertriglyceridemia	Highly effective in severe disease	Effective in severe disease
Not to be used in patients with hyperlipidemia No clinically significant effect on arthritis	No clinically significant effect on arthritis	Effective in arthritis	To some extent effective in arthritis

Nail psoriasis can impair the quality of life of psoriatics considerably. Systemic treatments, including MTX, cyclosporine, acitretin, and anti-TNF-α treatments, have been shown to be effective in nail psoriasis; in particular, cyclosporine and anti-TNF-α proved to have the most robust efficacy.

A considerable population of patients with moderate to severe psoriasis does exist that cannot be treated adequately with either phototherapy or classical systemic treatments and therefore can benefit from biologic therapies. Undertreatment of extensive chronic plaque psoriasis has a major impact on the progression of the course of psoriasis, with respect to quality-of-life issues, progression and permanent destruction of the joints for reason of arthritis, and progression of cardiovascular disease. Chronic inflammation resulting from active psoriasis may enhance the development of metabolic syndrome and the cardiovascular diseases, although the direct relevance of psoriatic inflammation for this aggravation remains to be substantiated. The association between severe psoriasis and cardiovascular problems may be explained by the lifestyles of psoriatic patients.

Therefore, advice has to be given beyond the systemic treatment.

Further reading

Chalmers, R.J., Kirby, B. and Smith, A. (2005) Replacement of routine liver biopsy by procollagen III aminopeptide for monitoring patients with psoriasis receiving long-term methotrexate: a multicentre audit and health economic analysis. *British Journal of Dermatology*, **152**, 444–450.

de Rie, M.A. and Bos, J.D. (1997) Cyclosporine immunotherapy. *Clinics in Dermatology*, **15**, 811–821.

Gisondi, P., Del Giglio, M., Di Francesco, V., Zamboni, M. and Girolomoni, G. (2008) Weight loss improves the response of obese patients with moderate-to-severe chronic plaque psoriasis to low-dose cyclosporine therapy: a randomized, controlled, investigator-blinded clinical trial. *American Journal of Clinical Nutrition*, **88**, 1242–1247.

Gollnick, H., Bauer, R., Brindley, C. *et al.* (1988) Acitretin versus etretinate in psoriasis. Clinical and pharmacokinetic results of a German multicenter study. *Journal of the American Academy of Dermatology*, **19**, 458–469.

Inzinger, M., Weger, W., Heschl, B., Salmhofer, W., Quehenberger, F. and Wolf, P. (2013) Methotrexate vs. fumaric acid esters in moderate-to-severe chronic plaque psoriasis: data registry report on the efficacy under daily life conditions. *Journal of the European Academy of Dermatology and Venereology*, **27**, 861–866.

Kirby, B., Fortune, D.G., Blushan, M. *et al.* (2000) The Salford Psoriasis Index: a holistic measure of psoriasis severity. *British Journal of Dermatology*, **142**, 728–732.

Miele, L., Vallone, S., Cefalo, C. *et al.* (2009) Prevalence, characteristics and severity of non-alcoholic fatty liver disease in patients with chronic plaque psoriasis. *Journal of Hepatology*, **51**, 778–786.

Mrowietz, U., Christophers, E., Altmeyer, P., for the German Fumaric Acid Ester Consensus Conference (1999) Treatment of severe psoriasis with fumaric acid esters: scientific background and guidelines for therapeutic use. *British Journal of Dermatology*, **141**, 424–429.

Mrowietz, U., Kragballe, K., Reich, K. *et al.* (2011) Definition of treatment goals for moderate to severe psoriasis: a European consensus. *Archives of Dermatological*, **303**, 1–10.

Pathirana, D., Ormerod, A.D., Saiag, P. *et al.* (2009) European S3-Guidelines on the systemic treatment of psoriasis vulgaris. *Journal of the European Academy of Dermatology and Venereology*, **23**, 1–70.

van Oosten, B.W., Killestein, J., Barkhof, F., Polman, C.H. and Wattjes, M.P. (2013) PML in a patient treated with dimethyl fumarate from a compounding pharmacy. *New England Journal of Medicine*, **368**, 1658–1659.

BIOLOGICS

Sandra Philipp

Psoriasis Research and Treatment Center, Charité University Medicine, Berlin, Germany

The term "biologics" is used as an abbreviation for biological medicinal products, substances that are derived from biological sources, such as cell lines from humans or animals, and are used as therapeutics. Many of them are biotechnologically engineered. In short, the genetic information of a specific protein is transferred into special cell lines, to induce the production of this protein (e.g. monoclonal antibodies or fusionproteins).

The respective substances used in psoriasis can be divided into three main groups: first, the TNF-α inhibitors that block the proinflammatory cytokine TNF-α, in alphabetical order, adalimumab, certolizumab pegol, etanercept, golimumab, and infliximab; second, the anti-p40 antibody ustekinumab that targets IL-12 and IL-23; and third, alefacept, a fusion protein of human IgG and leukocyte function adhesion molecule-3 that inhibits T-cell activation and depletes T-cells (Table 17.18).

Table 17.18 Biologics.

Biologics	• Indication: moderate to severe psoriasis, second line in the EU, first line in the US if patients are candidates for systemic therapy, and other medications seem less appropriate and/or psoriatic arthritis • Adverse events: ∘ upper-respiratory-tract infections, urinary-tract infections, rarely severe infections, including sepsis or opportunistic infections ∘ TNF inhibitors: immunogenicity: autoantibody development (antinuclear antibodies), very rarely development of lupus-like syndrom; paradoxical development of pustular psoriasiform eruptions, arthritis • Contraindications: ∘ severe chronic infections such as hepatitis B or HIV, malignancies ∘ TNF inhibitors: severe heart insufficiency (NYHA III/IV); medical history or family anamnesis of multiple sclerosis	
Substance	**Mechanism of action, elimination half life**	**Administration, dosage, adverse events, comments**
Etanercept (Enbrel®)	• TNF inhibition fusion protein of two TNF receptors (p55) and human immunoglobulin G • Half-life 3–4 days	• For plaque psoriasis recommended dosage initially 50 mg s.c. twice a week for max. 12 weeks; for psoriatic arthritis and during maintenance therapy 1 × 50 mg s.c. per week or 2 × 25 mg/week s.c. • Injection-site reactions are frequent, mainly mild; rarely increase in liver enzymes
Adalimumab (Humira®)	• TNF inhibition • Human monoclonal antibody against TNF-α • half-life 14 days	• For plaque psoriasis initially 80 mg s.c., after 1 week 40 mg s.c., then maintenance dose of 40 mg s.c. every second week • Injection-site reactions, mainly mild; hair loss, increase in liver enzymes
Certolizumab pegol (Cimzia®)	• TNF inhibition • Pegylated Fab′ fragment of humanized anti-TNF-antibody • Half-life 2 weeks	• Only approved for psoriatic arthritis • Initially 400 mg s.c. at weeks 0, 2, and 4 • Maintenance treatment with 200 mg s.c. every 2 weeks or 400 mg s.c. every 4 weeks • Headache, increase in liver enzymes, injection site reactions

Substance	Mechanism of action, elimination half life	Administration, dosage, adverse events, comments
Infliximab (Remicade®)	• TNF inhibition • Chimeric monoclonal antibody against TNF-α • Half-life 8–10 days	• IV application of 5 mg per kg body weight for 2 h, initially at weeks 0, 2 and 6, maintenance therapy in intervals of 8 weeks • Infusion reactions in about 10%, mainly mild reactions, but rarely anaphylactic reactions; premedication with paracetamol, or prednisolone and antihistamines may be considered • Increase in liver enzymes
Golimumab (Simponi®)	• TNF inhibition • Human monoclonal antibody against TNF-α • Half-life about 12 days	• Only approved for psoriatic arthritis • 50 mg s.c. every 4 weeks (>100 kg body weight 100 mg s.c.) • Injection-site reactions, increase in liver enzymes
Ustekinumab (Stelara®)	• Blockade of IL-12 and IL-23 • Human monoclonal antibody against p40 • Half-life 21 days	• 45 mg s.c. (>100 kg body weight 90 mg s.c.), initially at week 0, after 4 weeks, then during maintenance therapy every 12 weeks • Headache, rarely arthralgias
Alefacept (Amevive®)	• Inhibition of lymphocyte activation and depletion • Fusion protein of leukocyte-adhesion molecule-3 and human immunoglobulin G • Half-life 11 days	• Only approved for plaque psoriasis • 15 mg i.m. once a week for 12 weeks, multiple therapy cycles are possible • Injection-site reactions • Massive reduction of CD4+ T-cells; close control (weekly) during therapy cycle

Topic of interest—ending of biologic names

The formation of a biologic can be determined by the last syllable of its name. The ending -cept as in etanercept (ETA) or alefacept (ALE) implies that the substance is a fusion protein. Infliximab (IFX), which ends in -ximab, indicates a monoclonal chimeric antibody. This means that it consists of mouse variable domains and human constant domains. Certolizumab pegol (CZP), which ends in -zumab, is a humanized antibody (with mouse protein only at antigen-binding-site). Adalimumab (ADA), ustekinumab (UST), and golimumab (GO) are completely human monoclonal antibodies and therefore end in -mumab.

TNF inhibitors

TNF-α is a potent proinflammatory cytokine that plays a central role in chronic inflammatory diseases such as psoriasis (see Chapter 4). TNF-α exists as soluble cytokine and as a membrane-bound form, and mediates its activities via two different receptors, TNF-receptor 1 (p55) and TNF-receptor 2 (p75).

All TNF inhibitors bind both soluble and membrane-bound TNF- with high affinity and thus neutralize its biological activity. However, there are several differences that may partly explain their distinct safety and efficacy profile. In contrast to the fusion protein ETA, the antibodies (IFX, ADA, GO) are able to induce bridging of two transmembrane-TNF-molecules and thereby can cause apoptosis of these cells by reverse signaling. CZP lacks the Fc portion of an antibody and therefore is not able to induce antibody-dependent cellular cytotoxicity or complement activation. Furthermore, ADA, IFX, and CZP inhibit lipopolysaccharide-induced interleukin-beta release from monocytes in contrast to ETA. Conversely, only ETA binds to lymphotoxin-α3. Owing to their protein structures, all TNF inhibitors are not orally available and have to be administered parenterally.

Etanercept (ETA)

ETA, a fusion protein of two human TNF-receptors (p75) and constant domains of human immunoglobulin IgG1, is available as a syringe or injection pen with 25 mg or 50 mg for subcutaneous injections, which allow self-injections by patients after the necessary training. Interestingly, inflamed joints seem to react faster and also to lower dosages of ETA than the inflammatory skin reactions. Therefore, an initially higher dosage of ETA (2 × 50 mg/week s.c.) has been recommended in widespread skin disease. After 12 weeks the dose should be reduced to the maintenance dosage of 50 mg s.c. once a week or 25 mg s.c. twice a week. The elimination half-life is relatively short at about 3–4 days. The development of anti-ETA antibodies has been reported in 7–9% of patients, but as the antibodies are non-neutralizing and mainly transient, no associations with clinical response or adverse events have been found.

Clinical improvement in skin lesions can be expected after 6–12 weeks with a maximal response after 24 weeks. In clinical trials, treatment with ETA (25 mg biweekly or 50 mg weekly) resulted in PASI 75 responses in about one-third of patients (30–38%) at week 12, which further improved until week 24 in 44–71%. Initial higher dosages (50 mg s.c. biweekly) showed PASI 75 responses in about 50% (47–57%) of patients already at week 12. Long-term data (52–96 weeks) provide evidence for a sustained efficacy. Continuous treatment appears to lead to better results than intermittent treatment, but there is no evidence that patients show a loss of efficacy after treatment pauses.

Adalimumab (ADA)

ADA is a completely human IgG1 monoclonal antibody available as syringe and injection pen with 40 mg. Patients may self-inject after respective training. Initially, a dosage of 80 mg s.c. is recommended for the treatment of psoriasis, followed by 40 mg s.c. 1 week later. For maintenance therapy, a dose of 40 mg s.c. every 2 weeks is used. Dose adjustment according to weight is not recommended, though pharmacokinetic analyses revealed a trend toward higher apparent clearance with increasing body weight. Therefore, it might be of benefit to decrease the dosing intervals to 10 or 7 days in some patients showing insufficient treatment response for a limited period of time (off-label). A better option might be a combination of ADA with low-dose MTX (5–15 mg/week), as it has been shown that concurrent use of MTX has resulted in higher serum trough levels compared with monotherapy. The terminal elimination half-life is relatively long at 2 weeks.

In clinical studies, the prevalence of anti-adalimumab antibodies varies widely from 1–87%. In plaque psoriasis patients under monotherapy with ADA anti-ADA-antibody development has been reported in 8.4%. Formation of antibodies has been correlated with increased clearance (low serum trough levels) and loss off efficacy, but not with other adverse effects. This process was reduced when concomitant MTX was used.

ADA treatment frequently shows an improvement in clinical symptoms after 4–8 weeks, reaching its maximal efficacy usually after 16 weeks. In clinical trials, it has been reported that 71–80% of patients experience a PASI 75 response at week 16. Moreover, long-term data over 52–78 weeks provide evidence that the majority of responders show a sustained, good efficacy. Nevertheless, a small percentage of patients (about 5%) show loss of response.

Certolizumab (CZP)

CZP consists of the Fab′ fragment of a humanized monoclonal antibody against TNF conjugated with a 40 kDa polyethylene glycol (PEG) molecule (PEGylated Fab′ fragment). So far, it has been approved only for PsA. The pegylation increases the terminal elimination half-life to about 2 weeks.

CZP is available as a prefilled syringe with 200 mg. Initially, a dosage of 400 mg s.c. is recommended for the treatment of PsA at weeks 0, 2, and 4. For maintenance therapy, a dose of 200 mg s.c. every 2 weeks is used but can be changed to 400 mg s.c. every 4 weeks. Patients may self-inject after respective training. Combined treatment with MTX is recommended in PsA.

Preliminary data show evidence for its clinical efficacy in plaque psoriasis. In a phase II study, injections were given every second week until week 10. Eighty percent of patients (200 mg dose) and 84% of patients (400 mg dose), respectively, reached a PASI 75 response at week 12 in comparison with 4% of placebo patients. In responders, the median time to reach PASI 75 was 43–56 days. In a PsA study, the PASI 75 response rates at week 24 were 62.2% and 60.5% in patients treated with CZP 200 mg every second week and CZP 400 mg every 4th week, respectively, compared with 15.1% in the placebo group. The development of anti-CZP-antibodies has been reported in 11.7% of patients with PsA and has been associated with a reduced concentration of the substance in the blood.

Infliximab (IFX)

IFX is a chimeric antibody with human sequences in the constant region, whereas the variable regions are of murine origin. IFX should be administered as intravenous infusion with a recommended dosage of 5 mg/kg body weight initially followed by additional infusions at weeks 2 and 6 after the first application, then every 8 weeks thereafter for maintenance therapy. In some patients, a reduction in the infusion interval may be necessary to remain control of the disease (off-label), but it should not be reduced to less than every 4 weeks. In very good responding patients, the prolongation of infusion interval has been proposed, but due to a potential increased risk of antibody formation, this should be done with great caution and not exceed 10–12 weeks. Infusions should be given over a 2 h time period and patients should be observed for at least 1 h postinfusion for infusion-related reactions. If the infusions are well tolerated, the infusion period can be reduced to 1 h. Pretreatment may be considered with paracetamol, antihistamines, and/or glucocorticoids, particularly if infusion-related reactions have occurred previously. Limited data suggest a higher rate of infusion reactions with restart of treatment after therapy pauses, and it has been recommended that re-treatments should be begun not with induction dosing but directly with maintenance intervals of 8 weeks. The terminal elimination half-life ranges between 8 and 9.5 days, though complete elimination of the substance may need up to 6 months. In rheumatoid arthritis (RA) and Crohn's disease (CD) patients treated with infliximab, the prevalence of anti-infliximab antibodies varies greatly from about 6 to 60%. In psoriasis patients treated with IFX-monotherapy, about 15–28% developed antibodies to IFX. Antibody development has been associated with infusion-related reactions and with loss of efficacy. Additional administration of low-dose MTX (5–15 mg) can reduce the formation of antibodies to IFX and thereby may increase its plasma concentration. Therefore, a combination of IFX with MTX should be considered if there are no contraindications. Moreover, regular treatment regimens should be preferred to episodically applications. IFX often shows a fast clinical response with improvement of skin symptoms already after 1–2 weeks and a maximal response after 10 weeks. Patients treated with a dosage of 5 mg/kg body weight showed PASI 75 responses in 75.5–88% of cases after 10 weeks, and about two-thirds of patients showed a sustained good treatment response at week 52, though a certain number of patients experience a loss of efficacy under long-term treatment.

Golimumab (GO)

GO is a completely human IgG1 monoclonal antibody and so far only approved for the use in PsA. It is administered as subcutaneous injections. As it is available as a prefilled pen, patients may self-inject when they have received the respective training. The recommended dose is 50 mg s.c. applied once a month. If patients weigh more than 100 kg, the dose might be increased to 100 mg s.c. monthly. The terminal half-life has been estimated to be 12 ± 3 days. Antibodies to GO have been detected in 5% of patients, while concomitant use of MTX seems to reduce the antibody development. Treatment with GO 50 mg s.c. and 100 mg s.c. once per month has resulted in 40% and 58% of patients reaching PASI 75 response at week 14, and further improvements have been noted up to week 24 with 56% and 66%, respectively. In contrast to the joints, there might be evidence for a dose-dependent response of skin and nail affections.

Ustekinumab (UST)

UST has been approved for the treatment of plaque psoriasis in January 2009 and for the treatment of PsA in October 2013. It is a completely human IgG1 monoclonal antibody that binds with high affinity to the p40 subunit of IL-12 and IL-23, thereby inhibiting the attachment of both cytokines to their respective receptors on T-cell and natural killer cells. Thus, it results in impaired differentiation, proliferation, and survival of Th1- and Th17-cells, which play key role in psoriasis pathogenesis (see Chapter 4).

UST is given by subcutaneous injections, initially at week 0, followed by the next application after 4 weeks, and then every 12 weeks for maintenance treatment. It is available as a prefilled syringe with 45 mg or 90 mg of the substance. In general, patients receive a starting dose of 45 mg s.c., but if a patient weighs >100 kg, the dose may be increased to 90 mg s.c., as body weight has been found to affect the clearance of UST. In some patients showing only partial responses or regular recurrence of skin lesions before the next application, a reduction in the injection intervals to 10 or 8 weeks might be considered (off-label). The terminal elimination half-life is about 3 weeks. In clinical trials, around 6% of patients developed antibodies against UST, and preliminary data indicate that patients with poor responses showed more frequently neutralizing antibodies.

Clinical response can be expected after 6–12 weeks with maximal efficacy after 24 weeks. Treatment with either 45 mg or 90 mg dosages resulted in 66–79% of patients reaching PASI 75 responses at week 12. Long-term data (52–76 weeks) provide evidence for sustained efficacy during maintenance treatment, and first data suggest that interruption of treatment with a restart did not result in any significant loss of efficacy with 85.6% of patients achieving a PASI 75 within 12 weeks.

Alefacept (ALE)

ALE is a fusion protein consisting of the extracellular portion of human leukocyte function antigen-3 (LFA-3) and the Fc portion of human IgG1. By binding to lymphocyte antigen CD2, it inhibits the interaction of LFA-3 on dendritic cells and CD2 on T-lymphocytes (see Chapter 4), and thus blocks a costimulatory signal, which is particularly important for the reactivation of memory effector T-cells. Moreover, it can cause apoptosis of T- and NK-cells that are frequently found in psoriatic lesions and produce inflammatory cytokines. The recommended dose of ALE is 15 mg given once weekly as an intramuscular injection. One therapy cycle consists of a course with 12 weekly injections. Retreatment with an additional 12-week course may be initiated after a pause of 12 weeks. Data on re-treatment with more than two cycles are limited, but recent publications provide evidence for a good safety profile over five courses. The mean-elimination half-life following intravenous administration has been estimated to be about 11 days. In clinical studies, approximately 3% of patients treated with ALE developed low titers of antibodies to the substance; however, no influence on efficacy or safety has been reported so far.

Treatment with ALE either as an IV injection (7.5 mg/week) or as an IM application (15 mg/week) for one 12-week course resulted in PASI 75 responses in 14–33% and 21% of patients, respectively. The onset of response (PASI 50) begins about 8–9 weeks after the start of therapy. In the follow-up period after a course of 12 weeks, an additional 7–11% may reach PASI 75 response. Remarkably, patients treated with up to five consecutive 12-week courses demonstrated that the majority of responders showed consistent efficacy over multiple courses of treatment, and in those patients with very good improvement, additional courses resulted in remissions of up to 7 months.

Biologics and concomitant medications

Combinations of TNF inhibitors with MTX have been used successfully in rheumatology without an increased rate of adverse events. MTX seems not to influence the pharmacokinetics of ETA, but it has been reported that concomitant use of MTX reduced the apparent clearance of ADA and GO.

The metabolic drug–drug interaction between biologics and small molecules is low. The antibodies are believed to be eliminated by cells of the reticulo-endothelial system including interactions with Fc-receptors, and for ETA peptide and amino acid pathways have been suggested for metabolization with final elimination in bile or urine. In fact, small studies with ETA and concurrent digoxin and warfarin did not detect any clinically relevant interactions. In addition, in clinical studies, concomitant use of ETA with glucocorticoids, non-steroidal antirheumatics (NSARs), and analgesics did not show any interactions, with the exception of sulfasalazine, which resulted in a significant decrease in leukocytes. Similarly, analysis of frequently used concomitant medications in clinical studies with UST such as paracetamol, NSARs, or metformin and atorvastatin revealed no evidence for interactions. However, combinations of UST and further immunosuppressant agents have not been investigated. Simultaneous treatment of TNF inhibitors and anakinra (IL-1-receptor-anatgonist) or abatacept (inhibits costimulation) should be avoided, as combinations with ETA have resulted in an increased rate of serious adverse events. According to the European guidelines, sufficient data are available to allow potential combinations of ALE with MTX, cyclosporine, and retinoids in lower doses or sequential use, for example, as overlapping treatment when transitioning one patient from traditional agents to ALE for up to 12 weeks. A combination of ALE with UVB might be safely recommended to induce a potentially faster and improved response. Concurrent use of TNF inhibitors and UV therapy should be considered carefully for the potentially increased risk of nonmelanoma skin cancer. However, short-term combination of anti-TNF-agents with UVB might be an option in difficult-to-treat patients. Concerning UST, a synergistic effect of the combination with UVB could be shown in case series, but as is the case with anti-TNF agents, concurrent use should be considered carefully due to the potentially increased risk of non-melanoma skin cancer. Overall, one should keep in mind that combinations of several medications influencing the immune system might increase the risk of infections or malignancies. Therefore, combinations with immunosuppressant drugs should be used with caution, especially with regard to the still limited data in the long-term run.

Safety aspects of biologics and monitoring of therapy

Biologics show fewer organ toxicities than most traditional systemic therapies, but due to their protein structure and the potential influence on the immune system, they show a distinct safety profile (Tables 17.18 and 17.19). With respect to the possible immunomodulation, the potentially increased risk of infections and malignancies has been the focus of discussion.

Table 17.19 Recommendations for monitoring patients in case of therapy with biologics, modified after the German S3 guidelines for therapy of psoriasis vulgaris and the European S3 guidelines on the systemic treatment of psoriasis vulgaris.

Pretreatment:

- Screening for tuberculosis (chest X-ray, IGRA, in indeterminate cases additional PPD skin-test, according to local guidelines)
- Serologic test for hepatitis B + C, in patients with special risk factors or other evidence serologic tests for HIV
- Pretreatment pregnancy test might be advisable
- Important: As infections may show atypical courses (no fever, no increased CRP) or more serious courses, in case of signs for infections early consultation of medical professional, timely treatment, and potentially pause of therapy are warranted. Respective counseling of patients is advisable.
- Regular screening for nonmelanoma skin cancer

Substance	Time points	Monitoring
Infliximab	Pretreatment and before each infusion (IV application)	• Differential blood count, transaminases and γGT, creatinine according to the given time points of the respective substances • In case of altered values, controls may have to be done more often
Etanercept	Pretreatment, week 4, followed by every (2–)3 months	
Adalimumab	Pretreatment, week 4, followed by every (2–)3 months	
Certolizumab	Pretreatment, week 4, followed by every (2–)3 months	
Golimumab	Pretreatment, week 4, followed by every (2–)3 months	
Ustekinumab	Pretreatment, week 4, before each injection	
Alefacept	Pretreatment, week 4, followed by every (2–)3 months	Pretreatment (initially and before each treatment cycle) patients should have CD4+ T-cell counts in the reference range. During the 12-week treatment period, CD4+ T-cell counts have to be monitored weekly. If CD4+ T-cell counts fall below 250 cells/μL, dosing should be withheld. When the CD4+ T-cell count remains below 250/μL for 1 month, treatment should be discontinued.

There is some evidence that psoriasis patients suffering from moderate to severe disease have an increased risk of experiencing diseases belonging to the metabolic syndrome and therefore might be subject to an increased risk of cardiovascular events (see chapter 15). Although no official guidelines exist so far, it may be appropriate to control additionally (or initiate the control in cooperation with general practitioner) body weight and waist circumference, blood pressure, blood lipids as cholesterol (HDL, LDL), and triglycerides as well as fasting glucose level once yearly. Naturally, these general recommendations have to be adapted individually according to patients' distinct risk factors or already-known diseases as recommended by the respective guidelines.

TNF inhibitors

Most safety data are available for the TNF inhibitors, as they have been used worldwide in different indications. Several studies have shown evidence for an increased risk of infections of the upper respiratory tract, urogenital tract, or skin (e.g. herpes zoster, cellulitis) compared with controls. Interestingly, preliminary data indicate a higher risk of herpes zoster infections with the use of the monoclonal antibodies (IFX, ADA) compared with ETA. Though serious infections such as sepsis, invasive fungal, or opportunistic infections have been reported in treatment with all TNF inhibitors, the reported potential risk varies in the literature ranging from no increased risk to a doubled risk. Importantly, recent data have provided some evidence that the incidence might be highest during the first 6 months of treatment. The potential hazard of reactivation of latent tuberculosis by all TNF inhibitors is well known, although it may be greater with the monoclonal antibodies than with ETA. Therefore, before the start of treatment, a screening for tuberculosis infection is warranted, which should include a thorough medical history of risk factors (e.g. profession, travels), a chest-X-ray, and an interferon-gamma-release assay (IGRA-test; e.g. QuantiFERON®-TB-test or T-SPOT®.TB-test). A PPD-skin test (tuberculosis skin test) might additionally be used in unclear cases. If latent tuberculosis cannot be excluded, treatment with isoniazide tablets (5 mg/kg body weight/day, with a maximum dosage of 300 mg/day) has to be initiated 4 weeks in advance of the biologic therapy and maintained for 9 months. If isoniazide is not tolerated, rifampicin may be used (10 mg/kg body weight for 4 months).

Additionally, testing for potential hepatitis B and C infection should be done prior to any anti-TNF therapy due to observed reactivations of hepatitis B infections during treatment. There is some evidence that anti-TNF-therapy may be safe in patients with a previous, but not chronic hepatitis B infection (HBV-DNA negative); however, cooperation with a hepatologist is strongly recommended, and prophylactic antiviral therapy should be considered. In contrast to hepatitis B infection, in which TNF appears to be important for the virus elimination, TNF seems to play a different role in hepatitis C infection by favoring liver-cell destruction. In line with this observation, TNF inhibitors have been used successfully in patients suffering from chronic hepatitis C, also in combination with antiviral treatment.

Moreover, testing for HIV infection should be considered. Data on the use of TNF inhibitors in patients with HIV infection are limited. Several case reports with ETA and IFX indicate that the use may be possible in patients that are well controlled by antiretroviral therapy, but restrictive use and thorough clinical consideration on a case-by-case basis are strongly recommended.

Besides upper-respiratory-tract infections, the most common reported adverse events are injection-site reactions such as itching, swelling, or erythema, usually mild and transient, in up to 15% of patients depending on the distinct substances. Infusion reactions to IFX occurred in clinical studies in 10–18% of patients, especially in patients under monotherapy. Most infusion reactions are mild, but rare cases of anaphylaxis have been described. Additionally, delayed hypersensitivity reactions (myalgia, arthralgia, fever, or rash) under IFX have rarely been reported, with limited data suggesting an increased risk after treatment-free intervals.

Some further adverse events are viewed as class effects of anti-TNF therapy. These include hematological side-effects, such as thrombocytopenia and rare central or peripheral demyelinating events. Because of reports on new onset or exacerbation of multiple sclerosis, TNF inhibitors should not be given to patients with any history of multiple sclerosis or other types of demyelinating disease. Moreover, as TNF inhibitors have been reported to potentially worsen existing severe heart insufficiency, their use should be avoided in patients with heart insufficiency grade NYHA III-IV. Additionally, it has been reported that the use of TNF inhibitors could worsen preexisting interstitial lung disease.

Interestingly, although the data are still limited, there is evidence that a specific subgroup of patients may experience significant weight gain under TNF inhibitor treatment.

Another important safety topic involves the immunogenicity of biologics due to their protein structure. In addition to the development of antibodies against the distinct TNF-blocker, an increased incidence of autoantibodies such as anti-nuclear antibodies (ANA) or double-stranded DNA-antibodies (dsDNA) has been documented. Depending on the tests and the respective substances, ANA positivity has been found in 4% to nearly 50% of the patients and dsDNA in 3–17%. Yet, there have been only sporadic reports of patients developing clinical symptoms of lupus erythematodes or lupus-like syndrome. Nevertheless, if a patient develops clinical symptoms of lupus-like syndrome and is tested positive for double-stranded DNA autoantibodies, termination of treatment is recommended, which is usually followed by complete remission.

Psoriasis patients treated with TNF inhibitors may experience increases in the transaminases. However, although the increase may be significant, usually no severe liver damage occurs. Careful controls are recommended if aminotransferases are elevated more than three times above the upper limit, and discontinuation has to be considered in case of elevation higher than five times the upper limit or development of icterus.

So far, limited data do not allow assessment of definite conclusions about the potentially increased risk of developing malignancies with the use of biologics. In clinical trials, the incidence of malignancies was comparable with the expected risk in control populations. However, meta-analyses of clinical trials as well as observational studies and registries raised controversial results. While an observational investigation of rheumatologic patients in the US showed no evidence for an increased incidence of solid tumors or lymphoproliferative diseases, an increased risk of nonmelanoma skin cancers (NMSC) and melanomas has been found. In contrast, data from the Swedish registry did not reveal an increased risk for any malignancy. The British registry found no increased risk for solid cancers, but an increased risk for nonmelanoma skin cancer of RA patients treated with either disease-modifying antirheumatic drugs (DMARDs) or anti-TNF in comparison with the general population. In conclusion, at least it is important to recommend sun protection and regularly monitor the patients with respect to skin cancer. The fact that chronic inflammatory diseases might themselves predispose patients to an increased risk for lymphomas further complicates the situation. The French registry reported a two- to threefold risk for lymphomas in patients under TNF inhibitor therapy in comparison with the general population. Nevertheless, the reported risk has been comparable with the expected risk in a population with severe chronic inflammatory disease and was not increased in comparison with patients treated with traditional DMARDs. Recent data indicate a potential increased risk with monoclonal anti-TNF therapy (ADA, IFX) in comparison with ETA. Overall, it is recommended that one should avoid when possible, or at least consider carefully, the use of biologics in patients with existing malignancies or a history of malignancies (except basal cell carcinomas) in the last 5–10 years depending on the respective entity. Very limited and preliminary data indicate a potentially existing specific risk for patients with melanomas.

UST

First safety data about long-term use of UST over 5 years have been presented. The most common adverse effects include nasopharyngitis and upper respiratory tract infections. In clinical trials the rate of serious adverse events under UST short-term treatment has been reported comparable to placebo, and the rate of serious infections remained low in the long-term (about 1.1 events per 100 PY). However, there are reports of severe infections such as pneumonia or erysipelas as well as opportunistic infections and reactivation of tuberculosis. Therefore, monitoring recommendations in analogy to the TNF inhibitors are recommended (Table 17.19). Injection-site reactions are frequent, but mostly of mild character. Headache, myalgia and back pain are common. Data about an increased incidence of major adverse cardiac events in trials with another monoclonal antibody against the p40-subunit of IL-12 and IL-23 aroused concern of a possible class effect. Though this could so far not be confirmed for ustekinumab by the latest safety data over a period of 5 years, it might be reasonable for treating physicians to monitor patients with known cardiovascular risk factors. Considering safety data of 3117 patients with about 9000 PY of follow-up, the number of malignancies was low. The spectrum of malignancies as well as the incidence of malignancies other than NMSC was consistent with that expected in the general population.

The incidence of NMSC in ustekinumab-treated patients is comparable with or somewhat lower than the rates reported for anti-TNF agents in psoriasis. With respect to the limited data and the known immunomodulation an increased risk of malignancies cannot be ruled out.

ALE

Limited safety data are available for up to five repeated courses of ALE. Frequent adverse effects are mild injection-site reactions (16%) and headache. Clinical trials with ALE showed a slightly increased risk of infections. The most significant side effect consists in the reduction in the total lymphocyte count, especially the CD4+ and CD8+ T-cells. In a clinical trial 7.7% of the patients experienced CD4+ T-cell counts below 300/µL. Therefore, close monitoring of the CD4+ T-cells every second week during treatment is recommended. If CD4+ counts falls below 250/µL, injections have to be interrupted, and weekly controls should be initiated. If CD4+ counts stay low over 1 month, treatment has to be terminated. Moreover, an ALE treatment cycle should only be initiated if patients' lymphocyte and CD4+ T-cell counts are in the reference range.

In toxicity studies in nonhuman primates, a B-cell lymphoma and hyperplasia in B-cell-dependent areas have been observed, though the relevance for humans is unknown. Due to limited data and with regard to the known immunomodulation, an increased risk of malignancy cannot be excluded.

Further monitoring recommendations have been listed in Table 17.19. Though not mandatory, we suggest the same controls as those used for TNF inhibitors and UST.

In summary, the focus of monitoring should be on infections. Problems may result from the use of biologics altering the typical signs of infections such as fever or increases in C-reactive protein (CRP) with the risk of late diagnosis and possible septic courses. Therefore, patients should be advised to visit their respective doctors promptly when experiencing unspecific symptoms such as fatigue or feeling of illness. Patients should receive all necessary vaccinations, such as influenza vaccination, though concurrent application of live vaccines with all biologics should be avoided. Furthermore, besides MTX, combinations of biologics with different immunosuppressant agents have to be considered carefully, as this might increase the risk of infections.

Topic of interest—paradoxical skin reactions by TNF inhibitors

A relatively rare though well-known phenomenon is the paradoxical worsening or new onset of immune-mediated skin lesions during treatment with TNF inhibitors of patients suffering from chronic inflammatory diseases such as RA, chronic inflammatory bowel disease (IBD), spondylitis ankylosans, or PsA. The prevalence varies in different studies from 0.6 to 5.3%. The most frequently reported paradoxical skin reactions (about 80%) are psoriatic skin lesions, including plaque psoriasis, guttate psoriasis, and pustular psoriasis, especially palmoplantar pustulosis. The reason is still not fully understood, but a paradoxical production of IFN-α by plasmacytoid dendritic cells has been suggested. In many cases, respective treatment may allow continuation of the drug. Depending on the severity of the skin affection topical therapy, UV therapy, (topical) PUVA, or combinations with systemic treatments such as MTX, retinoids, or cyclosporine can be sufficient to control the skin lesions. However, in severe or recalcitrant cases, as well as in generalized pustular psoriasis, withdrawal of the drug is recommended. Switching to another TNF inhibitor can prove successful, though some patients may develop similar adverse skin reactions.

Besides psoriasis, eczemateous skin reactions have been reported repeatedly, particularly in patients with IBD, and more rarely alopecia areata, cutaneous vasculitis, vitiligo, granuloma anularis, lichen planus, morphea, or pemphigus. Whereas most of these skin affections can be managed by topical treatments, cessation of treatment should be considered in case of vasculitis or recalcitrant disease.

Indications—which patients are candidates for therapy with biologics?

All the above-mentioned substances are approved by the FDA and the EMEA for the treatment of moderate to severe plaque psoriasis and/or PsA (Table 17.18), with the exception of ALE, which is approved only in the US, Canada, and Switzerland. CZP and GO are approved only for patients with PsA. However, the use for psoriasis might be different in the US and the European Union. In the US, biologics are approved for first-line use in adult patients with moderate to severe psoriasis vulgaris and PsA if patients are candidates for systemic treatment or phototherapy, whereas in Europe, biologics are used only as second-line treatments, that is if traditional systemic treatments such as MTX, cyclosporine, and retinoids (and in Germany also fumaric acid esters) have been insufficient, caused side-effects, or are contraindicated. Similarly, in PsA at least one systemic basic treatment (e.g. MTX, leflunomide) has to be insufficient or excluded due to side effects or contraindications before biologics are indicated. The criteria that define moderate to severe disease and their limitations have already been discussed in detail in Chapter 14. Besides the so-called "rule of ten" (PASI > 10, BSA > 10%, DLQI > 10), other patient immanent factors, for example, affection of visible parts such as the face, or impairment of physical functions due to involvement of hands and feet, influence treatment decisions.

Although approval refers to plaque psoriasis, there is sufficient clinical experience to recommend the use of biologics also for other subtypes of the disease, especially in severely affected patients with erythrodermic psoriasis, pustular psoriasis, or nail affections. However, one has to consider that this might be regarded as "off-label" use.

Moreover, the choice of the respective substance is influenced not only by the severity and subtype of the disease but also by the distinct efficacy and safety profile of the substances.

Concerning skin involvement, ETA shows a slower onset of efficacy than IFX and ADA, though the number of responding patients increases further until week 24. In addition, with the initial use of 50 mg twice a week, one can accelerate the response rates. The sustained long-term efficacy and possibility of treatment interruptions without increased risk for loss of efficacy are favorable. IFX presents frequently with a very fast response, and the highest rates of patients with a PASI 75 improvement in the short-term. Therefore, it might be preferred in very severely affected patients who need prompt relief of symptoms, though when used for the long term, a certain number of patients show loss of efficacy. ADA demonstrated a high efficacy in the short-term as well as a good maintenance of response over a year of treatment, with about 5% of patients experiencing loss of response. UST proved highly efficacious with respect to skin affections, and the reported sustained efficacy appears promising. As data on potential intermittent treatment are still limited, so far maintenance treatment is recommended. Regarding ALE, about a third of patients show very good improvement with a specific subgroup even experiencing longstanding remissions. However, so far there exist no biomarkers to separate responders from nonresponders. Therefore, its relatively late onset of efficacy in a specific subpopulation of patients may nowadays limit its use for patients not responding to the other substances.

In contrast to the variable responses of the skin affections by different TNF inhibitors, all show comparably good efficacy in PsA with ACR 20 responses in about 60% of patients at week 12, and 52–72% at week 24.

Sustained long-term efficacy could be shown for ETA, GO, IFX, and ADA with inhibition of the radiographic progression over 2 years. First data from CZP at week 24 speak in favor of an inhibition of the radiographic expression, but further long-term data are needed. Therefore, if patients with plaque psoriasis suffer also from joint involvement, the use of TNF inhibitors can be strongly recommended. Furthermore, as TNF inhibitors in contrast to traditional DMARDs (e.g. MTX, leflunomide) appear to be efficacious in PsA with axial involvement, they have been proposed as first-line therapy in patients with axial involvement if NSARs are not sufficient. Recent data demonstrated also the efficacy of UST in PsA, ACR 20 responses have been reported in 42–49% of patients at week 24, and first data have demonstrated a significant and sustained inhibition of radiographic progression in active PsA after 52 weeks.

Additionally, severe nail disease may speak in favor of the use of biologics, with most efficacy data available for the TNF inhibitors, especially for IFX.

Concomitant chronic inflammatory diseases may additionally influence the choice of treatment. In patients with chronic IBD, ADA and IFX have proven to be effective and are approved for treatment. In clinical trials, efficacy could also be shown for GO in Crohn's disease, and first data indicate efficacy of certolizumab in ulcerative colitis. Concerning refractory uveitis, IFX and ADA have been shown to be rapidly effective, and first data show promising results for GO.

Last but not least, ETA may be of benefit in patients in whom a potential cessation of treatment is expected to be necessary due to its short half-life and the option of intermittent therapy, and the use appears to result in a lower risk for tuberculosis or herpes zoster infections compared with monoclonal antibodies.

In conclusion, biologics offer an effective treatment option for severely affected patients, with many different factors influencing the choice of the respective substances. If certain safety aspects are respected, the therapy seems to be reasonably safe. To facilitate the use of this new class of therapeutics, different evidence-based guidelines have been published, such as the European S3-guidelines, the BAD-guidelines from the Society of British Dermatologists, and, most recently, the updated German S3 guidelines.

Topic of interest: efalizumab

Efalizumab was the first biologic approved for plaque psoriasis in Europe in 2004. It is a humanized monoclonal antibody (-zumab) targeting CD11a, which is a subunit of leukocyte-function-adhesion-molecule-1, thereby inhibiting the migration of inflammatory cells from the blood into the tissue, and additionally reducing T-cell activation by impairing costimulatory signaling. In 2009, it was taken off the market, owing to an altered risk–benefit profile. The use of efalizumab has been associated with the occurrence of a rare and potentially life-threatening neurologic disease, the so-called progressive multifocal leukencephalopathy.

Further reading

Askling, J., van Vollenhoven, R.F., Granath, F. *et al.* (2009) Cancer risk in patients with rheumatoid arthritis treated with anti-tumor necrosis factor alpha therapies: does the risk change with the time since start of treatment? *Arthritis & Rheumatism*, **60**, 3180–3189.

Galloway, J.B., Hyrich, K.L., Mercer, L.K. *et al.* (2011) Anti-TNF therapy is associated with an increased risk of serious infections in patients with rheumatoid arthritis especially in the first 6 months of treatment: updated results from the British Society for Rheumatology Biologics Register with special emphasis on risks in the elderly. *Rheumatology*, **50**, 124–131.

Kimball, A.B., Gladmann, D., Gelfand, J.M. *et al.* (2008) National Psoriasis Foundation clinical consensus on psoriasis comorbidities and recommendations for screening. *Journal of the American Academy of Dermatology*, **58**, 1031–1042.

Mariette, X., Tubach, F., Bagheri, H. *et al.* (2010) Lymphoma in patients treated with anti-TNF: results of the 3-year prospective French RATIO registry. *Annals of the Rheumatic Diseases*, **69**, 400–408.

Nast, A., Boehncke, W.H., Mrowietz, U. *et al.* (2012) S3 guidelines for the treatment of psoriasis. *Journal der Deutschen Dermatologischen Gesellschaft*, **10** (Supplement 2), 1–95.

Pathirana, D., Ormerod, A.D., Saiag, P. *et al.* (2009) European S3-Guidelines on the systemic treatment of psoriasis vulgaris. *Journal of the European Academy of Dermatology and Venereology*, **23** (Supplement 2), 5–70.

Smith, C.H., Anstey, A.V., Barker, J.N.W.N. *et al.* (2009) British Association of Dermatologists' guidelines for biologic interventions for psoriasis. *British Journal of Dermatology*, **161**, 987–1019.

CHAPTER 18
Special therapeutic aspects

Wolfram Sterry
Department of Dermatology and Allergy, University Hospital Charité, Berlin, Germany

Psoriasis capitis

Psoriasis of the scalp is confined in most instances to the areas covered by hair, though psoriasis may transgress the frontline between hairy and nonhairy areas by 1 cm or even 2 cm. This causes specific problems in the treatment of scalp psoriasis: Most importantly, not all types of topical treatment are acceptable as they impair the aesthetics of the hair, for example by greasy ointments, exsiccating lotions, and discoloring agents such as anthralin (dithranol), or due to smell (e.g. from tar products) that is unacceptable in daily life. Furthermore, treatment options readily applicable on normal skin such as UV treatment are less easily used on the scalp. As the scalp is a visible area, both psoriatic involvement and treatment will be obvious to others, for example, family and friends, but also to persons in professional and social settings; therefore, this can have a high impact on a patient's quality of life. Finally, treatment of scalp psoriasis is difficult, since plaques on the scalp are among the most recalcitrant lesions, and relapses are frequent and fast. Consequently, an almost continuous treatment may be required in some patients. All of these aforementioned factors may have an important impact on treatment adherence as well.

While active agents of treatment should act on the skin of the scalp, the hair will absorb much of the applied substances; this will vary depending on the length and density of the hair. Treatment success will ultimately depend on the amount of active agent being available directly on the skin. Owing to the numerous sebaceous glands and the millions of hair channels, absorption of pharmaceuticals via the scalp is always an issue and needs to be considered carefully, particularly in lipophilic agents.

In patients who require systemic treatment, scalp lesions will normally respond as well, but in some, complete clearance of scalp lesions will not occur. Therefore, most patients with scalp psoriasis will require topical treatment, either as monotherapy or as combination treatment.

Psoriasis: Diagnosis and Management, First Edition. Edited by Wolfram Sterry, Robert Sabat, and Sandra Philipp.

The following classes of agents have been investigated with higher degrees of evidence:

1 keratolytics;

2 tar preparations;

3 anthraline;

4 topical glucocorticosteroids;

5 vitamin D_3 analogs.

Other procedures or devices such as simultaneous application of antimycotic agents, UV-combs, intralesional injection of crystalline glucocorticoid suspensions, or even X-ray irradiation have been studied to a lesser degree.

Keratolytics, such as salicylic acid, in concentrations of 3–5% may be applied for a few days at the beginning of the treatment to remove abundant and sticky scales. As the barrier function of psoriatic scales is low, one should not postpone specific treatment for more than a few days. Salicylic acid should not be used in children because of its toxicity.

Tar products have not been studied recently, and there is only a low level of evidence for their use. In the current German S3 guidelines for psoriasis, topical tar products are no longer recommended. Furthermore, the smell of tar is unpleasant and causes nonadherence.

Anthralin (0.5–3%) in biological wash oil is effective in scalp psoriasis and can be recommended at least in clinical settings and day-care units. However, irritation, hair discoloration, and staining of clothing make anthralin difficult to use in the outpatient setting.

Topical corticosteroids in different potencies and preparations have been studied extensively, and the efficacy has been widely documented. Regarding the vehicle, one should avoid alcoholic solutions that may cause additional exsiccation and thus pruritus of the scalp. Many commercial preparations have been developed as foams and shampoos, which cause less irritation. Initially, steroids may be used twice daily; for maintenance treatment, however, application once daily is recommended.

In patients with severe scalp involvement, we recommend a 3-day course of high-potency steroids in ointments over night; this can be done at weekends and will clear the scalp substantially, so that treatment can be continued with foams, shampoos, or ointments from then on. Atrophy, a common side effect of steroids in normal skin, is less frequently observed on the scalp; nevertheless, careful monitoring for steroid atrophy is important.

Vitamin D_3 analogs are useful for scalp psoriasis; both calcipotriol and tacalcitol have been studied and are effective. Their efficacy is less strong than that of high potency steroids such as clobetasol but present with less potential adverse reactions as well. They can be prescribed alone or in combination with betamethasone; combinations are preferred as induction treatment, while monotherapy with vitamin D_3 analogs is used for maintenance therapy.

Intertriginous psoriasis

Intertriginous areas require a different therapeutic approach as well. While certain treatment options cannot be properly applied such as UV therapy, others are just not suitable because of an increased irritability in these locations such as anthralin, tar, or tazaroten, or because of a higher risk of adverse reactions due to an increased absorption of highly active agents such as potent corticosteroids. This is due to the thin stratum corneum found in intertriginous areas with a low barrier function, and also due to occlusion effects coming from the direct skin-to-skin contact. To add to the complexity, intertriginous areas show a higher degree of microbial colonization that may act as a trigger factor, and reduction in the microbial colonization is frequently regarded as a mainstay of treatment in these areas.

Randomized and controlled studies are rare, and treatment relies on the clinical experience. Topical agents that are used in intertriginous areas are as follows:

1 corticosteroids;
2 vitamin D_3 analogs;
3 calcineurin inhibitors.

It is important to use only corticosteroids of low or medium potency, as the risk of skin atrophy is high due to the thin, horny layer. In severe cases, high-potency steroids may be used for a few days at the beginning. The response is usually good, but obviously, corticosteroids are not used on a long-term basis but are used for acute phases and as an induction treatment. The duration of use should not exceed 4 weeks, and application should be performed only once daily.

Vitamin D_3 analogs, alone or in combination with corticosteroids (for induction), are efficacious and safe but may be irritating in some patients; therefore, patients should be informed about this possibility and be advised to stop treatment in case of irritation. Calcineurin inhibitors have a firm place in topical treatment of intertriginous psoriasis, even over prolonged periods, as they do not induce atrophy or confer other known adverse drug reactions.

The choice of vehicle is important, as greasy vehicles may induce occlusion and thereby promote microbial growth. Many individual prescriptions rely on soft pastes as vehicles.

Simultaneous treatment or prophylaxis against *Candida* infection or bacterial colonization may be used in the form of antifungals (such as nystatin or clotrimazol) or antiseptics, and physical measures against humidity such as linen wraps may be a helpful adjunctive measure.

Guttate psoriasis

For guttate psoriasis, which mainly affects children and young adults, systemic treatments are less commonly applied, while topical therapy and UV therapy are preferred. As guttate psoriasis is a rather superficial form of psoriasis, both anthralin treatment and UV therapy induce quick responses. Regarding UV therapy, there is a general consensus that psoralen + UVA therapy should not be used in children; rather, 311 nm narrow-band UV treatment should be applied.

On the other hand, as guttate psoriasis reflects a systemic immune response, its interruption may be advantageous also with respect to the long-term course of psoriasis. Furthermore, guttate psoriasis frequently affects larger areas of the body, thus limiting the use of corticosteroids, vitamin D_3 analogs, and calcineurin inhibitors. Therefore, systemic treatments may have to be used.

In children and young adults, one can consider all treatment options that are registered for adults. This holds true for acitretin, methotrexate, and cyclosporine, which are regarded safe in children if used in appropriate dosages. For cyclosporine, a dose of 1–5 mg/kg per day is used for both maintenance and induction therapy. However, we recommend dosing according to ideal, rather than actual, body weight to avoid overdosing and subsequent kidney damage in obese individuals. Methotrexate is regarded as a useful intervention for severe cases of guttate psoriasis in children (defined as a Psoriasis Area and Severity Index score of >10, with disseminated widespread lesions that are unresponsive to antibiotics, topical treatment, and UV therapy). A dose of 0.3 mg/kg per week is preferred (regardless of age) without exceeding the maximum standard dose of 22.5 mg per week. Methotrexate treatment may be combined with folate supplements, for example, 2 days after every methotrexate dose or daily except on the day of methotrexate therapy. Acitretin therapy is rarely performed under the age of 10. In girls after pubarche, acitretin must be used together with oral contraceptives, and further controls are necessary to monitor blood lipids and premature closure of bone epiphyses.

Among the biologics, etanercept has been registered in children and allows effective and safe treatment also in this age group. Although etanercept has been registered specifically for plaque psoriasis in children, many experts nevertheless regard etanercept as a treatment of first choice in patients with active and widespread guttate psoriasis. Etanercept 0.8 mg/kg body weight s.c./week (max. 50 mg s.c./week) would be an appropriate dose for children and young adults with guttate psoriasis.

Erythrodermic psoriasis

Erythrodermic psoriasis represents an emergency situation. Therefore, effective systemic treatment should be initiated, and preference is given to those therapies that have a rapid mode of onset and high efficacy.

Cyclosporine A at a dose of 3 mg per kg body weight would be an option that can be started immediately following exclusion of any contraindication for cyclosporine (see Chapter 17). A response would be expected after several days, and after 1–2 weeks at the latest. Alternatively, a potent and fast-acting tumour necrosis factor (TNF) blocker would be an appropriate option; here, infliximab would be the treatment of choice as the application via infusion allows high plasma levels and a rapid onset of action. Again, contraindications have to be checked carefully before the start of treatment.

Retinoids work well in experienced hands. The general rule is to use acitretin 0.3 mg/kg body weight daily for 3–4 weeks, divided into two doses per day; this will avoid exfoliation and retinoid dermatitis in most cases. Thereafter, this can be increased to 0.5 mg/kg body weight daily.

Along with systemic treatment, patients need emollients for skin care, several times per day, warm rooms to reduce the thermal loss via the dilated capillaries of the skin, and further systemic medical workup to detect and control systemic complications such as cardiac failure, protein loss, or signs of malabsorption.

As a rule, patients with erythrodermic psoriasis require hospitalization.

Pustular psoriasis

Pustular psoriasis may present in different forms, which will require different treatments. *Annular pustular psoriasis,* including *annular pustular psoriasis in pregnancy (impetigo herpetiformis),* requires special measures, as this variant of psoriasis is highly inflammatory. Annular pustular psoriasis is observed during flares and irritation of psoriasis vulgaris, and can be controlled sometimes by wet bandages or application of zinc oil, which may calm down irritated psoriasis. Also, application of topical steroids can be useful, but one should be aware of possible rebounds after stopping the steroids. In more chronic and recalcitrant cases, systemic therapy is required; the choice of active agent will depend on other factors such as the extent and severity of psoriasis, contraindications, and personal situation of the patient.

Impetigo herpetiformis is a severe manifestation of pustular psoriasis in pregnancy, often associated with systemic complications (see chapters 13 and 22). Systemic corticosteroids (prednisone) are the treatment of choice for patients with impetigo herpetiformis. One should start with a low dose of 15–30 mg/day, but it may become necessary to increase the dose to 60 mg/day to control the disease. Oral cyclosporine is an effective second choice of treatment of impetigo herpetiformis. TNF blockers may be considered if the above-mentioned therapies are ineffective or contraindicated; case reports on safe and successful administrations of TNF blockers in impetigo herpetiformis have been published. Finally, close cooperation with the obstetrician is required.

Generalized pustular psoriasis often complicates erythrodermic psoriasis and should be treated along the same rules as have been recommended for erythrodermic psoriasis itself. Addition of systemic retinoids, in particular acitretin, is recommended by many experts, but this should be added to another systemic therapy like e.g. infliximab and should not be used as a single therapy. Acitretin is given in doses of 20–30 mg/day; for contraindications and monitoring, see Chapter 17.

Psoriasis pustulosa palmoplantaris is a severe and chronic variant of psoriasis causing major distress and morbidity for the patient. Topical treatment will not be sufficient to control more severe cases, and systemic therapy has to be initiated. Acitretin may be used as one of the first options, but all other systemic treatments have been shown to be effective in case reports or case series, although loss of efficacy is not rare, requiring a rotation to other treatments. Fumarates, cyclosporine A, methotrexate, etanercept, infliximab, adalimumab, and ustekinumab can be effective, and the choice of agent should be made while considering other manifestations and aspects of psoriasis and other health problems of the patients, particularly when considering contraindications.

Acrodermatitis continua suppurativa is a chronic, aggressive, destructive form of pustular psoriasis that may lead to loss of nails, atrophy, and even loss of finger tips. Systemic treatment is invariably required. Choice may depend on other potential manifestations of psoriasis as well as the health status of the patient.

Nail psoriasis

Nail psoriasis represents a heavy burden for the patient given the manifold functions of the nails from aesthetics to their function in manual activities, as well as to counterpoint the sensitivity of the fingertips. Nail psoriasis is a manifestation of the nail matrix, which is hidden partly below the proximal nail and for the most part below the proximal nail fold, and the skin distal to the proximal nail fold. The nail matrix is thus several millimeters below the surface and because of the limitations in penetration, topical treatment has at best very limited efficacy, although many topical treatments are promoted.

There are two approaches for the treatment of nail psoriasis:

1 Injection of crystalline suspensions of corticosteroids directly above the nail matrix. This procedure is somewhat painful but with some dermatological experience, this can be an effective measure. The nail will improve after several weeks, when the matrix has restarted to produce a normal nail. After several months, the effect is lost, and treatment has to be repeated. The treatment requires an experienced dermatologist to outweigh the risk of skin atrophy and maintenance of the success of treatment, but in the hands of experts it is a very valuable tool. Similarly, methotrexate has been used for intralesional therapy of nail psoriasis, but only a few case reports are available.
2 The other treatment option is systemic treatment. For several drugs, prospective randomized trials have been performed that showed improvement of the condition of the nails and quality of life as well. Such trials have been published for methotrexate, cyclosporine A, etanercept, adalimumab, and infliximab. Case reports have been published for ustekinumab. However, nails often respond after a delay and may not recover their full integrity, even after prolonged periods of treatment, thus representing an unmet need in the field of psoriasis treatment.

Further reading

Paul, C., Gallini, A., Maza, A. *et al.* (2011) Evidence-based recommendations on conventional systemic treatments in psoriasis: systematic review and expert opinion of a panel of dermatologists. *Journal of the European Academy of Dermatology and Venereology*, **25** (Supplement 2), 2–11.

Sanchez-Regan, M., Sola-Ortigosa, J., Alsina-Gibert, M., Vidal-Fernandez, M. and Umbert-Millet, P. (2011) Nail psoriasis: a retrospective study on the effectiveness of systemic treatments (classical and biological therapy). *Journal of the European Academy of Dermatology and Venereology*, **25**, 579–586.

Ståhle, M., Atakan, N., Boehncke, W.H. *et al.* (2010) Juvenile psoriasis and its clinical management: a European expert group consensus. *Journal der Deutschen Dermatologischen Gesellschaft*, **8**, 812–818.

Thaci, D., Paetzold, S. and Kaufmann, R. (2003) Treatment of intertriginous and genito-anal psoriasis. *Aktuelle Dermatologie*, **29**, 207–215.

Wozel, G. (2008) Psoriasis treatment in difficult locations: scalp, nails, and intertriginous areas. *Clinics in Dermatology*, **26**, 448–459.

Wozel, G., Klein, E., Mrowietz, U., Reich, K., Sebastian, M. and Streit, V. (2011) Scalp psoriasis. *Journal der Deutschen Dermatologischen Gesellschaft*, **10**, 70–74.

CHAPTER 19
Combination treatments

Peter C.M. van de Kerkhof
Department of Dermatology, Radboud University Nijmegen Medical Centre, Nijmegen, Netherlands

Why combination treatment of psoriasis?

The aim of combination treatment is to enhance the efficacy of treatments while reducing side effects. The rationales for combination treatment are as follows:

1 combining treatments with a different mode of action;
2 side effect profiling;
3 systemic treatment with topical treatment;
4 bridging slow-onset treatment.

For safety reasons, some combinations have to be avoided.

Beneficial combinations

Topicals in combination treatment

The mode of action of the combination of a topical corticosteroid and calcipotriol has been studied extensively. The mode of action of vitamin D treatments and corticosteroids is entirely different. In a comparative in vivo study, it was shown that the vitamin D analog, calcipotriol, has a major effect on epidermal proliferation (Ki-67) and epidermal differentiation (keratin 10), whereas the effect on T-cells was more selective and restricted to a reduction of CD45RO and CD8 cells. In contrast, betamethasone dipropionate resulted in normalization of epidermal differentiation without any significant effect on epidermal proliferation. The effect of the corticosteroid on T-cells was focused on CD94 and CD161 cells, which are receptors of natural killer cells. The combination of both treatments did not affect epidermal proliferation and keratinization beyond the effect of calcipotriol, but virtually all T-cell subsets were reduced past the effect of monotherapies.

The combination of calcipotriol with betamethasone dipropionate has been shown to be more effective than either treatment as a monotherapy, whereas

Psoriasis: Diagnosis and Management, First Edition. Edited by Wolfram Sterry, Robert Sabat, and Sandra Philipp.

the combination of calcipotriol plus low-strength corticosteroids did not have a substantial additive effect compared with each as a monotherapy. However, the irritation caused by calcipotriol can be reduced by the addition of medium-strength corticosteroids. A two-compound formulation of calcipotriol and betamethasone dipropionate is commercially available and is applied once daily as ointment for chronic plaque psoriasis and as gel for scalp psoriasis. The efficacy of this combination is superior to monotherapies and is well tolerated. Long-term efficacy and safety have been shown for a treatment duration of 52 weeks. In facial psoriasis, the combination of calcipotriol with hydrocortison proved to be more effective and better tolerated than monotherapy with calcipotriol.

Some studies suggest that the combination of calcipotriol and photo(chemo) therapy may be useful. Combining TL01 phototherapy with topical calcipotriol cream has a UVB-sparing effect. The combination of calcipotriol and psoralen + UVA (PUVA) is characterized by a marked reduction in the cumulative dose of UVA and an enhanced efficacy, compared with the respective monotherapies. The combination of phototherapy with dithranol and the combination of phototherapy with tar are time-consuming therapies. However, if phototherapy is optimized by using near-erythematogenic doses, the additive effect of dithranol or tar above that of phototherapy is unsubstantiated; remission periods following the combination of dithranol and optimized phototherapy are prolonged.

Improved efficacy has also been observed with the combination of calcipotriol–cyclosporine and calcipotriol–acitretin, compared with each as a monotherapy. Again, the mode of action of calcipotriol (affecting epidermis with a selective effect on T-cells) is different from that of cyclosporine (strong immunosuppressive effect) and from acitretin (opposite effect on epidermal differentiation). Indeed, with low-dose cyclosporine (2 mg/kg/day), a marked improvement or clearing was seen in 90% of the patients who received the combination. The combination may be of importance to reduce the dose of this strong immunosuppressive treatment and to increase the safety of cyclosporine. In a case report, the superior efficacy at the calcipotriol-treated side was clearly shown in a patient suffering from psoriatic erythroderma treated with cyclosporin (5 mg/kg; Figures 19.1 and 19.2). In a dose-escalating study of acitretin, the combination of calcipotriol and acitretin was more effective and permitted a lower dose of both acitretin and calcipotriol as compared with each as monotherapy. Recently, the combination of topical calcipotriol/betamethasone with adalimumab was studied. This combination resulted in more rapid and higher efficacy within the first 4 weeks; thereafter, the trend was towards a higher response with adalimumab monotherapy.

Topical corticosteroids are frequently combined with other antipsoriatic treatments. Although reduction in the duration of subsequent remission periods has been claimed, controlled studies are required to substantiate these claims.

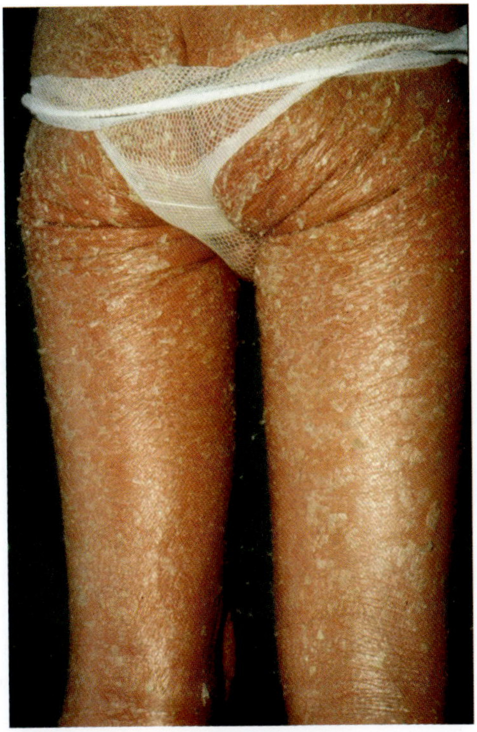

Figure 19.1 Erythrodermic psoriasis before treatment.

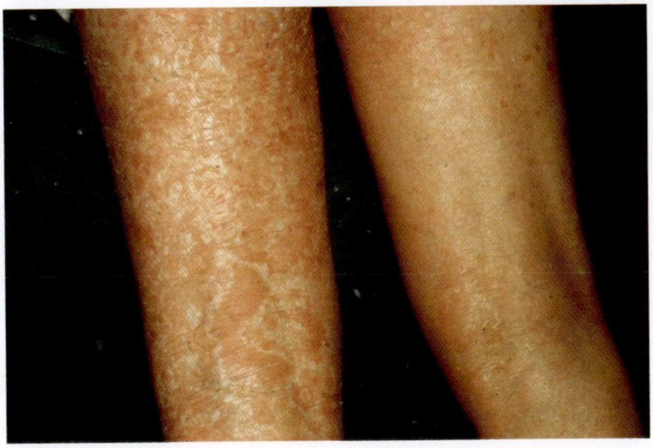

Figure 19.2 Eythrodermic psoriasis after 4 weeks' treatment with cyclosporine (5 mg/kg) and calcipotriol ointment on the right-hand side.

Photo(chemo) therapy in combination treatment

Photo(chemo)therapy can be combined with topicals (see above), and several combinations with systemic treatments are highly effective and safe. The combination with fumarates is possible, although no information on efficacy and safety is available from comparative studies. The combination of UVB with methotrexate has been reported to result in a rapid clinical improvement. Additional studies are needed before these combinations can be recommended. The combination of UVB with acitretin and photo(chemo)therapy with acitretin are time-honored principles. Anecdotal evidence is available for the combination of UVB phototherapy and etanercept. UVB-irradiated body halves showed an average reduction in Psoriasis Area and Severity Index score of 89% versus a reduction of 68% on nonirradiated body halves in patients treated with etanercept.

Systemic therapy in combination treatment

As acitretin is not an immunosuppressive treatment, its combination with other classical treatments is of interest. The combination with methotrexate has been reported to be effective in some cases, although hepatoxicity is a safety concern. Some reports on optimization of efficacy are available on the combination of acitretin with fumarates and cyclosporine.

The combination of acitretin and etanercept (25 mg twice weekly) has been shown to be as effective as etanercept 50 mg twice weekly. Again, the entirely different mode of action may be relevant for this added therapeutic effect and for improving the safety of etanercept. This combination results in a substantial reduction in costs, as less etanercept is administered. The combination of methotrexate and cyclosporin has been used with success by rheumatologists, and in recalcitrant psoriasis, the combination proved to be very effective without any major side effects. The combination of low-dose cyclosporin and etanercept has been described as very effective in seven patients with recalcitrant disease.

The combination of methotrexate and anti-TNF-α drugs has been shown to have an excellent efficacy. In patients on methotrexate, etanercept has been shown to increase efficacy, and vice versa, adding methotrexate to etanercept also increased the efficacy. Furthermore, methotrexate inhibits the formation of antibodies to anti-TNF-α drugs, which is relevant to infliximab and adalimumab, as reduced clinical efficacy has been observed due to neutralizing antibodies in patients treated with monotherapy with these TNF-α antibodies.

Contraindicated combinations and combinations for restrictive use

The combination of coal tar with PUVA is contraindicated, as it may induce significant phototoxic responses. Methotrexate has immunomodulatory properties and might increase the occurrence of UVB- or PUVA-induced cutaneous malignancies. However, the combination of narrowband UVB and methotrexate has been used with success in patients with treatment-resistant psoriasis, and so far there is no evidence that malignancies are induced during methotrexate therapy. Although a combination of methotrexate and PUVA has been reported to be safe, additional long-term studies are needed.

An increased occurrence of squamous cell carcinomas has been observed in patients treated with the combination of cyclosporine and PUVA, either simultaneously or sequentially. Therefore, the combination of cyclosporine and photo(chemo)therapy is contraindicated. The combination of acitretin and cyclosporine carries the risk of accumulation of cyclosporine, because cyclosporine is inactivated by the cytochrome P450 system, which is inhibited by acitretin.

The combination of methotrexate and acitretin has been used in those patients in whom all treatments have failed. Although this combination can be very effective, severe hepatotoxicity has been reported; therefore, careful monitoring of liver functions remains mandatory. The combination of cyclosporine and methotrexate has been viewed as contraindicated because both are immunosuppressants. However, in patients with severe psoriasis, the combination has been shown to be the "ultimum refugium."

The combination of biologics and cyclosporine is relatively contraindicated, as both treatments have immunosuppressive properties.

How to use combination treatment in practice

In real clinical life, the treatment of psoriasis is individualized to the needs and possibilities of the patient, reconciling the fact that patients have used treatments for a long time. This has implications for cumulative toxicity of a treatment but also for the acceptance of a treatment by the patient.

The evidence for increased efficacy/safety is not available for all combinations, and the preference for a combination is largely experience based. Based on available evidence and experience, Table 19.1 lists several recommendations for combinations.

Evidence for an added value to combine biologics with topicals is sparse. In some patients, it may be useful to add a topical treatment to a biologic in order to gain some improvement in the first 2–3 months when the systemic treatment is not yet fully effective, although the evidence from studies for such value is limited. Anti-TNF drugs in combination therapy with methotrexate, and in combination with acitretine, may be beneficial. Classical systemic and photo(chemo)therapy may benefit from the combination with a topical. The combination of acitretin and phototherapy is a well-established beneficial combination. With respect to the combination of topicals, the combination of calcipotriol and a corticosteroid is, based on evidence and experience, the first-line topical treatment.

Table 19.1 Combination of treatments in psoriasis.

	Topical vitamin D_3	Topical corticosteroid	Tarazotene	Dithranol	Fumarates	UVB	PUVA	Methotrexate	Cyclosporin	Acitretin
Biologics	+	+	+/–	+ +	+/–	+ +	–	+ + +	+/–	+++
Acitretin	+ + +	+	+/–	+ +	+/–	+ + +	+ + +	+/–	+/–	
Cyclosporin	+ + +	+	+ /–	+ +	+/–	–	–	+/–		
Methotrexate	+ + +	+	+ /–	+ +	+/–	+/–	+/–			
PUVA	+ +	+/–	+	+	+/–	–				
UVB	+	+/–	+	+ + +	+/–					
Fumarates	+ +	+	+ /–	+ +						
Dithranol	+ +	+ +	+							
Tarazotene	+	+ + +								
Topical corticosteroid	+ + +									

–: not recommended; ++: moderate; +: poor; +++: excellent.

Further reading

Gisondi, P., Del Giglio, M., Cotena, C. and Girolomoni, G. (2008) Combining etanercept and acitretin in the therapy of chronic plaque psoriasis: a 24-week, randomized, controlled, investigator-blinded pilot trial. *British Journal of Dermatology*, **158**, 1345–1351.

Grossman, R.M., Thivolet, J., Claudy, A., *et al.* (1994) A novel therapeutic approach to psoriasis with combination calcipotriol ointment and very low-dose cyclosporin: result of multicenter placebo-controlled study. *Journal of the American Academy of Dermatology*, **31**, 68–74.

Guenther, L., Cambazard, F., van de Kerkhof, P.C., *et al.* (2002) Efficacy and safety of a new combination of calcipotriol and betamethasone dipropionate (once or twice daily) compared to calcipotriol (twice daily) in the treatment of psoriasis vulgaris: a randomized, double blind, vehicle controlled clinical trial. *British Journal of Dermatology*, **147**, 316–323.

Hendriks, A.G., Keijsers, R.R., de Jong, E.M., Seyger, M.M. and van de Kerkhof, P.C. (2013) Efficacy and safety of firstline topical treatments in chronic plaque psoriasis: a systematic literature review. *Journal of the European Academy of Dermatology and Venereology*, **27**, 931–951.

Mahajan, R., Kaur, I. and Kanwar, A.J. (2010) Methotrexate/narrowband, UVB phototherapy combination vs. narrowband, UVB phototherapy in the treatment of chronic plaque-type psoriasis—a randomized single-blinded placebo-controlled study. *Journal of the European Academy of Dermatology and Venereology*, **24**, 595–600.

Roenigk, H.H. Jr. (1999) Acitretin combination therapy. Journal of the American Academy of Dermatology, **41**, *18–21.*

Thaçi, D., Ortonne, J.P., Chimenti, S., *et al.* (2010) A phase, IIIb, multicentre, randomized, double-blind, vehicle-controlled study of the efficacy and safety of adalimumab with and without calcipotriol/betamethasone topical treatment in patients with moderate to severe psoriasis: the, BELIEVE study. *British Journal of Dermatology*, **163**, 402–411.

van de Kerkhof, P.C., Cambazard, F., Hutchinson, F., *et al.* (1998) The effect of the addition of calcipotriol ointment (50 µg/g) to acitretin therapy in psoriasis. *British Journal of Dermatology*, **138**, 84–89.

Wolf, P., Hofer, A., Legat, F.J., *et al.* (2009) Treatment with 311-nm ultraviolet B accelerates and improves the clearance of psoriatic lesions in patients treated with etanercept. *British Journal of Dermatology*, **160**, 186–189.

Woo, W.K. and McKenna, K.E. (2003) Combination, TL01 ultraviolet B phototherapy and topical calcipotriol for psoriasis: a prospective randomized placebo-controlled clinical trial. *British Journal of Dermatology*, **149**(1), 146–150.

Zachariae, C., Mørk, N.J., Reunala, T., *et al.* (2008) The combination of etanercept and methotrexate increases the effectiveness of treatment in active psoriasis despite inadequate effect of methotrexate therapy. *Acta Dermato-Venereologica*, **88**, 495–501.

CHAPTER 20

Optimizing adherence to treatment

Frank Bachmann
Department of Dermatology and Allergy, University Medicine Charité, Berlin, Germany

In medicine, adherence describes the degree to which a patient correctly follows medical advice. Adherence is one of the major problems in effective delivery of healthcare. The complexity of treatment regimens, poor "health literacy" and lack of comprehension of treatment benefits, the occurrence of unexpected adverse drug reactions, the cost of prescription medicine, and poor patient–physician communication or lack of trust are among the most important factors negatively influencing treatment adherence, especially in chronic diseases. Furthermore, efficacy and safety are key contributors. Lack of efficacy is particularly contributory to nonadherence, and the preferences and views of others may have an additional impact on nonadherence.

Nonadherence may result in poorer prognosis, more frequent hospitalizations, and significantly higher healthcare costs. It is said that every 10% decrease in adherence to topical treatment may result in a one-point increase in disease severity on a 9-point scale.

In dermatology, most problems with adherence are encountered in topical treatment regimes for different reasons: (1) topical treatment is time-consuming, inconvenient, and more or less messy; and (2) treatment success is rather limited and demands considerable effort. Additionally, cost of treatment and unclear or complicated instructions might contribute to nonadherence. In fact, topical treatment is considered to be one of the most negative aspects of psoriasis.

For systemic treatment, the situation is somewhat different. For different reasons, the patient is more successfully linked to the treating physician: (1) treatment response is good to excellent in most cases, and (2) systemic therapy requires regularly blood controls and more frequent visits. On the other hand, systemic treatment is often perceived to carry a greater potential for a severe adverse reaction, wherefore patients may be more reluctant to start systemic treatment.

One might believe that disease severity improves adherence to treatment; interestingly, patients with more severe psoriasis are actually less likely to use their medications than patients with milder disease. Patients with severe disease are often less satisfied with their treatment leading to a vicious circle where those with

Psoriasis: Diagnosis and Management, First Edition. Edited by Wolfram Sterry, Robert Sabat, and Sandra Philipp.

more severe disease, worse quality of life, and poor treatment satisfaction may be less likely to adhere to treatment regimens. Furthermore, most of them present with a long history of rather frustrating treatment attempts. Because of this, it is of upmost importance that the patient knows what to expect from the treatment in order to prevent disappointment if treatment response is slow or rather limited.

Adherence to treatment seems best in patients still suffering from symptoms but experiencing substantial relief and improvement in symptoms and quality of life. On the other hand, adherence is worse if the response is lacking. Compliance may also deteriorate in patients in long-term remission by simply forgetting the impact of disease and the necessity of maintenance therapy.

Recommendations on improving patients' adherence to treatment (modified from the recommendation of the International Psoriasis Council: Feldman *et al.* 2008) are as follows:

1. Physician–patient relationship. A strong physician–patient relationship establishes trust. Such a relationship does not depend solely on the treating physician but starts with the friendliness and professionalism of the clinic staff as well as the clinical setting. Patients should feel comfortable. Attentive listening is a key to create a positive relationship and, therewith, is critical for adherence and good outcomes. Patients should have the feeling that they are listened to. Physical contact such as palpating the skin and commenting on its characteristics helps further to create a good relationship and indicates thoroughness of examination. Simultaneously, physical contact reduces patients' sense of stigmatization. Try to use understandable language that relates to the patients' educational level. Using the patients' own words and language significantly increases patient satisfaction. Encourage open exchange and participation. Ask questions and allow the patients to talk about their psychosocial concerns, which may be particularly important and increases patients' satisfaction. In general, patient satisfaction correlates with patients' perception of physicians' concerns for their health, the quality of explanations, and the quality of the answers to their questions.
2. Patient's preference. It is difficult to predict patients' preferences. Therefore, we encourage open discussion of this issue. Preferences for certain vehicles affect use, efficacy, and thus adherence. Preferences and views of others such as family or friends may have a further impact on adherence. Family members, however, can be advocates for treatment adherence as well. They may assist with treatment applications, help to remember dosing schedules, and provide a support network.
3. Choosing the right vehicle. A wide range of vehicles are available for delivery of topical medications. The location and extent of disease may influence the choice of vehicle. While white petroleum might work for a localized, severely infiltrated plaque, for example, on the lower leg, patients will usually not accept the same for the whole body surface. However, explaining why and for

how long a certain vehicle may be necessary improves adherence, even if it is perceived as bothersome. Patients may frequently require more than one vehicle for more extensive disease. Choose vehicles that can be applied easily. Interval therapies may be beneficial in order to reduce repeated application of active agents such as highly potent steroids. If the vehicle does not moisturize sufficiently, overly frequent application or application of unwanted products may result. Therefore, make sure that you provide or recommend adjusted topical treatment regimes including moisturizers that do not reduce the desired treatment effects. Adjust topical therapy to temperature and climate by using lotions or creams rather than ointments in warm seasons and vice versa. Traditionally, ointment vehicles have been recommended because of their perceived greater potency and their greater ability to moisturize. Nonetheless, if a patient expresses dislike for ointment vehicles, other choices may be more appropriate. New data suggest that newer formulations such as gel formulations, lotions, or foams show a similar efficacy, are well accepted, and, therefore, may improve adherence and thus efficacy. Try to adjust products to the needs and wishes of the patient. In general, the best vehicle to prescribe to a patient is the vehicle that a patient is willing to use.

4. Appropriate application may require special instructions. Upon introduction of treatment regimens, explain to the patient when and how to use each of the components. Encourage note-taking or hand out written instructions. Patients will benefit from practical demonstrations. Instruction programs provided by specialized nurses may further improve adherence. Clear instructions and treatment-specific individual dosing devices or the use of the fingertip unit concept may help dose and apply topical treatment correctly.
5. Complexity of treatment regimens. Simplify treatment as much as possible and try to prescribe a regimen that is practical. Individualizing the treatment and minimizing its complexity will likely encourage adherence. Therefore, we recommend a regime with one or only few products that can be applied for many if not all of the affected locations. Simple dosing routines such as twice or preferably once daily are more likely to increase adherent behavior. Limit twice-daily application to a short period of time. Some patients may not improve even with appropriate treatment. In these cases, address difficulties with treatment adherence rather than introducing more complex or more potent regimens. The initial treatment may have been too complex or perceived as too risky. Consequently, try to simplify treatment regimen. In these patients, instruction programs may be of benefit.
6. "Health literacy." Patient education is critical in optimizing psoriasis management, treatment adherence, and thus safety and efficacy. Patients should feel that they have been informed adequately concerning safety and risks, efficacy and benefits, as well as alternatives to the regimen suggested to them. Do not overload patients with data that the average patient cannot understand. Use the patient's language (if appropriate). Be clear and refrain

from vague statements. Encourage and allow time for questions. Ensure that you have been understood, and if in doubt, ask the patient to explain the regimen to you. Provide patients with take-home messages and written instructions or references if necessary. Try to evaluate the patient's learning upon revisit if appropriate. However, never embarrass the patient by pointing out shortcomings or difficulties in comprehension. Instead, slow down and take extra time for explanation.

- Health risk associated with severe psoriasis. Psoriasis is barely an inflammation of the skin alone but a systemic inflammation with associated diseases, higher risks of cardiovascular complications, and eventually reduced life expectancy if untreated. Provide patients with information necessary to understand the need for treatment. Nevertheless, do not scare or threaten patients, and adjust the amount of information to the needs and wishes of the individual patient.
- Available treatment regimens. To allow informed consent for any treatment suggested, provide enough information and explain the advantages as well as the disadvantages of the available treatment options. You might want to explain why you choose one treatment over the other and what might be the next step.
- Comprehension of treatment benefits. Explain the general benefits of the treatment such as a risk reduction for certain comorbidities, improvements in health-risk parameters, such as insulin resistance, and positive impacts on quality of life.

7 Efficacy of treatment. It is important to point out that treatment response cannot be expected immediately—neither for potent topical nor for systemic therapy. For better adherence, give a time frame in which one will expect initial signs for improvement and explain that a full evaluation of response will be carried out after 3 months of treatment. In addition, explain to the patient that on-and-off therapies may result in a loss of efficacy. In many clinical controlled trials, continuous therapy was better than intermittent therapy.

8 Safety concerns. Any therapy implies potential safety risks and adverse drug reactions. Explain (1) the potential risks, (2) how to recognize and minimize them, and (3) what your and the patient's parts for prevention and early recognition are. For most patients, systemic therapy presents with more pronounced safety concerns, while others are reluctant to apply topical steroids. In these patients, one must carefully explain the reasons for and against that particular therapy. Patients feel safer the more you are sure and convinced about your choice. Here again, limiting the time of any treatment perceived as potentially harmful increases treatment adherence, safety, and efficacy. On the other hand, some patients do not care at all about safety risk. These patients are at higher risks for overly frequent or incorrect use of therapy. Here, it might be appropriate to emphasize and point out the potential risks related to therapy and encourage proper use. In general, try to instill an attitude free of fear but with regard to potential adverse drug reactions and safety concerns.

9 Occurrence of unexpected adverse drug reactions. Unexpected adverse drug reactions may occur at any time during the course of treatment. In these cases, enable the patient to contact you or other health authorities immediately in order to guarantee safety and confidence in you and others. If possible, provide an emergency contact number or refer to appropriate emergency departments.

10 Adherence to treatment tends to decline with time. In chronic diseases such as psoriasis, patients tend to adhere less with treatment over time. Even in controlled clinical trials, compliance can decrease by up to 40% after only 8 weeks. Therefore, health providers must motivate not only the patients to accept and adhere to therapy but also their support network for example, family and friends. Return visits shortly after beginning treatment may reduce the perception of burden. If early return visits are not practical, a scheduled telephone or e-mail contact may offer the same benefits. More frequent visits and interaction with the treating physician positively contribute to adherence. Again, instruction programs with specialized nurses and other patient-oriented programs may help to prevent or lessen nonadherence over time.

Further reading

Bewley, A. and Page, B. (2011) Maximizing patient adherence for optimal outcomes in psoriasis. *Journal of the European Academy of Dermatology and Venereology*, **25** (Supplement 4), 9–14.

Carroll, C.L., Feldman, S.R., Camacho, F.T. and Balkrishnan, R. (2004) Better medication adherence results in greater improvement in severity of psoriasis. *British Journal of Dermatology*, **151**, 895–897.

Carroll, C.L., Feldman, S.R., Camacho, F.T., Manuel, J.C. and Balkrishnan, R. (2004) Adherence to topical therapy decreases during the course of an 8-week psoriasis clinical trial: commonly used methods of measuring adherence to topical therapy overestimate actual use. *Journal of the American Academy of Dermatology*, **51**, 212–216.

Feldman, S.R., Horn, E.J., Balkrishnan, R. *et al.* (2008) Psoriasis: improving adherence to topical therapy. *Journal of the American Academy of Dermatology*, **59**, 1009–1016.

Richards, H.L., Fortune, D.G. and Griffiths, C.E. (2006) Adherence to treatment in patients with psoriasis. *Journal of the European Academy of Dermatology and Venereology*, **20**, 370–379.

CHAPTER 21
Psoriasis therapy in children

Sandra Philipp
Psoriasis Research and Treatment Center, Department of Dermatology and Allergy/Institute of Medical Immunology, University Hospital Charité, Berlin, Germany

The treatment of pediatric psoriasis is a complex and challenging task, including not only the choice of the best and safest treatment option for the individual patient, but also special counseling of both patients and parents, to minimize the negative impact of the disease on the development of the child, to help the patient to cope with the disease, and to prevent potential complications. In contrast to the variety of approved treatment options for adult patients suffering from psoriasis, data regarding their use in children are rare and often based on case reports or small case series. This results in a lack of official guidelines and often determines use out of current license. The great need for information led to two recent publications by European and German experts that combined the currently available published data with their clinical expertise (Ståhle *et al.* 2010; Sticherling *et al.* 2011).

An important therapeutic aspect of pediatric psoriasis is the early detection of potential infections. In particular, infections with group A hemolytic streptococci have been associated with the elicitation of psoriasis, and so microbial swabs of the throat, anal cleft, or ano-genital region or streptococci-specific antibody titers are recommended. Routine use of antibiotics is not advisable, but treatment should be initiated in cases of a positive microbial swab or may be considered in guttate psoriasis. The most commonly used antibiotics in children are penicillin V, first generation cephalosporins and erythromycin. Consultation with an otorhinolaryngologist might be helpful in children with more than three recurrent infections and a positive streptococcal swab to consider a potential tonsillectomy.

Topical treatment

The basis of any treatment strategy regardless of age and disease severity is the use of emollients to minimize symptoms such as pain, itching, or dryness (the Koebner phenomenon). In common usage are lipophilic ointments to which additional substances might be added: polidocanol 3–5% can be chosen in case of pruritus, urea 3–10% for dryness of skin (e.g. face 3%; body 3–5% <10 years,

Psoriasis: Diagnosis and Management, First Edition. Edited by Wolfram Sterry, Robert Sabat, and Sandra Philipp.

5–10% >10 years), or antimycotics such as clotrimazol 1% if the genitoanal area is affected. Additionally, oil baths can be used. If scales are dominant, keratolysis might be necessary. Yet, in contrast to adults, the use of salicylic acid should be limited due to the potential risk of salicylic intoxication. Since children's skin has a greater permeability and covers a greater surface in relation to body weight, this results in increased absorption of topical substances. Therefore, if at all, only localized short-term use is recommended at concentrations not exceeding 3%, and in children below school age, a concentration of 0.5% has been proposed. As an alternative, a hydrophilic emulsifying cream with the addition of lactic acid 3% may be applied. In scalp psoriasis, the use of olive oil or a hydrophilic emulsifying cream overnight followed by washing off with a shampoo containing pyrithion has been used successfully.

The most frequently used topical preparations in pediatric psoriasis are locally applied corticosteroids and vitamin D analogs. Although two studies with vitamin D analogs (calcipotriol + calcitriol) raised no safety concerns, only the ointments have been licensed for use in pediatric psoriasis. Yet, the different preparations allow for the adjusted use according to different locations, such as emulsion for the face or flexures, or solution for the head. Depending on the substance, application should not exceed 15–30% of body surface area, so as to prevent any alterations to calcium metabolism (Table 21.1). The most frequent adverse effects include irritation and itching. The response onset is expected after 2 weeks, reaching a maximum efficacy after 6–8 weeks. Initial short-term combination of vitamin D analogs with betamethasone (also available as a fixed combination) is common.

Corticosteroids are especially useful in highly inflammatory and itchy lesions, but use should be restricted with respect to area and time to prevent skin atrophy (striae distensae) and limit systemic absorption. Nowadays, modern substances such as mometasonfuroat, methylprednisolone aceponat, or prednicarbat are preferred over traditional class II or III glucocorticoids (German/Nordic classification, see Chapter 17) owing to their better risk–benefit ratio (fewer adverse effects such as atrophy). The use of highly potent (Class III and IV, German/Nordic classification, see Chapter 17) glucocorticoids should best be avoided in children, and on the face, flexures, or intertriginous areas. If the use is deemed necessary it has to be restricted with respect to area and time (Table 21.1). Abrupt application cessation should be avoided by tapering and/or possible combination with vitamin D analogs. From long-term experience, dithranol (anthralin) can still be considered as a first-line topical treatment for pediatric patients, though the use may be limited due to its irritant potential and the brownish staining of skin and textiles. Respective training of patients and parents, and close control by a physician are important. Short-term contact therapy with preparations that do not stain when washed off with cold water may be used in an outpatient setting (Table 21.1), whereas classical long-term therapy generally involves a hospital setting. The calcineurin inhibitors tacrolimus and pimecrolimus are both used to treat plaque psoriasis in children, though they are only licensed for atopic dermatitis. Efficacy

Table 21.1 Selected topical treatments for pediatric psoriasis.

Calcipotriol	Only ointment approved ≥6 years (50 g/week 6–12 years, 75 g/week 12–18 years), max. 8 weeks, max. 30% of BSA Solution (scalp), emulsion (face, flexures), cream: not licensed in children (below 18)
Tacalcitol	Ointment from 12 years on 10 g/day max. 8 weeks; max. 15% BSA Emulsion from 12 years on (face, flexures), <70 mL/week
Calcitriol	Not licensed in children, rarely used, max. 35% of BSA, max. 6 weeks
Betamethasone/calcipotriol fixed combination	Not licensed in children, short-term, max. 4 weeks
Methylprednisolone aceponat	Cream: ≥3 years (atopic dermatitis, eczema) Milk: >4 months, but careful consideration below 3 years Ointment, greasy ointment: no restriction in children or neonates
Mometason furoat	Rich cream: ≥2 years (all inflammatory skin diseases) ointment, solution: ≥6 years, max. 3 weeks, <10% of BSA
Prednicarbat	Cream, ointment, greasy ointment: no restriction, but only exceptional in neonates
Class II, e.g. triamcinolonacetonid 0.1%	Infants and children with inflammatory skin diseases for which moderately GCS are indicated, short-term and limited area
Class III, e.g. betamethasonvalerate	Chronic inflammatory diseases for which high-potent GCS are indicated, >1 year, restricted to area <10% of BSA, max. 1 week
Class IV exceptional: e.g. clobetasolproprionate	3–12 years only in exceptional cases, restricted to area <10% of BSA, only short term (max. 1 week), not in flexures or face
Dithranol (anthralin)	No restriction, preparations (0.065–3%), mainly long-term application in a hospital setting. Fixed preparations are available (0.5–3%), some contain urea, and some contain salicylic acid. The latter should not be used in children below school age (attention: salicylic intoxication)
Micanol cream 1% or 3%	No restriction, special formulation prevents or reduces brownish staining when washed off with cold water; short-contact therapy (5–20 min)
Tazarotene	Rarely used due to its irritating potential; in some countries only available by international pharmacy
Coal tar	Preparations with 5–8%, limited by its odour
Tacrolimus	Ointment 0.03% licensed in children with atopic dermatitis ≥2 years twice daily, max. 3 weeks, then tapering (0.1% ≥16 years)
Pimecrolimus	Cream 1%, licensed in children with atopic dermatitis ≥2 years

BSA: body surface area; GCS: glucocorticoids.

has been shown especially for use on the face and intertriginous areas with the advantage of not showing atrophogenic potential. Moreover, they may be considered to reduce the need for glucocorticoids. The most frequent adverse effect is a burning sensation after application, especially at the beginning of treatment. Widespread use should be avoided due to potential absorption, and combination with UV therapy is contraindicated for an increased risk of UV-related skin tumors. The use of tar compounds is limited owing to the undesirable odour and the potential carcinogenicity, though the latter is still controversial. Topical retinoids (e.g. tazarotene) are rarely applied, because of their irritating potential.

UV-light-therapy and systemic treatment

However, topical treatment might not be sufficient in children with widespread disease. Narrow-band UVB is the most frequently prescribed form of UV therapy in pediatric psoriasis and is considered to be especially appropriate in older children (>10 years) with skin type III and IV according to Fitzpatrick. Nevertheless, caution is recommended, and exposure should be limited when possible. UVB should not be used in fair-skinned children. The most common side effect is solar dermatitis (erythema), albeit mostly mild in severity. A few small studies have shown a good efficacy and safety profile for the short-term treatment with narrow-band UVB in children. The frequency of treatments ranges from two to five times weekly. The initial dosage should be adjusted according to skin type (e.g. UVB 0.03 J/cm^2 in skin type I and II or UVB 0.05 J/cm^2 in skin type III and IV, see chapter 17) with an increase in dosage of about 10–20% in the subsequent session depending on tolerability. Long-term data are lacking, and the potential carcinogenicity of UVB is still controversial. Dosage should be chosen carefully, as the number of cases of sunburn in childhood appears to be a risk factor for increased incidence of melanoma. Documentation of the number of sessions and the cumulative dosage is recommended. Combinations of UVB and anthralin or vitamin D analogs are possible. In contrast to UVB, the use of photochemotherapy with psoralen in combination with UV-A (PUVA) should be avoided in children, as oral PUVA has been shown to increase the risk of nonmelanoma skin cancers. A potential exception may be topical PUVA (cream- or bath PUVA) for cases of severe pustular psoriasis of hands and feet.

Systemic treatment in children might be considered in severely affected children with either widespread or recurrent disease or involvement of the joints. Treating physicians must thoroughly weigh up the potential benefits and risks of the various treatments, with a special emphasis on safety. Intensive counseling of patients and parents is of upmost importance, with respect to use, possible side effects, and potential lack of licensure. The best clinical experience on use in children is available for methotrexate, cyclosporine, and etanercept, but still there are only limited data, particularly regarding the long-term use.

Methotrexate

Methotrexate has recently been approved for the treatment of juvenile idiopathic arthritis including pediatric psoriatic arthritis. Although not licensed for plaque psoriasis, it has been frequently used in pediatric psoriasis resulting in valuable clinical experience. In children with widespread disease that is unresponsive to topical therapy or UV treatment, methotrexate may be considered as a first-line therapy. If children suffer from psoriatic arthritis, methotrexate is the therapy of choice if nonsteroidal anti-inflammatory drugs and/or local glucocorticoids have failed. The recommended dosage is 0.3 mg/kg body weight once a week orally, subcutaneous or intramuscular regardless of age or weight, though the dosage of 22.5 mg should not be exceeded. In a recent consensus paper of pediatric rheumatologists, a dose of 10–15 mg/m^2 surface area once a week has been recommended. Folate supplementation is advised, either as a 5 mg tablet 2 days after each methotrexate application, or as a daily administration of folate 1 mg except on the day of methotrexate intake. Efficacy is often quite good with a favorable side-effect profile in children compared with adults. The most common adverse effects are gastrointestinal complaints (nausea, aversion to taking the medication). Regular blood analysis is recommended (white and red blood cell count, liver enzymes, creatinine, and urea) to monitor hepatotoxicity or potential bone marrow suppression.

Cyclosporine

Regarding cyclosporine, limited evidence (case reports) is available for the use in pediatric psoriasis, though more experience exists in children with atopic dermatitis or organ-transplant recipients. Therefore, in case of severe psoriasis flairs, cyclosporine seems to be an appropriate treatment option in children. Regardless of age, a dosage of 1–5 mg/kg body weight per day is given in two applications. To avoid overdosing and subsequent kidney toxicity, the dose is best adjusted according to ideal rather than actual body weight. When the response is reached and stable, the dose may be slowly reduced again. Clinical response has been reported between 2 and 8 weeks. Treatment should not be interrupted abruptly to prevent rebound, and it is recommended that one should use the lowest possible maintenance dose and shortest treatment period necessary. A prolonged treatment exceeding 6 months should be administered only with great caution. Side effects such as nephrotoxicity and hypertension are dose-dependent and usually reversible after discontinuation, so control is important. Monitoring involves blood pressure, blood analysis, especially creatinine, and CsA levels under certain circumstances. Cyclosporine is available as a solution, which might be preferable in children. Concurrent phototherapy is not recommended due to the potentially increased risk of developing skin cancer.

Acitretin

Acitretin, though approved for children with severe psoriasis, is only rarely used in childhood, in particular in cases of pustular psoriasis or erythrodermic psoriasis, and mainly in children older than 10 years. Its efficacy as monotherapy for plaque psoriasis is rather limited. Commonly, a dosage of 0.3–0.5 mg/kg per day is used; in exceptional cases, the dose may be increased to 0.75 or 1.0 mg/kg if tolerated (max. 35 mg/day). Depending on the response, tapering to 0.2 mg/kg may be applied. The treatment is limited due to its side effects such as dryness and irritation of skin, potentially impairing compliance, as well as its influence on bone metabolism. In adolescents, the application may be limited due to teratogenicity. Pubertal girls should use contraception during and after treatment for 1–2 years. In view of the potential precedent epiphyseal closure, an X-ray of growing bones should be considered.

Fumaric acid esters

In Germany, fumaric acid esters (FAEs) are considered first-line therapy in adults with psoriasis, and sustained efficacy with good long-term tolerability has recently been shown in a retrospective study. However, concerning children, only two case reports have been published so far. The most common adverse effects, particularly at the beginning, are gastrointestinal complaints (bowel pain, nausea, and diarrhea) and flushing. To minimize these side effects, an initial dosage scheme has been introduced, starting with tablets containing 30 mg per day and slowly increasing the dose to three tablets per day before switching to one tablet with 120 mg. The dosage then can be raised to a maximum of six tablets per day (2–2–2), though usually a mean maintenance dose of three tablets (360 mg) is sufficient to treat psoriasis effectively. Monitoring should include regular blood analysis (red-blood-cell count, differential blood count, liver enzymes, and creatinine). FAEs can decrease the number of lymphocytes, and in rare cases where the leukocyte count falls below 3000/μL and the lymphocyte count falls below below 500/μL, treatment termination should be considered. Regarding the favorable safety profile of FAEs, treatment in children may be reasonably safe on a case-by-case basis; yet, because of the dose increments and gastrointestinal side effects, treatment of small children might be limited. Previous experience with FAE treatment in adolescents has proven successful, and a clinical trial in children aged 12-17 is ongoing.

Biologics

So far, etanercept may be considered as a first-choice biologic for use in pediatric psoriasis. In Europe, it has been approved for children aged 6 years or older who are inadequately controlled by, or are intolerant to, other systemic therapies or phototherapies. However, some experts even suggest first-line use in severely affected children. Etanercept is applied as a subcutaneous injection at a dosage of 0.8 mg/kg body weight once a week (max. 50 mg/week). One randomized placebo-controlled study in 211 children (4–17 years of age) suffering from psoriasis showed a good efficacy with PASI 75 responses in 57% of patients after 12 weeks and sustained efficacy until week 96. Etanercept was generally well tolerated with the most common reported adverse effects being upper-respiratory-tract infections, nasopharyngits, streptococcal pharyngitis, headache, and sinusitis. Neither opportunistic infections nor malignancies have been observed. Screening includes exclusion of tuberculosis by interferon-γ-release assay, and the vaccination status should be updated. Monitoring involves regular blood analyses, and special attention should be focused on potential infections. Regarding infliximab, licensure for children suffering from psoriasis is pending. However, clinical experience on the use in children is available from other indications, as infliximab has already been approved for children suffering from juvenile idiopathic arthritis or Crohn's disease. The primary side effect was an increased risk of infection, as it is common with all tumour necrosis factor (TNF) inhibitors. There are several case reports in the literature on the successful use of infliximab in pediatric psoriasis at a dosage of 5 mg/kg body weight at weeks 0, 2, and 6, thus providing evidence for its excellent efficacy. Infliximab may be considered especially in pustular and erythrodermic forms of pediatric psoriasis, or if a rapid response is warranted to control the disease.

Reports on the use of adalimumab in pediatric psoriasis are scarce, though there is limited experience in children treated with adalimumab for juvenile idiopathic arthritis or Crohn's disease. The most common adverse effects were infections and injection-site reactions with no opportunistic infections or malignancies reported, and the efficacy was good. Dosage was weight-adjusted every second week 0.4 mg/kg body weight subcutaneously. A trial for the use of adalimumab in children and adolesecents suffering from psoriasis is ongoing. So far, there are no published data available on the use of alefacept or ustekinumab in children, but regarding ustekinumab, a clinical trial for use in children aged 12–17 years is currently running.

Overall, experience with the use of TNF inhibitors for psoriasis in childhood is still limited, and recent reports about potential cutaneous malignancies and lymphomas have to be considered when choosing the therapy. Rare reports of malignancies, particularly lymphomas in children and adolescents treated with TNF-antagonists either for Crohn's disease or for juvenile idiopathic arthritis have raised concerns. For children and adolescents with inflammatory bowel disease treated with infliximab or adalimumab combined with azathioprine or 6-mercaptopurine, rare fatal cases of hepatosplenic T-cell lymphoma have been observed. However, one should take into consideration that patients suffering from systemic chronic inflammatory diseases have an increased lymphoma risk compared with the general population. Therefore, long-term data are still very much needed, and registries of children treated with TNF inhibitors are strongly recommended.

Further reading

Benoit, S. and Hamm, H. (2007) Childhood psoriasis. *Clinics in Dermatology*, **25**, 555–562.

Gerdes, S., Domm, S. and Mrowietz, U. (2011) Long-term treatment with fumaric acid esters in an 11-year-old male child with psoriasis. *Dermatology*, **222**, 198–200.

Morris, A., Rogers, M., Fischer, G. and Williams, K. (2001) Childhood psoriasis: a clinical review of 1262 cases. *Pediatric Dermatology*, **18**, 188–198.

Niehues, T., Horneff, G., Michels, H., Sailer Höck, M. and Schuchmann, L. (2005) Evidence-based use of methotrexate in children with rheumatic diseases: a consensus statement of the Working Groups Pediatric Rheumatology Germany (AGKJR) and Pediatric Rheumatology Austria. *Rheumatology International*, **25**, 169–178.

Paller, A.S., Siegfried, E.C., Langley, R.G. *et al.* (2008) Etanercept treatment for children and adolescents with plaque psoriasis. *New England Journal of Medicine*, **358**, 241–51.

Ståhle, M., Atakan, N., Boehncke W-H. *et al.* (2010) Juvenile psoriasis and its clinical management: a European expert group consensus. *Journal der Deutschen Dermatologischen Gesellschaft*, **8**, 812–818.

Sticherling, M., Augustin, M., Boehncke W-H. *et al.* (2011) Therapy of psoriasis in childhood and adolescence—a German expert consensus. *Journal der Deutschen Dermatologischen Gesellschaft*, **9**, 815–823.

Wright, N.A., Piggott, D.S. and Eichenfield, F. (2010) The role of biologics and other systemic agents in the treatment of pediatric psoriasis. *Seminars in Cutaneous Medicine and Surgery*, **29**, 20–26.

Zamberk, P., Velázquez, D., Campos, M., Hernandez, J. and Lázaro, P. (2010) Paediatric psoriasis—narrowband UVB treatment. *Journal of the European Academy of Dermatology and Venereology*, **24**, 415–419.

Zappel, K., Sterry, W. and Blume-Peytavi, U. (2004) Therapie-optionen der psoariasis im kindes- und jugendalter. *Journal der Deutschen Dermatologischen Gesellschaft*, **2**, 329–342.

CHAPTER 22

Therapy of psoriasis during pregnancy

Sandra Philipp

Psoriasis Research and Treatment Center, Department of Dermatology and Allergy/Institute of Medical Immunology, University Hospital Charité, Berlin, Germany

Management of psoriasis in pregnancy

Managing psoriasis in pregnancy (see Figures 22.1 and 22.2) involves not only the choice of treatment, which is restricted to avoid potential harm to the fetus, but also counseling of patients with regard to the course of disease, the potential influences on pregnancy, or vice versa, as well as about comorbidities along with lifestyle factors that might have a negative impact (see Chapters 13 and 15). Whereas it is still recommended that systemic drug exposure be avoided during pregnancy when possible, this may not be feasible in widespread disease. Anticipatory management of psoriasis is advisable to induce a period of remission or optimize the control of the disease before conception to prevent or minimize flare-ups during pregnancy, including consideration of the necessary washout periods of the respective substances. In addition, prior planning in case of a worsening condition after delivery may help to control the disease without affecting nursing.

Treatment options during pregnancy

Topical treatment

Topical treatment with emollients and topical glucocorticoids are considered first-line therapy for psoriasis in pregnancy. Mild to moderate *glucocorticoids* are preferred to potent or very potent ones, as the latter have been associated with a potential risk of fetal growth restriction. However, women can be reassured that there is no significantly increased risk of orofacial cleft, preterm delivery, or fetal death when using topical corticosteroids within restricted areas in pregnancy. In addition, a favorable side-effect profile has been suggested for newer lipophilic substances with a good therapeutic index (see Table 22.1). Data on anthralin use during pregnancy in humans are missing.

Psoriasis: Diagnosis and Management, First Edition. Edited by Wolfram Sterry, Robert Sabat, and Sandra Philipp.

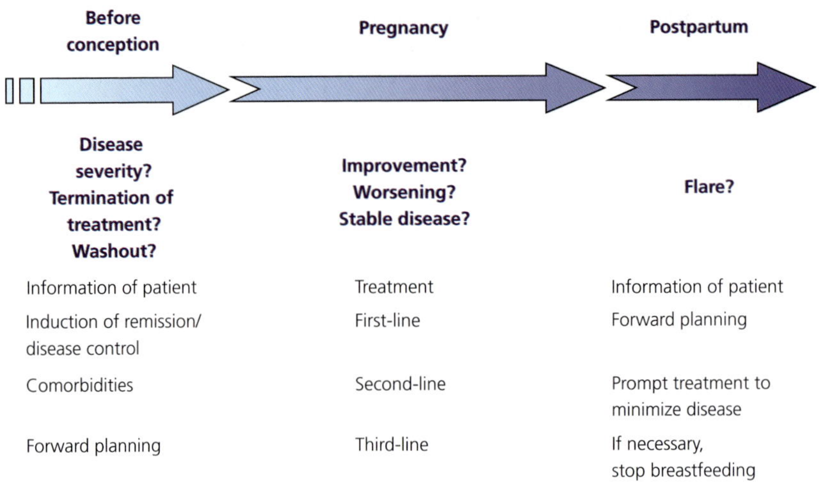

Figure 22.1 Therapeutic management of psoriasis in pregnancy.

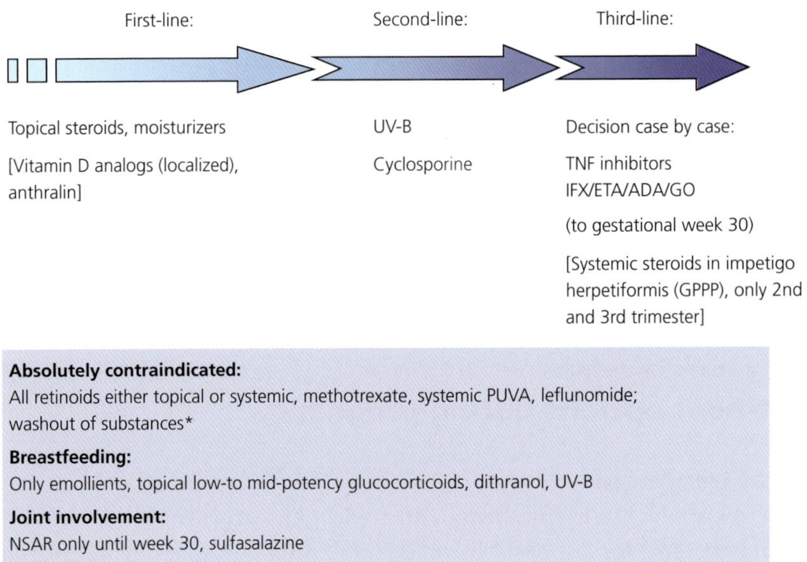

Figure 22.2 Therapeutic options of psoriasis in pregnancy. *Washout-periods: systemic retinoids 2 years; methotrexate 3–5 months, leflunomide either 2 years or washout with colestyramine.

Nevertheless, as there is no evidence of systemic absorption from topical application, treatment might be considered safe in pregnancy (CAVE:only preparations without salicylic acid).

If deemed necessary, localized use of topical vitamin D analogs may be considered during pregnancy, and in specific cases restricted application of topical tacrolimus might be possible when no alternative exists.

Table 22.1 Examples of mild to very potent topical corticosteroids (adapted from Chi *et al.* 2011).

Mild to moderate glucocorticoids	Potent and very potent glucocorticoids
Hydrocortisone 0.1–2.5%	Fluticasone propionate 0.005–0.05%[a]
	Hydrocortisone butyrate 0.1%[a]
	Mometasone furoate 0.1%[a]
	Methylprednisolone aceponate 0.1%[a]
Fluocortolone 0.25%	Diflucortolone valerate 0.1–0.3%
Betamethasone valerate 0.025%	Betamethasone dipropionate 0.05%,
	Betamethasone valerate 0.1%
Clobetasone butyrate 0.05%	Clobetasol propionate 0.05%
	Triamcinolone acetonide 0.1%

[a]Substances with a good therapeutic index, that is, drugs considered to be of high potency with regard to efficacy while showing fewer adverse effects.

Though manufacturers recommend restrictive use of vitamin D analogs during pregnancy, topical *calcipotriol* is likely safe for the treatment of localized psoriasis in pregnancy. In animal studies, high subcutaneous doses have resulted in decreased weight gain, and high oral doses have led to skeletal abnormalities, but when the ointment is applied to psoriatic plaques, only about 6% is absorbed systemically; therefore, significant fetal exposure is unlikely to occur when they are used within a restricted area.

Although topical *tacrolimus* is not approved for psoriasis, it has been shown to be effective in special locations such as the face or intertriginous areas. Systemic tacrolimus used during pregnancy may result in fetal malformations or preterm deliveries. However, the bioavailability of topical tacrolimus is estimated at less than 5% of the oral drug, and the localized topical use has not been associated with systemic effects. Therefore, restricted topical treatment might be reasonably safe during pregnancy, for example, when a reduction of topical glucocorticoids is necessary.

Salicylic acid, used as a keratolytic agent in concentrations of 2–5%, usually shows low systemic absorption, but rare case reports describe systemic salicylate poisoning due to prolonged and widespread use. As maternal intake of oral salicylates has been associated with an increased risk of gastroschisis in early pregnancy and impaired homeostasis within a week of delivery, as well as oral cyclo-oxygenase inhibitors in late pregnancy with constriction of the fetal ductus arteriosus, the use of topical salicylic acid should at best be avoided.

The safety of *coal tar products* is still a matter of debate. Topical application may result in systemic absorption of potentially mutagenic polycyclic aromatic hydrocarbons, and animal studies have suggested teratogenicity, whereas this has not been reported in humans. However, treatment in pregnancy cannot be recommended. When considering treatment options, special attention should be given during first trimester (development of embryo) and late pregnancy. To prevent increased systemic absorption occlussive dressings or combinations with other substances should be avoided.

Phototherapy

In pregnant patients with widespread disease that cannot be managed with topical treatment, *UVB therapy* is regarded as a safe and effective therapeutic option. UVB cannot penetrate beyond the superficial skin, and so it is not thought to be harmful for the fetus. As phototherapy may worsen melasma, covering of face is advisable. In case of higher cumulative doses administration of folate may prevent folate deficiency, and as such the risk of neural tube defects.

Systemic *PUVA* treatment is contraindicated in pregnancy due to its mutagenic potential, as photoactivation of psoralens may induce sister chromatid exchanges. However, so far, no adverse fetal outcomes have been reported for women becoming pregnant during treament with PUVA. With respect to topical PUVA, small studies have revealed no detectable blood levels after localized application on the palms and soles, and absorption might be additionally minimized by washing the skin after topical PUVA treatment. Subsequently, fetal exposure is unlikely with restricted use of topical PUVA. In conclusion, when PUVA is deemed to be necessary, topical PUVA should be favored, although since there is insufficient evidence, its use cannot be recommended.

Systemic treatment

If systemic treatment is needed to control disease, *cyclosporine* (CyA) should be considered first. Most data on safety during pregnancy are derived from pregnant women who have been treated with CyA for prevention of organ-transplant rejection. Several studies have indicated an increased risk of premature birth or low birth weight, but neither major malformations nor specific birth defects have been reported. Moreover, although T-, B-, and NK cell numbers are significantly lower than in controls, the immune functions of newborns seem not to be impaired. It is evident that thorough clinical considerations of the impact on the health of the mother and child have to precede the use of CyA, but in severe psoriasis the benefits may outweigh the risks.

All *retinoids* are potent teratogens, especially when used in the first trimester, and may lead to a characteristic pattern of malformations involving craniofacial, cardiac, thymic, and central nervous system structures. Therefore, both, oral and topical retinoids are contraindicated in pregnancy, despite the limited bioavailability of the latter. Since acitretin may be converted into etretinate with a half-life of about 80–100 days, especially in the presence of ethanol, a washout period of at least 2 years is needed before conception is considered safe. Therefore, effective birth control is important during treatment and for 2 years thereafter in women of childbearing potential.

Similarly, *methotrexate* (MTX) is contraindicated during pregnancy due to its teratogenic potential. MTX has been linked to miscarriages as well as to a specific pattern of malformation in infants, which includes cleft palate, ocular hypertelorism, or micrognathia, limb defects, and mental retardation. There is some evidence that a dosage greater than 10 mg/week is required to induce fetal abnormalities with a critical exposure period of 6–8 weeks after conception, but there are insufficient data to determine an exact threshold dose. However, the potential dose dependency might be helpful in counseling patients.

As MTX can cause chromosomal aberrations in human cells, it may theoretically also affect spermatogenesis, although it is not known whether the affected spermatozoa are still capable of fertilization. Therefore, the current guidelines recommend both women of childbearing potential and men whose partner may become pregnant to delay conception during and 3 months after treatment with MTX.

Fumaric acid esters (FAEs) are widely used in Europe, particularly in Germany. Animal studies on FAEs with rabbits and rats did not reveal any signs of teratogenicity or mutagenic potential. However, data on the use of FAEs during pregnancy in humans are lacking. Therefore, treatment during pregnancy cannot be recommended. When deemed necessary, FAEs should be used only cautiously on a case-by-case basis and with individual patient counseling.

Biologics

Manufacturers of all approved TNF inhibitors for psoriasis [infliximab (IFX), adalimumab (ADA), etanercept (ETA), certolizumab (CZP), and golimumab (GO)] as well as of ustekinumab (UST) or Alefacept (ALE) advise avoidance during pregnancy and recommend washout periods for the single substance before it is considered safe to conceive (IFX 6 months, ADA 5 months, ETA 3 weeks, GO 6 months, CZP 5 months, UST 15 weeks, ALE 2 months). However, no toxicity or teratogenicity has been reported in animal studies. Although preclinical data are restricted due to limited cross-reactivity with TNF-α or IL-12/IL23 from species other than humans and/or the formation of neutralizing antibodies in rodents, developmental toxicity studies with analog antibodies conducted in mice and rats or studies in cynomolgus monkeys have revealed no maternal toxicity, embyotoxicity, or teratogenicity with the exception of a reduced number of pregnant mice in a fertility and general reproductive function study with anti-TNF. Published studies on TNF inhibitors are mainly based on patients with arthritis and inflammatory bowel disease. Overall, 650 live births have been recorded, including rarely occurring congenital anomalies such as Fallot's tetralogy or intestinal malrotation in infants from mothers exposed to infliximab and VACTERL syndrome (vertebral anomalies, anal stenosis, tracheoesophageal fistula and radial anomalies) after potential exposure to etanercept.

Data from registries and case series in gastroenterology or rheumatology have not shown any increased risk of birth defects in women exposed to infliximab, adalimumab, or etanercept during pregnancy. In addition, an ongoing prospective study of the American Organization of Teratology Information Specialists has shown no excess of major birth defects in comparison with control groups. However, between 1999 and 2005, the FDA received 24 reports of congenital anomalies belonging to the VACTERL spectrum that have been linked to the use of IFX, ADA, and ETA. As the rate is higher than expected compared with historical controls, this has raised concerns about a possible causative association. In most cases, exposure to TNF inhibitors occurred unintentionally around the time of conception or in the first trimester, and there are only about 33 published reports on continuous use in the second or third trimester. This might be of importance as the transplacental transport of IgG is poor up to the late second or third trimester, and therefore there may be only limited transport across the placenta by the substances in early pregnancy.

In conclusion, although absolute safety is still difficult to ascertain, the available safety data suggest that women who conceive while unintentionally exposed to infliximab or other TNF inhibitors may be reassured that termination of the pregnancy is not required. However, data with respect to intentional use during pregnancy are still rare, and if the use is deemed necessary to control the disease, this should be decided on a case-by-case basis with individual patient counseling. Concerning infliximab, it may be favorable to stop treatment around gestational week 20 (if necessary in special situations week 30) to minimize the exposure to the newborn. In case of long-term exposition, *in utero*, vaccination of the child with life vaccines should be postponed (>6 months of life). So far, there are insufficient data on the use of ustekinumab in pregnant women. Regarding alefacept, the interruption of an unintended pregnancy is not recommended, but if a patient becomes pregnant, the inclusion in a registry is strongly recommended.

Management of psoriasis postpartum/breastfeeding

More than half of patients experience a flare-up within 6 weeks of delivery. In nursing mothers, first-line treatment options are primarily restricted to emollients, moderate- to low-potency topical steroids, and dithranol. It is advisable to apply the medications after breastfeeding and then wash them off before the next feed. Limited use of calcipotriol or salicylic acid may be considered. The next treatment option is UV-B treatment. Systemic treatment with acitretin, methotrexate, cyclosporine, and fumaric acid ester is contraindicated while breastfeeding, as the substances may be excreted in human milk and absorbed by the infant. Therefore, nursing should be stopped if these therapies are required. Concerning biologics, it is not known whether the different TNF inhibitors or ustekinumab are excreted in human milk or absorbed systemically after ingestion. In animal models, ETA, GO, and UST were detectable in breast milk, but absorption of the large molecules is still questionable. Interestingly, small case series with infliximab administered up to gestational week 30 and then again after delivery resulted in no detectable levels in breast milk or sera of the newborn, whereas application about 30 days before delivery led to detection of infliximab in the sera of the newborn, which speaks in favor of placental transfer instead of being excreted in breast milk. Nevertheless, as data are still limited, and human immunoglobulins in general can be excreted in milk, it is recommended that women should stop breast-feeding if treatment with biologics is necessary.

Topic of interest—treatment of GPPP

As generalized pustular psoriasis of pregnancy (annular pustular psoriasis) can show a serious course of disease with potential risk to the mother and child, prompt recognition and treatment are important.

The first choice of therapy is topical and/or systemic glucocorticoids. Often 15–30 mg/day (prednisolon-equivalent) is sufficient, though rarely an increase to 40–60 mg/day may be necessary to control the disease. Adverse effects on pregnant women are considered comparable with nonpregnant patients, though pregnancy-associated osteoporosis, diabetes, or hypertension might be aggravated. The use of prednisone, prednisolone, and methylprednisolone is preferable, because the substances are metabolized by the placenta, and so the fetus will receive less than 10% of the maternal dose. Systemic glucocorticoids in high doses have been associated with low birth weights. In animal models, cleft palates have also been reported, but not in humans.

Several publications have reported the successful use of cyclosporine; therefore, it is considered a second-line systemic treatment in GPPP. One recent case report suggested the potential use of infliximab in therapy-resistant GPPP. In addition, close monitoring and supportive therapy with fluids and electrolytes may be requested, as well as correction of potential hypocalcemia. Antibiotics may be used in cases of superinfection. In very severe cases, early delivery should be taken into consideration.

In the postpartum period, retinoids and methotrexate have been used effectively but clearly are not indicated during pregnancy for their teratogenic potential. In breastfeeding women, low-dose glucocorticoids are reasonably safe, though they are excreted minimally into breast milk. To reduce exposure to the newborn, breastfeeding should be avoided during the first 4 h after intake.

Further reading

Chi, C-C., Kirtschig, G., Aberer, W. *et al.* (2011) Evidence-based (S3) guideline on topical corticosteroids in pregnancy. *British Journal of Dermatology*, **165**, 943–952.

Kane, S., Ford, J., Cohen, R. and Wagner, C.J. (2009) Absence of infliximab in infant sera and breast milk from nursing mothers receiving therapy for Crohn's disease before and after delivery. *Journal of Clinical Gastroenterology*, **43**, 613–616.

Lam, J., Polifka, J.E. and Dohil, M.A. (2008) Safety of dermatologic drugs used in pregnant patients with psoriasis and other inflammatory skin diseases. *Journal of the American Academy of Dermatology*, **59**, 295–315.

Puig, L., Barco, D. and Alomar, A. (2010) Treatment of psoriasis with anti-TNF drugs during pregnancy: case report and review of the literature. *Dermatology*, **220**, 71–76.

Rosmarin, D.M., Lebwohl, M., Elewski, E. and Gottlieb, A.B. (2010) Cyclosporine and psoriasis: 2008 National Psoriasis Foundation* Consensus Conference. *Journal of the American Academy of Dermatology*, **62**, 838–853.

Roth, M.M., Feier, V., Cristodor, P. and Moguelet, P. (2009) Impetigo herpetiformis with postpartum flare-up. *Acta Dermatoven*, **18**, 77–82.

Salmon, J.E. and Alpert, D. (2006) Are we coming to terms with tumor necrosis factor inhibition in pregnancy? *Arthritis & Rheumatism*, **54**, 2353–2355.

Tauscher, A.E., Fleischer, A.B., Kathy, C. Phelps, K.C. and Feldman, S.R. (2002) Psoriasis and pregnancy. *Journal of Cutaneous Medicine and Surgery: Incorporating Medical and Surgical Dermatology*, **6**, 561–570.

Weatherhead, S., Robson, S.C. and Reynolds, N.J. (2007) Management of psoriasis in pregnancy. *British Medical Journal*, **334**, 1218–1220.

CHAPTER 23

Recent and future developments in targeted therapy

Caitriona Ryan and Alan Menter

Department of Dermatology, Baylor University Medical Center, Dallas, TX, USA

The serendipitous discovery of cyclosporine for the treatment of psoriasis in 1979 transformed the field of psoriasis research from a presumed hyperproliferative, keratinocyte-driven disorder to a T-cell-mediated, immune-driven disease. The efficacy of anti-TNF-α therapies for psoriasis was again a fortuitous finding that helped to further unravel the immunopathogenesis of psoriasis, paving the way for the biologic revolution in psoriasis. Over the past decade, the delineation of new cellular and molecular pathways important in disease pathogenesis, particularly the role of the T helper 17 cell/interleukin-23 axis, has facilitated the development of more selective biologic agents, many of which are now in the advanced stages of clinical development. Although T-cells are certainly central to the pathogenesis of psoriasis, the potential roles of keratinocytes or leukocytes such as dendritic cells and macrophages have also been suggested in murine models of psoriasis. Increased knowledge of the role of leukocyte subsets, keratinocytes, cytokines, chemokines, growth factors, adhesion molecules, neuropeptides, and angiogenesis in disease pathogenesis will allow the identification of novel therapeutic targets and pharmacological modulation of these dysregulated pathways. Psoriasis is being increasingly used as a paradigm for autoimmune diseases in studies of targeted biologic therapies due to easy accessibility to the skin and the ability to objectively measure disease severity and treatment response. Hence, psoriasis patients are often the first to experience the benefits of emerging targeted biologic treatments.

Current and emerging biologic therapies

Anti-TNF-α agents

Although infliximab, etanercept, and adalimumab continue to be the main anti-TNF-α agents used for the treatment of moderate-to-severe psoriasis (see Chapter 17), other TNF-α inhibitors are in development or licensed for other

Psoriasis: Diagnosis and Management, First Edition. Edited by Wolfram Sterry, Robert Sabat, and Sandra Philipp.

indications. Golimumab (Centocor), a fully human IgG1/κ anti-TNF antibody, is licensed for the treatment of psoriatic arthritis but not cutaneous disease alone. In a study of 405 patients with psoriatic arthritis (PsA), 48% of all patients receiving golimumab achieved an ACR-20 response at week 14, compared with 9% of patients receiving placebo ($p<0.001$ for all comparisons) with clinical improvements sustained for up to 2 years. Of the patients who had a minimum of 3% body surface area (BSA) affected by psoriasis at baseline, 40% of those in the golimumab 50 mg group and 58% of those in the golimumab 100 mg group had a Psoriasis Area and Severity Index (PASI)-75 response at week 14 compared with 3% of placebo-treated patients. There are no studies to date in psoriasis patients with purely cutaneous disease. Golimumab is licensed for the treatment of PsA in the US and Europe. Another anti-TNF-α agent, certolizumab-pegol (UCB), is the Fab segment of an anti-TNF-α antibody, which is pegylated to allow a longer half life. This agent does not fix complement or cause antibody-dependent cell-mediated cytotoxicity due to the absence of the Fc region. It is licensed for use in rheumatoid arthritis and in Crohn's disease but has also shown efficacy in the treatment of psoriasis in a phase 2 study of 176 patients. In this study, 82.8% of those receiving certolizumab 400 mg every other week and 74.6% of those receiving certolizumab 200 mg every other week achieved a PASI-75 response at 12 weeks compared with 6.8% of those receiving placebo. In a phase 3 study of 409 patients with PsA, an ACR-20 response was achieved in 58% of patients treated with 200 mg every other week, in 51.9% of patients treated with 400 mg every 4 weeks, and in 24.3% of patients treated with placebo at week 12. In patients with greater than 3% BSA involvement, 46.7% of patients were treated with 200 mg every other week, 47.4% were treated with 400 mg every 4 weeks, and 14% of placebo-treated patients achieved a PASI-75 response at 12 weeks.

Agents targeting the Th17 axis

One of the most crucial advances in psoriasis research has been the identification of the central role of the Th17-cells in disease pathogenesis. Formerly considered to be purely a Th1-cell-mediated disease, the crucial function of Th17-cell/IL-17 paradigm in the immunopathogenesis of psoriasis has become increasingly apparent over the past 5 years. Th17 cells express the IL-23 receptor (IL-23R), which mediates IL-23-triggered differentiation, cytokine production in these cells, and their survival (see Chapter 4). There is increased expression of IL-23 and its downstream Th17 cytokines, IL-17A, IL-17 F, and IL-22 but not IL-12 in the lesional skin of psoriatic patients (see Chapter 4).

Ustekinumab is a fully human IgG1/κ monoclonal antibody, which binds to the shared p40 subunit of IL-12 and IL-23 with high affinity and prevents its interaction with IL-12Rβ1, thus inhibiting the activity of both interleukins. As discussed previously (see Chapter 17), ustekinumab has been licensed for 4 years for the treatment of chronic plaque psoriasis and in 2013 for PsA in adults in the United States, Europe, and many other areas around the world.

Table 23.1 Drugs currently in development for the treatment of psoriasis.

Drug name	Mechanism	Pharmaceutical company
Injectable biologic agents		
Golimumab	Fully human IgG anti-TNF-α antibody	Centocor
Certolizumab-pegol	Fab segment of an anti-TNF antibody that is pegylated to allow a longer half life	UCB
Brodalumab (AMG- 827)	Fully human IgG antibody to IL-17RA	Amgen
Secukinumab (AIN-457)	Fully human IgG antibody to IL-17A	Novartis
Ixekizumab (LY2439821)	Fully human IgG antibody to IL-17	Eli-Lilly
ILV-094	Fully human IgG antibody to IL-22	Pfizer
MK-3222	Fully human IgG antibody to IL-23p19	Merck
Guselkumab (CNTO 1959)	Fully human IgG antibody to IL-23p19	Jansen
BI655066	Fully human IgG antibody to IL-23p19	Boehringer Ingelheim
AbGn-168H	Humanized IgG to P-selectin glycoprotein ligand (PSGL-1)	AbGenomics
Abatacept	Fully human fusion protein of the extracellular domain of CTLA-4 bound to Fc portion of IgG1	Bristol-Myers Squibb
BT-061	T-helper-cell-inhibiting agent	Biotest
Oral systemic agents		
Aminopterin	Antifolate	Syntrix Biosystems
Voclosporin	Calcineurin inhibitor	Isotechnika
Tofacitinib	JAK inhibitor	Pfizer
ASP-015K	JAK inhibitor	Astellas
Baricitinib (LY3009104)	JAK inhibitor	Eli Lilly
CEP-071	Fms-like receptor tyrosine kinase-3 (FLT-3) inhibitor	Cephalon
CC-10004	Phosphodiesterase-4 inhibitor	Celgene
BMS-582949	P38-mitogen-activated protein kinase inhibitor	Bristol-Myers Squibb
AEB-071	Protein kinase C inhibitor	Novartis
CF-101	Adenosine receptor agonist	Can-Fite BioPharma
VB-201	Synthetic oxidized phospholipid analog	Vascular Biogenics
ACT-128800	Sphingosine-1-phosphate receptor agonist	Actelion
Talarozole	All-*trans* retinoic acid metabolism blocking agent	Barrier Therapeutics/ Stiefel
AE-941	Naturally occurring inhibitor of vascular endothelial growth factor and matrix metalloproteinase	Aeterna Laboratories
Doxercalciferol	Synthetic oral vitamin D_2 prohormone	Genzyme
Topical therapies		
LEO-80185	Vitamin D analog	LEO
LEO-80190	Vitamin D analog	LEO

(Continued)

Table 23.1 (*Continued*)

Drug name	Mechanism	Pharmaceutical company
CD-2027	Vitamin D analog	Galderma
COL-121	Vitamin D analog	Galderma
M518101	Vitamin D derivative	Maruno
INCB-018424	JAK inhibitor	Incyte
Tofacitinib	JAK inhibitor	Pfizer
AN2728	Phosphodiesterase-4 inhibitor	Anacor Pharmaceuticals
MK-0873	Phosphodiesterase-4 inhibitor	Merck
CT-327	Pegylated nerve growth factor receptor blocker	Creabilis SA
IP10.C8	Combined inhibition of dipeptidyl peptidase IV and aminopeptidase N	Immune Technologies and Medicine GmbH

There are at least six different isoforms of the IL-17 molecule, all of which have different affinities for the IL17 receptors. IL-17A and IL-17F share the same receptor composed of two chains: IL-17RA and IL-17RC. These chains are ubiquitously expressed on numerous cell types, including keratinocytes, endothelial cells, fibroblasts, chondrocytes, macrophages, and dendritic cells. IL-17 can stimulate the production of antimicrobial peptides and inflammatory mediators in these cells. Several agents blocking IL-17 and the IL17 receptors have shown very promising results in phase 2 and 3 clinical trials, and approval of these agents for clinical use is expected in late 2014 and 2015.

Secukinumab (AIN 475, Novartis) is a fully human monoclonal IgG1 monoclonal antibody to IL-17A. The initial phase 2a study of AIN457 in 36 psoriasis patients showed superiority over placebo, with a 63% decrease in PASI relative to baseline 12 weeks after a single 3 mg/kg intravenous dose of AIN-457 compared with a 9% decrease in placebo-treated patients, and no significant increase in adverse events ($p=0.0005$). In a phase 2, dose-ranging study, 125 patients were randomized to receive placebo, 25 mg of secukinumab once only, 25 mg of secukinumab at weeks 0, 4, and 8, 75 mg of secukinumab at weeks 0, 4, and 8, or 150 mg of secukinumab at weeks 0, 4, and 8 subcutaneously. The proportion of patients achieving a PASI-75 response was significantly higher in the 150 mg (81%) and 75 mg arms (57%) compared with the placebo arm (9%). In a post-hoc analysis of the dose-ranging phase 2 study, the effect of secukinumab in a subgroup of subjects with moderate-to-severe palmoplantar psoriasis was examined. This subgroup of patients had a baseline hand/foot 5-point static IGA score of ≥2. The palm or sole most seriously affected at baseline was assessed. The percentage of patients achieving an IGA response of 0 (clear) or 1 (almost clear/minimal) and a ≥2-point improvement on the 5-point hand/foot IGA scale compared with baseline at week 12 appeared higher in the 150 mg secukinumab group compared with placebo (71.4% vs 20.0%, $p=0.074$). As there were only seven patients in this group, statistical significance was not achieved. A larger phase 3 study is currently under way to determine the therapeutic effect of secukinumab in this recalcitrant psoriasis patient population.

In another phase 2 study, 404 patients were randomized to receive 150 mg of secukinumab once only, on weeks 0, 1, 2, and 4 ("early"), and on weeks 0, 4, and 8 ("monthly"), or placebo subcutaneously. At week 12, the PASI-75 response was statistically higher in the "early" and "monthly" group at 55% and 42% respectively, compared with 2% in the placebo arm. The FIXTURE (Full year Investigative eXamination of Secukinumab vs eTanercept Using 2 dosing Regimens to determine Efficacy in Psoriasis) study was a multicenter, phase 3, randomized, double-placebo-controlled trial of 1306 patients, comparing 300 mg and 150 mg doses of secukinumab, 50 mg of etanercept weekly, and placebo. At week 12, a PASI-75 response was achieved in 77.1% of the secukinumab 300 mg arm, 67% of the secukinumab 150 mg arm, 44% of the etanercept arm, and 4.9% of the placebo arm. A PASI-90 response was achieved by 54% of patients receiving secukinumab 300 mg by week 12 compared with 21% of etanercept patients, and complete clearance (PASI-100 response) was achieved in 24% versus 4% of these groups, respectively. Secukinumab efficacy was sustained over a full year of follow-up. The SCULPTURE (Study Comparing Secukinumab Use in Long-term Psoriasis maintenance therapy: Fixed regimens vs reTreatment Upon start of RElapse) study was another phase 3 study of long-term maintenance therapy with secukinumab, comparing a fixed regimen with retreatment upon relapse. This showed that patients who initially achieved PASI-75 at week 12 were more likely to maintain their response if they received secukinumab at fixed monthly intervals, compared with treatment only on the "start of relapse." The results of five more phase 3 studies in chronic plaque psoriasis are awaited, and other phase 3 studies are examining the use of secukinumab in palmoplantar psoriasis, generalized pustular psoriasis, and moderate-to-severe nail psoriasis. Open-label extension studies of more than 3300 patients treated with secukinumab will provide long-term safety and efficacy data for secukinumab.

A phase 2, 24-week study compared the use of two injections of 10 mg/kg of secukinumab with placebo in 42 patients with active PsA. The ACR-20 responses achieved in secukinumab-treated patients versus placebo-treated patients were 39% versus 15% at week 12 and 43% versus 18% at week 24. Phase 3 studies of secukinumab in PsA are currently ongoing.

Brodalumab (AMG-827, Amgen) is a fully human Chinese hamster ovary cell-derived IgG2 monoclonal antibody to IL-17RA, thus antagonizing the effects of IL-17A, IL-17F, IL-17A/F, and IL-25 (IL-17E). A phase 2, dose-ranging study of brodalumab compared treatment with 70 mg, 140 mg, or 210 mg of brodalumab at day 1, weeks 1, 2, 4, 6, 8, and 10, or 280 mg monthly with placebo in psoriasis patients. A PASI-75 response was achieved by 67%, 82%, 77%, and

33% of patients treated with the 280 mg, 210 mg 140 mg, and 70 mg doses, respectively, compared with 0% in the placebo arm. At week 12, 38.5% of those receiving 140 mg of brodalumab achieved a PASI-100 response (complete clearance) compared with 62.5% of the 210 mg group. The rate of adverse events also appeared to be dose-related, with two cases of neutropenia reported in the 210 mg group. In the open-label extension phase of this study, all patients received 210 mg of brodalumab every other week. Upon receiving treatment, prior placebo patients showed a rapid response with a PASI-75 response achieved in all patients. The PASI-75 response was maintained in 95% of patients through week 48. Two current phase 3 studies are comparing 210 mg and 140 mg doses of brodalumab with ustekinumab and placebo. Another phase 3 study is examining the withdrawal of brodalumab and retreatment following relapse with 140 mg and 210 mg dose regimens. A phase 2 study has also evaluated the use of brodalumab 140 mg and 210 mg compared with placebo for the treatment of PsA.

Ixekizumab (LY2439821, Eli Lilly) is another humanized anti-IL-17 monoclonal antibody currently under evaluation. In a phase 2, placebo-controlled trial, 142 patients were randomized to receive subcutaneous injections of 10, 25, 75, or 150 mg of ixekizumab or placebo at 0, 2, 4, 8, 12, and 16 weeks. A PASI-75 response was achieved in 82.1% of patients taking 150 mg of ixekizumab, 82.8% of patients taking 75 mg of ixekizumab, and 76.7% of patients taking 25 mg of ixekizumab, compared with 7.7% of patients in the placebo arm. A PASI-90 response was achieved in 71.4%, 58.6%, and 50.0% of these groups, respectively versus 0% of the placebo arm ($p<0.001$ for each comparison). Complete clearance (PASI-100) was achieved in 39.3% of the 150 mg group and 37.9% of the 75 mg group compared with 0% of the placebo group ($p<0.001$ for both comparisons). Clinically significant differences occurred as early as 1 week and were maintained through 20 weeks. Several phase 3 studies are currently in progress—two studies comparing treatment with 80 mg of ixekizumab, 50 mg of etanercept and placebo, an open-label study in Japanese patients, and an open-label study evaluating the 80 mg dose of ixekizumab administered with a prefilled syringe compared with an auto-injector. In addition, a phase 3 study comparing ixekizumab, adalimumab, and placebo is currently in progress.

Several IL-23 blocking agents are now also in development. MK-3222 (SCH900222, Merck) is a humanized IgG1 antibody to the p19 subunit of IL-23. In a phase 2b, dose-ranging study of 339 patients, patients were treated at week 0 and week 4 with placebo, or with 5 mg, 25 mg, 100 mg, and 200 mg of MK-3222. A PASI-75 response was achieved in 33.3%, 64.4%, 66.3%, and 74.4% of patients treated with 5 mg, 25 mg, 100 mg, and 200 mg, respectively, compared with 4% of patients in the placebo arm. Two placebo-controlled phase 3 studies evaluating the 100 mg and 200 mg doses are currently ongoing, one of which is comparing MK-3222 to etanercept and placebo.

Guselkumab (CNTO 1959, Jansen Pharmaceutical) is another humanized monoclonal antibody to IL-23p19. A phase 2 study comparing 5 mg, 15 mg,

50 mg, 100 mg, and 200 mg of guselkumab with adalimumab and placebo has been completed with results awaited. Another phase 2 study of this agent is examining its use in the treatment of palmoplantar psoriasis. A separate phase 1 study is examining single rising intravenous and subcutaneous doses of BI655066 (Boehringer Ingelheim), another humanized IgG1 monoclonal antibody to the IL-23p19 subunit.

Levels of IL-22 are increased in psoriatic lesions and peripheral blood, making this another putative target for psoriasis therapies. IL-22 is expressed by activated T-cells and acts through its receptor on keratinocytes, hepatocytes, and fibroblasts to stimulate production of antimicrobial peptides such as beta-defensins and S100A7 as well as some chemokines (see Chapter 4). The antimicrobial proteins may also act as chemoattractants of neutrophils, monocytes, and T lymphocytes. IL-22 regulates local tissue inflammation by its action on nonimmune cells. The use of a IL-22 neutralizing antibody blocked the progression of disease in a mouse model of psoriasis. ILV-094 (Pfizer), a fully human monoclonal IgG1 antibody to IL-22, has previously been evaluated for use in psoriasis among other indications. A phase 1 study was completed in January 2010 with no further studies planned.

Other biologic agents

Studies evaluating the antagonism of several other inflammatory mediators with a putative role in psoriasis pathogenesis have also been performed. It has been postulated that IFN-α plays a pivotal role in the development of early psoriasis lesions. However, a phase 1 study of MEDI-545 (Medimmune), an anti-IFN-α monoclonal antibody, did not show efficacy in the treatment of psoriasis and failed to inhibit the type I interferon gene signature in lesional skin. Inhibition of other putative key proinflammatory cytokines involved in the psoriasis inflammatory cascade such as IFN-γ, IL-21, and IL-6 is yet to be evaluated. Isolated case reports have suggested a potential therapeutic role for tocilizumab in PsA, a monoclonal antibody to the IL-6 receptor.

AbGn-168H (AbGenomics) is a humanized IgG4/κ antibody directed against P-selectin glycoprotein ligand-1 (PSGL-1; CD162), an adhesion molecule that induces apoptosis of activated T-cells while sparing the resting T-cell population and other inflammatory cells. This agent does not interfere with P-selectin-mediated tethering or rolling of leukocytes or trigger production of inflammatory cytokines. The selectivity for activated T-cells, with sparing of naive and resting memory T-cells, suggests that this drug may be less immunosuppressive than other T-cell depleting agents. A phase 2a, randomized, double-blind, placebo-controlled, multicenter study is currently evaluating this agent for use in the treatment of psoriasis.

The blockade of costimulatory signals can also serve to inhibit recruitment of inflammatory cells. CTLA-4 (CD152) is a costimulatory molecule that has immunosuppressive qualities and induces tolerance (see Chapter 4). Abatacept

(BMS188667, Bristol-Myers Squibb) is a fully human fusion protein of the extracellular domain of CTLA-4 bound to a modified Fc portion of human IgG1, which selectively inhibits T-cell activation by competitive binding of CD28/CD152 to CD80 or CD86. This, in turn, leads to decreased levels of cytokines and inflammatory mediators implicated in inflammatory diseases such as psoriasis and PsA. In a 26-week, phase 1, open-label, dose-escalation study of abatacept in 43 psoriasis patients, 46% of patients had at least a 50% improvement in clinical disease activity, as determined by the physician's global assessment of disease severity, with a dose–response relationship observed at higher doses and a sustained clinical improvement in some cases for up to 147 days after the final dose. Clinical improvement was associated with the reduction of intralesional T-cells. In a phase 2 study, 170 patients with PsA were randomized to take abatacept 3, 10, and 30/10 mg/kg (two initial doses of 30 mg/kg followed by 10 mg/kg) or placebo on day 1, 15, and 29, followed by every 28 days; 19%, 33%, 48%, and 42% of patients receiving placebo, abatacept 3, 10, and 30/10 mg/kg achieved ACR20, respectively, with significantly higher improvements in those receiving abatacept 10 mg/kg ($p=0.006$) and 30/10 mg/kg ($p=0.022$) compared with placebo. Improvements in PASI of greater than 50% were observed in all abatacept groups. A phase 2 study is planned to determine if the use of abatacept subsequent to a course of ustekinumab will prevent relapse in patients with psoriasis. Abatacept is not currently approved for the treatment of psoriasis or PsA.

BT-061 (Biotest) is a CD4+ T-cell-inhibiting agent that has completed phase 2 studies for use in psoriasis. Teplizumab (MGA-301, Macrogenics/Eli Lilly) is an anti-CD3 monoclonal antibody that has been studied for use in those with recently diagnosed type 1 diabetes mellitus to arrest the loss of beta-cell function. A phase 2 study of this agent for use in psoriasis was terminated due to injection-site reactions.

Oral systemic treatments in development

Antifolate therapies

There are several emerging oral systemic treatments in the late stages of development or in clinical trials for the treatment of psoriasis. Methotrexate (MTX) has been the first-line systemic agent for psoriasis for over 50 years, but its use is limited by unpredictable response and potential toxicity. Up to 30% of subjects with moderate-to-severe plaque psoriasis discontinued oral MTX because of intolerance to the drug. The large interindividual variability in clinical response to oral MTX has been attributed to significant differences in oral bioavailability between subjects and may be related to genetic polymorphisms in MTX metabolic pathways. Other antifolate therapies are now being studied for use in psoriasis as an alternative to MTX.

Aminopterin (4-amino-pteroyl-glutamic acid) is an antifolate that is structurally very similar to MTX and differs from folic acid by only two atoms.

Aminopterin was used between 1953 and 1964 for the treatment of pediatric acute leukemia and was the initial antifolate drug used to treat over 3500 psoriatic patients, prior to the advent of MTX. However, this agent was discontinued for what appeared to have been manufacturing preferences by Lederle for MTX. Animal and human clinical studies comparing aminopterin and MTX show that aminopterin has improved mean oral bioavailability, is more actively and completely taken up by cells, accumulates less in the cerebrospinal fluid, has less of an effect on erythropoiesis, and causes fewer increases in serum liver transaminases. As a result, aminopterin is now being studied again for use in psoriasis and other inflammatory conditions such as rheumatoid arthritis, transplantation, systemic lupus erythematosus, polymyositis, and inflammatory bowel disease. A phase 1 randomized crossover study was performed to examine the pharmacokinetics of 0.25 mg and 1.0 mg aminopterin tablets in psoriasis patients who were on stable-dose MTX for at least 3 months' duration up to the commencement of the study (Syntrix Biosystems in collaboration with the National Institute of Allergy and Infectious Diseases of the National Institutes of Health). Currently, a phase 2 study is in the early stages of development.

Purine nucleoside phosphorylase deficiency leads to profound suppression of T-cell immunity that results in severe combined immunodeficiency in humans. R3421 (Hoffmann-La Roche) is a potent purine nucleoside phosphorylase inhibitor that inhibits lymphocyte proliferation and induces apoptosis in T-, B-, and NK-cells, and has been examined in a phase 2 study of psoriasis.

Calcineurin inhibitors

Cyclosporine, although effective for the treatment of psoriasis, is limited by adverse effects such as nephrotoxicity and hypertension, which preclude its long-term use. A similar calcineurin inhibitor, voclosporin (ISA 247, Isotechnika), with a modification of the first amino acid residue, has been studied in psoriasis. A phase 3 study showed it to be less nephrotoxic, but slightly less effective, with 47% of patients receiving the highest dose achieving PASI 75 at week 12, compared with 4% of the placebo group. This medication has not been approved for the treatment of psoriasis.

Oral small molecule therapies

Janus kinases (JAK) are a family of protein tyrosine kinases that are activated by cytokines that target STAT (Signal Transduction And Transcription) transcription factors. Several oral and topical JAK inhibitors are currently in trial for the treatment of psoriasis and rheumatoid arthritis, and for immunsuppression in transplant recipients. Janus kinases are activated by a cytokine such as IL-2, IL-4, and IL-12, and so their blockade would inhibit the activation, proliferation, and homeostasis of T-cells.

Tofacitinib (CP-690,550, Pfizer) is a potent JAK inhibitor with selectivity for JAK1 and JAK1/JAK3, developed as an immunosuppressive agent for the prevention of transplant rejection and for the treatment of autoimmune diseases. A study of 59 psoriasis patients compared the effect of 5, 10, 20, 30, and 50 mg twice-daily oral tofacitinib or 60 mg tofacitinib once daily with that of placebo for 14 days. There was a dose-dependent improvement in Psoriatic Lesion Severity Sum (PLSS) score from baseline to day 14 for all tofacitinib doses except the 5 mg twice-daily group ($p<0.01$ vs placebo), while 37.5% of patients in the highest dose group (50 mg twice daily) reduced their PLSS scores to 0. In a further phase 2b dose-ranging study of 197 patients, 25%, 40.8%, and 66.7% of those taking 2, 5, and 15 mg of tofacitinib twice daily achieved a PASI-75 response compared with 2% of placebo-treated patients. Four phase 3 RCTS studies of tofacitinib, including a comparator study comparing tofacitinib, etanercept, and placebo, have been completed, and a long-term open-label extension study for participants of these studies is currently ongoing. The results of these phase 3 studies are eagerly awaited. Tofacitinib is also in late-stage development for use in PsA as well as for use as a topical agent in psoriasis.

ASP-015K (Astellas Pharma) is another JAK inhibitor with activity against JAK 1, 2, 3, and Tyk2. A phase 2a dose-escalation study in 124 psoriasis patients examined the efficacy of 10 mg, 25 mg, 60 mg, or 100 mg of ASP015K twice daily, 50 mg of ASP015K daily or placebo for 6 weeks. The change in PASI score from baseline to end of treatment was significantly higher for those treated with ASP015K compared with placebo ($p<0.0001$), with reductions of 11.9 for the 100 mg twice-daily group, 6.4 for the 10 mg twice-daily group, and 4.2 for the placebo group. A phase 2b study of Baricitinib (LY3009104, Eli Lilly), another JAK inhibitor that preferentially inhibits JAK2 over JAK1 and JAK3, has also been completed with results pending.

The fms-like receptor tyrosine kinase-3 (FLT-3) is important for the normal development of hematopoietic stem cells and cells of the immune system. Dendritic cells are known to be important in both the initiation and maintenance of psoriasis lesions (see Chapter 4), and FLT-3 is known to have a role in dendritic cell development. Lestaurtinib (CEP-701, Cephalon) is a multitargeted tyrosine kinase inhibitor that potently inhibits FLT-3. In a mouse model of autoimmune encephalitis, lestaurtinib resulted in decreased secretion of TNF-α, IL-6, and IL-23 by dendritic cells, alongside a decrease in the expression of costimulatory molecules and a decrease in the levels of signaling molecules such as phospho-Stat1, Stat3, Stat5, and NF-κB. A phase 2 study has evaluated the use of lestaurtinib in psoriasis.

Phosphodiesterase-4 (PDE-4) is the main cyclic adenosine monophosphate (cAMP)-degrading enzyme in T-cells, macrophages, neutrophils, keratinocytes, and fibroblasts, suggesting a role for PDE-4 inhibitors as anti-inflammatory agents in psoriasis. Apremilast (Celgene, CC-10004) is an oral PDE-4 inhibitor that has shown efficacy in the treatment of psoriasis. In a study of 259 psoriasis patients, 24.4% of patients treated with 20 mg of apremilast twice daily achieved PASI 75 after 84 days, compared with 10.3% of those treated with placebo. Another phase

2b study of 352 psoriasis patients comparing the efficacy, safety, and pharmacokinetics of 10 mg, 20 mg, and 30 mg of apremilast and placebo twice daily showed a PASI 75 response in 11%, 29%, 41%, and 6% of these groups, respectively. Three phase 3 multicenter studies have examined the safety and efficacy of 30 mg apremilast twice daily, the results of which will soon be available. Another phase 3 study has compared the efficacy of apremilast with that of etanercept and placebo. Patients from these studies are enrolled in an open-label extension study that will continue until June 2016 to allow for long-term evaluation of the agent. Apremilast has also shown efficacy in the treatment of PsA. In a phase 2 study of 204 patients with PsA, 43.5% of patients receiving apremilast 20 mg twice daily and 35.8% of those receiving 40 mg daily achieved an ACR20 response at week 12, compared with 11.8% of those receiving placebo. Three phase 3 studies are further evaluating its efficacy in the treatment of PsA.

Mitogen-activated protein kinases (MAPK) are a family of Ser/Thr protein kinases that are involved in many cellular programs such as cell proliferation, cell differentiation, inflammation, and apoptosis. P38-MAPK triggered cascades are activated in keratinocytes and other inflammatory cells in response to TNF-signaling. Conversely, anti-TNF-α therapy reduces p38 MAPK phosphorylation in psoriatic skin leading to reduced expression of p38 MAPK regulated genes including IL-1β, IL-8, IL-17C, and IL-20. Previous p38 inhibitors resulted in adverse effects such as hepatotoxicity and neurotoxicity due to the ubiquitous activity of p38 MAPK. A new p38 inhibitor that does not cross the blood–brain barrier, BMS-582949 (Bristol-Myers Squibb), has been studied in phase 2 trials for psoriasis. This study compared the effect of 10 mg, 30 mg, or 100 mg of BMS-582949 twice daily with placebo in 99 psoriasis patients with results not yet available.

Sotrastaurin (AEB071, Novartis Pharmaceuticals) is an oral protein kinase C (PKC) inhibitor that indirectly inhibits T-cell proliferation and prevents the production of inflammatory cytokines by activated T-cells, keratinocytes, and macrophages through selective inhibition of the α, β, and θ-PKC isoforms. This agent is currently being studied for the treatment of psoriasis alongside multiple other studies in ulcerative colitis, uveitis, and postorgan transplantation. A study of 32 psoriasis patients compared the effect of treatment with ascending doses of AEB071 (from 25 mg to 300 mg twice daily) with that of placebo for 14 days. There was a 69% improvement in PASI in the group receiving the 300 mg twice-daily group after 2 weeks of treatment. Long-term studies are ongoing to determine the safety and efficacy in larger cohorts of patients.

The A3 adenosine receptor (A_3AR) is a Gi protein-coupled cell surface receptor that belongs to the adenosine receptor family. CF101 (Can-Fite BioPharma) is an A_3AR agonist that mediates anti-inflammatory effects through downregulation of protein kinases B/Akt and NF-κB, leading to the inhibition of TNF-α and CCL3, and apoptosis of inflammatory cells. A phase 2 study compared 1 mg, 2 mg, or 4 mg twice-daily dosages of CF101 versus placebo for the treatment of psoriasis. A statistically significant improvement was demonstrated in the 2 mg arm only, with 35.3% of patients achieving a PASI-50 response at week 12. A phase 2/3 study of 2 mg twice daily is near completion.

The targeting of chemokine receptors is another potential means of inhibiting leukocyte recruitment and subsequent inflammation. CXCR1 and CXCR2 are G protein-coupled receptors expressed on neutrophils and monocytes that mediate the activities of CXCL. Sch527123 (Schering Plough) is a potent oral CXCR1/CXCR2 antagonist, which inhibits chemokine activation of these receptors, thus inhibiting neutrophil chemotaxis and myeloperoxidase release, which has been studied in a phase 2 study of psoriasis. Results in psoriasis studies have not yet been made available.

Although oxidized phospholipids are generated at sites of inflammation, recent studies have shown that these molecules also display anti-inflammatory properties such as impaired Th1/Th17-cell differentiation, inhibition of p40, and TNF-α secretion by activated dendritic cells and decreased expression of costimulatory molecules such as CD80 and CD86. VB-201 (Vascular Biogenics) is an oral synthetic oxidized phospholipid analog that has anti-inflammatory activity and is currently being evaluated in phase 2 trials for use in psoriasis.

Sphingosine-1-phosphate (S1P) is a lysophospholipid that mediates its activity through five specific G-protein coupled receptors numbered S1P1 to S1P5. Agonists of the S1P1 receptor inhibit the egress of T-cells from the thymus and lymphoid organs and so potentially may be useful in the treatment of autoimmune disease. ACT128800 (Actelion), a potent, oral S1P receptor agonist, has been evaluated in two phase 2 studies of psoriasis patients, with results awaited.

Antiglycemic agents

As discussed earlier (Chapter 15), there is a large and growing body of evidence that patients with moderate-to-severe psoriasis have a clinically significant increased risk of various aspects of the metabolic syndrome, including cardiovascular disease, diabetes mellitus, and obesity, compared with the general population. Further research is needed to determine how to maximize the primary prevention of cardiovascular events in patients with psoriasis and to develop agents that not only mitigate but also reverse cardio-metabolic risk while improving psoriasis, particularly in those patients with metabolic syndrome.

In a preliminary study, liraglutide, a glucagon-like peptide-1 analog, typically used to reduce weight and improve glycemic control in patients with type 2 diabetes, appeared to produce an improvement in the severity of psoriasis. In this study of seven psoriasis patients, liraglutide treatment produced significant changes in PASI and Dermatology Life Quality Index at 10 weeks, along with an increase in circulating invariant natural killer T-cells and a nonsignificant decrease (53%) in the proportion of circulating TNF-α-producing monocytes. Further studies are now ongoing in multiple centers. Similarly, isolated case reports have suggested that sitagliptin, a dipeptidyl peptidase-IV (DPP-IV) inhibitor, typically administered for control of blood glucose in type 2 diabetes, also produced an improvement in psoriasis. A phase 2 randomized placebo-controlled trial to compare the effect of sitagliptin and glipazide on psoriasis severity is due to commence shortly in psoriasis patients with concomitant type 2 diabetes.

Retinoid therapies

Oral retinoids have been used to treat psoriasis since the early 1980s. While their mechanism of action in psoriasis is not fully understood, they are known to decrease epidermal proliferation and have anti-inflammatory properties. As a monotherapy, acitretin is less effective than other systemic agents with approximately 25% of patients achieving a PASI 75-response. Retinoic acid metabolism blocking agents (RAMBAs) are agents that increase the levels of endogenous alltrans-retinoic acid (ATRA) by inhibiting the cytochrome P450-dependent ATRA-4-hydroxylase enzymes responsible for ATRA metabolism. Talarozole (R115866/Rambazole/Liarazole, Barrier Therapeutics/ Stiefel) is a new-generation all-*trans* RAMBA, highly specific against the retinoic acid 4-hydroxylase. This agent has been shown to reduce hyperproliferation and normalize differentiation of the epidermis in animal models of psoriasis. An open-label, phase 2 trial examined the safety and efficacy of 1 mg/day of R115866 for 8 weeks in 19 psoriasis patients (of whom only 14 completed the study). A PASI-50 response was achieved in 26% of the patients, with further improvement noted in the 2-week follow-up period where 47% of the patients showed a PASI-50 response. The most common adverse events were similar to those of acitretin, including pruritus, xerosis, cheilitis, and an increase in blood triglycerides. A dose-ranging, phase 2 study of 176 psoriasis patients has since evaluated the use of 0.5 mg, 1 mg, and 2 mg of talarozole daily compared with placebo for the treatment of psoriasis, with results currently not available.

Antiangiogenic therapies

Upregulation of angiogenesis is a feature of psoriasis lesions, and overexpression of vascular endothelial growth factor (VEGF) isoforms can even be detected in uninvolved skin compared with that of healthy donors (see Chapter 4). Polymorphisms of VEGF are associated with an increased susceptibility to psoriasis, while transgenic overexpression of VEGF in keratinocytes in mice induces a psoriasiform phenotype. In line with this, anti-VEGF antibody treatment in psoriasis mice models results in clinical improvement of psoriasiform disease. The *VEGF*–460C>T polymorphism has also been shown to play a role in predicting response or nonresponse of psoriasis to acitretin. Furthermore, psoriasis patients treated with anti-VEGF therapies for cancer such as bevacizumab have shown complete clearance of their disease. Tie2 transgenic mice, which have overexpression of Tie2, the receptor for angiopoietin-1 and -2, also display psoriasisform skin inflammation. Thus, neutralizing antibodies and soluble receptors to angiopoietins such as VEGF, fibroblast growth factor-2 and angiopoetin-1 and -2 may have a therapeutic benefit in psoriasis. AE-941 (Neovastat; Aeterna Laboratories) is a naturally occurring inhibitor of angiogenesis derived from shark cartilage, which inhibits both VEGF and matrix metalloproteinase, activators of angiogenesis. A randomized phase 1/2 trial compared the efficacy of oral AE-941 in 49 patients with psoriasis. Improvement in PASI was observed in 50%, 41.7%, and 30.8% of the patients receiving 240, 120, and 60 mL/day, respectively. Nonserious gastrointestinal and cutaneous adverse effects were reported.

Vitamin D therapies

Vitamin D_3 is a potent antiproliferative and prodifferentiation factor for keratinocytes, modulating immunological processes such as T-cell activation, cytokine secretion, and dendritic cell maturation. Studies have shown that NB-UVB affects vitamin D status while clearing psoriasis, suggesting that the increase in serum vitamin D could partly account for the beneficial effect of phototherapy in psoriasis. A phase 2 trial evaluated doxercalciferol (Genzyme), a synthetic oral vitamin D_2 prohormone for the treatment of psoriasis. Results have not been made available, and no further studies are planned.

Neuropeptide inhibition

The potential role of neuropeptides and cutaneous neurogenic inflammation has been studied in the pathogenesis of psoriasis. The symmetrical distribution of psoriatic plaques possibly reflects the anatomical distribution of cutaneous nerves suggesting that sensory nerves and their secretory products may form part of a neuroimmunomodulatory network, contributing to the development of psoriasis. Numerous reports of increased levels of substance P, somatostatin, nerve growth factor, vasoactive intestinal peptide, and calcitonin gene-related peptide in lesional psoriatic skin support this theory. The resolution of psoriatic plaques in areas of denervated skin shows the importance of neuronal input in the maintenance of psoriasis. Elevated stress levels are a well-recognized trigger for exacerbations of psoriasis, and neuropeptides may mediate this process. Thus, the use of neuropeptide modulating agents may present a potential therapeutic option for the treatment of psoriasis. K252a, a high-affinity nerve growth factor receptor blocker, produced both clinical and histological improvement of psoriasis in a xenotransplant model. CT 327 (Creabilis SA) is a pegylated derivative of K252a which has been evaluated for the topical treatment of psoriasis in two phase 2 studies, the results of which are not currently available.

Future topical therapies

The main advantage of topical therapy is the avoidance of significant systemic side effects and immunosuppression, although many will argue that psoriasis is a systemic disease with associated comorbidities that warrant systemic therapy in moderate-to-severe cases. However, the majority of psoriasis patients are in the mild-moderate category, making topical therapy the mainstay of treatment. Currently, glucocorticoids, vitamin D analogs and tar-based treatments are the predominant agents used in psoriasis topical therapy. Several new vitamin D analogs (LEO 80185, Leo Pharmaceuticals; LEO 80190, Leo pharmaceuticals; CD2027, Galderma; COL121, Galderma) or derivatives (M518101, Maruho Co.) are under investigation in or have completed phase 2 and phase 3 trials. In a randomized controlled trial of combination therapy with topical niacin (nicotinamide) and calcipotriene in 168 patients, 50% of patients using the combination therapy achieved clearance or near-clearance, compared with 18.8% of patients randomized to placebo, 25% of patients treated with nicotinamide alone or 31.5% of patients treated with calcipotriene alone. This product is not commercially available.

Newer more targeted agents are now also in development for topical treatment. WBI-1001 (isopropyl-5-[(E)-2-phenylethenyl] benzene-1,3-diol) is a nonsteroidal agent derived from metabolites of bacterial symbionts of nematodes, which inhibits TNF-α and INF-γ secretion from activated T-cells. In a phase 2, randomized, placebo-controlled study of 61 patients, 67.5% of patients treated with WBI-100 achieved a PGA of clear or almost clear, with a mean improvement in BSA affected of 79.1%, compared with 4.8% ($p<0.0001$) and an increase of 9.4% ($p<0.0001$), respectively, for patients randomized to placebo.

Several topical agents directed at small molecules described earlier, such as JAK1/2 inhibitors (INCB 18424, Incyte Corporation), JAK3 inhibitors (Tofacitinib, Pfizer), and PDE4 inhibitors (AN2728, Anacor Pharmaceuticals; MK0873, Merck), have been investigated for use in psoriasis and may have a larger role to play in future topical therapy in psoriasis. INCB018424 (Incyte Corporation) is a selective topical JAK1/2 inhibitor that potently inhibits cytokine-induced JAK signaling. In a study of 29 patients, both the 1% cream and the 1.5% cream improved lesion thickness, erythema, and scaling, and reduced lesion area compared with placebo; the composite lesion score decreased by more than 50% with the efficacious doses compared with 32% for vehicle controls. Two 2% tofacitinib ointment formulations in different vehicles were evaluated in a phase 2, multicenter, double-blind, vehicle-controlled trial of 71 patients over 4 weeks. Each formulation and corresponding vehicle control was administered twice daily for 4 weeks to a single fixed 300 cm^2 treatment area containing a target plaque. There was a statistically significant improvement in percentage change from baseline in the Target Plaque Severity Score at week 4 with one of the tofacitinib formulations compared with its vehicle control and the other formulation.

IP10.C8 (Immune Technologies & Medicine GmbH) is a T-cell-inhibiting topical gel that works by the synergistic inhibition of dipeptidylpeptidase IV and aminopeptidase N. Inhibition of these postproline splitting peptidases leads to immunosuppression by inhibiting the proliferation of lymphocytes, decreasing the production of inflammatory cytokines from Th1- and Th17-cells and inducing immunosuppressive cytokines, such as TGF-β1 and IL-1RA. A phase 2 trial was commenced in 2009, but results have not been made available. Neuropeptide inhibitors such as CT327 (Creabilis SA), described previously, are also in clinical development and clinical trials.

Research has shown that transgenic mice overexpressing hyaluronidase have a significant decrease in the number of dermal dendritic cells in their skin. A phase 2 study evaluating the effect of weekly subcutaneous injections of recombinant human hyaluronidase into psoriatic plaques over a 4-week period is due to commence shortly.

Advances in topical drug-delivery technologies and newer formulations utilizing vesicular and particulate colloidal drug-delivery systems such as liposomes, transferosomes, niosomes, ethosomes, solid lipid nanoparticles, microspheres, micelles, and dendrimers may facilitate the development of more effective topical psoriasis therapies. In this regard, topical cyclosporine has finally been developed in a hyaluronic acid base with better transepidermal penetration and release. Proof-of-concept studies will be initiated in early 2014. Transdermal gene therapy has been used to effectively deliver IL-4 using ultraderformable cationic liposome in the K14-VEGF transgenic psoriasis mouse model. Although it will be many years before we see transdermal gene therapy in clinical practice, this method of gene therapy is an attractive candidate for the future treatment of psoriasis.

Personalized medicine

Current systemic and biologic treatments used for the treatment of moderate-to-severe psoriasis show significant variability in efficacy and are associated with varying degrees of toxicity and cost. As a result, there is a great need for biomarkers to predict treatment outcomes and individualize care for psoriasis patients, particularly for drugs with significant side effects or a low rate of response. This would allow the identification of patients less likely to respond to particular treatments and those at increased risk of adverse drug reactions, reducing unnecessary exposure to treatment toxicity and resulting in significant health-related savings. The science of individualizing treatment using molecular profiling and clinical phenotyping is gaining momentum. Psoriasis results from a complex interplay between both genetic and environmental factors, and although clinical phenotype is likely most strongly influenced by genotype, it is also modulated by environmental influences and extracutaneous factors, including smoking status, alcohol intake, body mass index, and comorbidities. As a result, predictive models or algorithms of treatment response in psoriasis must combine pharmacogenomic approaches with comprehensive clinical characterization for the development of truly "personalized" medicine.

Until now, pharmacogenomic studies in psoriasis have been underpowered to produce reliable results, and the majority have not recorded treatment response or treatment toxicities prospectively in an objective and reproducible manner. Validation of results in distinct, adequately powered patient cohorts is therefore essential before pharmacogenomic markers can be used to predict treatment response in the clinical setting. The analysis of genetic variation and transcriptional profiling as part of large-scale phase 3 or 4 clinical drug trials could facilitate great advances in the field of pharmacogenomics of psoriasis and of autoimmune diseases in general. The genetic profiling of patients in registries for systemic and biologic treatments, which accrue comprehensive demographic and phenotypic information and prospectively record treatment response and toxicities over time in a standardized fashion, could play a valuable role in advancing the field of pharmacogenomics of psoriasis. Biostatistical data-modeling techniques could be employed to integrate longitudinal data collected from these patients such as genetic polymorphisms, gene-expression profiling, epigenetic, proteomic, and metabolomic studies, in association with comprehensive clinical phenotyping to construct models predictive of treatment response with more far-reaching applicability.

Conclusion

Borne from a translational approach, newly developed treatments are becoming more targeted, with science driving pharmacological advances rather than serendipity. The potential for patients with psoriasis to achieve long-term clinical remission with targeted biologic therapy is thus becoming very promising. With increasing efficacy of these new treatments, PASI-90 is becoming the measure of optimal response rather than PASI-75. The ultimate "cure" for psoriasis, however, is still many years away. This will most likely involve gene therapy or modulation of the immune response to prevent initial sensitization or to induce desensitization to the antigenic triggers that are initiating and maintaining the disease.

Despite revolutionary advances in the therapy of psoriasis, our long-term experience of these compounds is still very limited, and robust evidence of long-term safety is still an absolute necessity with newly developed drugs. A salutary lesson was the finding of three cases of progressive multifocal leukoencephalopathy in patients treated with the approved CD11a inhibiting agent, efalizumab, shortly after a very reassuring postmarketing 3-year safety study report was published. The very short time frame of current placebo-controlled phases (typically 12–16 weeks) greatly hinders the statistical power to make conclusions with regard to safety. Phased approval, mandating the continued collection of comprehensive safety data in postmarketing, and observational pharmacoepidemiologic studies are potential means of addressing this need. The use of carefully constructed registries, commonplace for the TNF inhibitors, is essential to monitor the long-term safety of new agents under development.

One final aspect that could revolutionize our future targeted therapy is the advent of biosimilar drugs, the first of which was approved by the European Medicines Agency in 2013 (infliximab). Having biosimilar agents available to all our known TNF-α agents currently in the marketplace for moderate-to-severe psoriasis at a cheaper price could allow millions of patients access to biologic therapies. An exciting prospect indeed!

Further reading

Ahern, T., Tobin, A.M., Corrigan, M. *et al.* (2013) Glucagon-like peptide-1 analogue therapy for psoriasis patients with obesity and type 2 diabetes: a prospective cohort study. *Journal of the European Academy of Dermatology and Venereology*, **27**, 1440–1443.

Bissonnette, R., Bolduc, C., Maari, C. *et al.* (2012) Efficacy and safety of topical WBI-1001 in patients with mild to moderate psoriasis: results from a randomized double-blind placebo-controlled, phase II trial. *Journal of the European Academy of Dermatology and Venereology*, **26**, 1516–1521.

Clinicaltrials.gov. [WWW document] URL http://www.Clinicaltrials.Gov/ct2/results?Term=psoriasis [accessed on 8 July 2012]

David, M., Akerman, L., Ziv, M. *et al.* (2011) Treatment of plaque-type psoriasis with oral cf101: Data from an exploratory randomized phase 2 clinical trial. *Journal of the European Academy of Dermatology and Venereology*, **26**, 361–367.

Gottlieb, A., Menter, A., Mendelsohn A. *et al.* (2009) Ustekinumab, a human interleukin 12/23 monoclonal antibody, for psoriatic arthritis: randomised, double-blind, placebo-controlled, crossover trial. *Lancet*, **373**, 633–640.

Hueber, W., Patel, D.D., Dryja, T. *et al.* (2010) Effects of AIN457, a fully human antibody to interleukin-17A, on psoriasis, rheumatoid arthritis, and uveitis. *Science Translational Medicine*, **2**, 52ra72.

Kavanaugh, A., McInnes, I., Mease, P. *et al.* (2009) Golimumab, a new human tumor necrosis factor alpha antibody, administered every four weeks as a subcutaneous injection in psoriatic arthritis: Twenty-four-week efficacy and safety results of a randomized, placebo-controlled study. *Arthritis & Rheumatism*, **60**, 76–86.

Mease, P.J., Fleischmann, R., Deodhar, A.A. *et al.* (2014) Effect of certolizumab pegol on signs and symptoms in patients with psoriatic arthritis: 24-week results of a Phase 3 double-blind randomised placebo-controlled study (RAPID-PsA). *Annals of the Rheumatic Diseases*, **73**, 48–55.

Menter, A., Thrash, B., Cherian, C. *et al.* (2012) Intestinal transport of aminopterin enantiomers in dogs and humans with psoriasis is stereoselective: evidence for a mechanism involving the proton-coupled folate transporter. *Journal of Pharmacology and Experimental Therapeutics*, **342**, 696–708.

Nishioka, T., Shinohara, M., Tanimoto, N., Kumagai, C. and Hashimoto, K. (2012) Sitagliptin, a dipeptidyl peptidase-IV inhibitor, improves psoriasis. *Dermatology*, **224**, 20–21.

Ortonne, J.P., Sterry, W., Tasset, C. and Reich, K. (2007) Safety and efficacy of subcutaneous certolizumab pegol, a new anti-TNF-alpha monoclonal antibody, in patients with moderate-to-severe chronic plaque psoriasis: preliminary results from a double-blind, placebo-controlled trial. *Journal of the American Academy of Dermatology*, **56** (Supplement 2), AB6.

Papp, K., Bissonnette, R., Rosoph, L. *et al.* (2008) Efficacy of ISA247 in plaque psoriasis: A randomised, multicentre, double-blind, placebo-controlled phase III study. *Lancet*, **371**(9621), 1337–1342.

Ports, W.C., Khan, S., Lan, S. *et al.* (2013) A randomized phase 2a efficacy and safety trial of the topical Janus kinase inhibitor tofacitinib in the treatment of chronic plaque psoriasis. *British Journal of Dermatology*, **169**, 137–145.

Punwani, N., Scherle, P., Flores, R. *et al.* (2012) Preliminary clinical activity of a topical JAK1/2 inhibitor in the treatment of psoriasis. *Journal of the American Academy of Dermatology*, **67**, 658–664.

Ryan, C., Abramson, A., Patel, M. and Menter, A. (2012) Current investigational drugs in psoriasis. *Expert Opinion on Investigational Drugs*, **21**, 473–487.

Ryan, C., Leonardi, C.L., Krueger, J.G. *et al.* (2011) Association between biologic therapies for chronic plaque psoriasis and cardiovascular events: A meta-analysis of randomized controlled trials. *Journal of the American Medical Association*, **306**, 864–871.

Index